Statistics and Computing

Series Editors:

J. Chambers

D. Hand

W. Härdle

For other titles published in this series, go to
http://www.springer.com/series/3022

Roberto Baragona · Francesco Battaglia · Irene Poli

Evolutionary Statistical Procedures

An Evolutionary Computation Approach to Statistical Procedures Designs and Applications

Springer

Prof. Roberto Baragona
Sapienza University of Rome
Department of Communication
and Social Research
Via Salaria 113
00198 Rome
Italy
roberto.baragona@uniroma1.it

Prof. Francesco Battaglia
Sapienza University of Rome
Department of Statistical Sciences
Piazzale Aldo Moro 5
00100 Roma
Italy
francesco.battaglia@uniroma1.it

Prof. Irene Poli
Ca' Foscari University of Venice
Department of Statistics
Cannaregio 873
30121 Venice
Italy
irenpoli@unive.it

Series Editors:

J. Chambers
Department of Statistics
Sequoia Hall
390 Serra Mall
Stanford University
Stanford, CA 94305-4065

D. Hand
Department of Mathematics
Imperial College London,
South Kensington Campus
London SW7 2AZ
United Kingdom

W. Härdle
C.A.S.E. Centre for Applied
Statistics and Economics
School of Business and
Economics
Humboldt-Universität zu Berlin
Unter den Linden 6
10099 Berlin
Germany

ISSN 1431-8784
ISBN 978-3-642-16217-6 e-ISBN 978-3-642-16218-3
DOI 10.1007/978-3-642-16218-3
Springer Heidelberg Dordrecht London New York

Cover design: SPI Publisher Services

Printed on acid-free paper

Springer is part of Springer Science+Business Media (www.springer.com)

Preface

In many application fields, artificial intelligence, data mining, pattern recognition operations research, to name but a few, often problems arise that may be reduced at their very essence to optimization problems.

Unfortunately, neither the objective function nor the solution search space display that nice properties that may be conveniently exploited by widespread familiar numerical analysis tools. Though these latter offer powerful devices to cope with a great deal of both theoretical and practical problems in so many disciplines, the hypotheses on which they rely are far from being fulfilled within the frameworks that so often constitute the background of the application fields we mentioned so far. Here well behaved analytic functions and compact domains are not commonplace and only raw hazardous simplifying assumptions may constrain so many classes of problems in such a way they may be treated by means of comfortable numerical procedures.

It may happen that too much simplification does not allow the actual problem to be solved satisfactorily, that is we obtain useless though well grounded solutions. Heuristic methods have been developed to yield reliable solutions to many particular problems, but only the development of general heuristics offered a theoretical framework for dealing with a large class of problems.

One outstanding approach in this kind of methods proved to be evolutionary computing. This rapidly growing research field came nowadays to a well established discipline on its own enjoying solid theoretical foundations and large evidence of effectiveness as far as complex non conventional optimization problems are concerned. History dates back to the fifties and since then an enormous body of theory has been developed which makes evolutionary computing a suitable framework for building applied methodology while it is an active and thriving research field. Its influence spread out through so many disciplines, from biology to informatics and engineering and to economics and social sciences.

We shall try to make an account of the influence of evolutionary computing in Statistics and close related fields. Evolutionary computation is particularly useful in Statistics, in all cases when the statistician has to select, inside a very large discrete set just one element, be it a method, a model, a parameter value, or such.

Therefore a common application of evolutionary computation is to the selection of variables, both in regression problems and in time series linear models. In time series analysis it has been proposed also for building non linear models. For the same reason, evolutionary computation may be employed in the problem of outlier detection, and several papers were published both for the independent observations case and for time series.

A recent, very promising application is in the design of experiments, where the optimal choice of a combination of factors, and their levels, is needed, and cost constraints are very strong.

Finally, a typical field of application of evolutionary computation to Statistics is cluster analysis. Here, the use of an evolutionary algorithm provides a valid alternative when the number of units and variables is large, and the standard cluster techniques allow only approximate solutions.

This book brings together most literature on the use of evolutionary computation methods in statistical analysis, and contains also some unpublished material. It is based on the over 15 years experience and research work of the authors in this field.

This book requires a basic knowledge of mathematics and statistics, and may be useful to research students and professionals to appreciate the suitability for solving complex statistical problems of evolutionary computation. We believe that these algorithms will become a common standard in Statistics in a few years.

Much of the research work included in this book has been possible due to generous funding from Institutions that we are happy to acknowledge with thanks. F. Battaglia and R. Baragona gratefully acknowledge funding from MIUR, Italy (PRIN 2007) and European Commission through Marie Curie Research and Training Network COMISEF – Computational Methods in Statistics, Econometrics and Finance (contract MRTN-CT-2006-034270). I. Poli also would like to acknowledge the MIUR for the PRIN 2007 project, the European Commission for the PACE integrated project (IST-FET, www.istpace.org), and the Fondazione di Venezia for the DICE project. She also would like to thank the researchers at the European Centre for Living Technology for the very fruitful collaboration at the development of the evolutionary perspective in Statistics, in particular Davide de March, Debora Slanzi, Laura Villanova, Matteo Borrotti, Michele Forlin.

We are willing to express our gratitude to many colleagues who commented on large parts of the manuscript letting some obscurities and subtleties be disclosed. In particular we need to mention Antonietta di Salvatore and Domenico Cucina who patiently and carefully read all of the versions of the manuscript, and Debora Slanzi who provided us with lot of computer programs and graphical displays, specially as regards design of experiments. We are indebted for useful and animated discussions to Matt Protopapas, specially concerned with issues related to non linear time series, and to Sanghamitra Bandyopadhyay and Ujjwal Maulik who pointed out in particular some important aspects related to multiobjective optimization and cluster analysis. We have to thank the Springer Editors who successively took care of the manuscript for their assiduous assistance and encouragement, Lilith Braun and Peter

Niels Thomas. Also our thanks are deservedly due to the Desk Editor Alice Blanck for her accurate preparation of the final version of the manuscript, and to Samuel Roobesh, Project Manager at Integra Software Services Pvt. Ltd., for his attentive care in handling the production of this book.

Rome, Italy — Roberto Baragona
Rome, Italy — Francesco Battaglia
Venice, Italy — Irene Poli
September 2010

Contents

Chapter 1
Introduction

Abstract A new line of research has started since the fifties originated by a new awareness in scientific community that natural and biological mechanisms could provide not only the traditional object of study but suggest new disciplines theories and methods by themselves. We may cite the Rosenblatt's perceptron, one of the first examples of a learning machine, and the Box's evolutionary approach to industrial productivity, an early attempt to modeling a process using the concepts of evolutionary behavior of living creatures. This short introduction aims at highlighting the basic ideas that led to an unprecedented enlargement of the guidelines for developing theoretical and applied research in a large body of scientific disciplines. An outline of the present book as far as the impact of the new research technologies on statistics and strictly related subjects is concerned is given with special emphasis on methods inspired by natural biological evolution.

1.1 Bio-inspired Optimization Methods

Since the fifties a new idea has started its way in the real world and academic problem solving domain. The core of this point of view resides in developing bio-inspired methodologies for handling issues that received not entirely satisfactory treatment by means of current to date procedures. Well known examples are the Rosenblatt's perceptron (Rosenblatt, 1958) and Box's evolutionary approach to industrial productivity (Box, 1957).

Box discussed the evolutionary approach as regards the improvement of the output of a plant at minimum or no cost at all. This is well distinguished from the innovation, that is a significant change in the production process, and quality control, which aims at ensuring that the product properties satisfy pre-specified standard. Evolutionary operation includes two features that outline a unique specific activity, (i) variation, and (ii) selection. The process has to be monitored as usual without the intervention of specialized plant personnel. Unlike laboratory experiments, the process itself performs ordinary production and yields information to give hints for improving the product. If unrecorded this information will be lost. By using the evolutionary operation approach both input and output of the process have to be recorded and a committee of three/four people may examine this information at

R. Baragona et al., *Evolutionary Statistical Procedures*, Statistics and Computing,
DOI 10.1007/978-3-642-16218-3_1,

regular intervals, once a month, for instance, to discover the variant, if any, which has been able to yield a better output. This way an evolution process may develop which adopts the good variants and discards those that yielded material of inferior quality.

The outstanding characteristic of such approach that an automatic activity may evolve itself by learning from its own past performances is present in the perceptron mechanism as well.

At the time of their appearance such proposals had to face on one hand the limited computational resources and on the other hand the widespread confidence in well established analytical tools. Nevertheless, complexity of real world called soon for complex models founded on a solid theoretical background. As a matter of fact, oversimplification does not help to get a really useful representation of many phenomena. High complex models are needed to properly handle hard problems. Unfortunately, these latter often result to be analytically intractable. An outstanding example is meteorological forecasting. The relatively simple models developed some decades ago were able to account for the overall dynamics of weather changes for small areas and short time span. However, forecasts proved to be almost useless as but a small improvement with respect to random guess. At present large high complex models allow forecasts to be delivered reliable enough to short-medium term. Such complicated models may be managed only by the nowadays high speed parallel computers. Only the lack of computing power prevented using appropriate models and providing people with useful forecasts. High complex models prompted for using evolutionary computing and large computer resources allowed the evolutionary algorithms to be developed. This does not mean that evolutionary computing is to be considered the best available problem solver. There are instances for which algorithms developed within a different framework may yield far better results. Moreover, researchers and practitioners are aware that a general purpose evolutionary algorithm will perform worse than any problem – oriented algorithm. On the other hand, fine tuning may improve the performance of an evolutionary algorithm so that it turns to be the best choice for some particular instance of a problem. This circumstance offers the main motivation for introducing the so – called hybrid methods. Hybridization may take place either between an evolutionary algorithm and an algorithm founded on analytical premises or between an evolutionary algorithm and a meta – heuristic algorithm. In the former case, the evolutionary algorithm is generally given the task of exploring the search space while the support algorithm refines the solution. In the latter case, it is the searching mechanism itself that is improved by features offered by the meta – heuristic. At present this seems the most promising approach and a line of active research. It is interesting to note that diffusion of evolutionary computing has been not quite uniform in application fields. Evolutionary algorithms have become standard tools for solving some classes of problems while there are domains where they are virtually unknown. For example, the traveling salesman problem is maybe the first application of evolutionary computing as favorite (or at least among the best choices) problem solver.

The problem is well known, in its simplest formulation it consists in finding the shortest route to visit each and every location in a given set only once. Constraints may be added and more complicated problems of this kind may arise. If labels $\{1, 2, \ldots, n\}$ identify the locations (towns, for instance) then the permutation that satisfies the constraints and optimizes the objective function (cost, distance, ...) yields the solution. Permutations, however, are known to grow large fast. So complete enumeration, exact/heuristic algorithms, meta heuristic methods have to be used in this order as far as the computing devices available at the moment allow their practical feasibility.

It is extremely difficult to predict if an evolutionary algorithm will succeed in handling a given problem. In general, evolutionary computing is to be considered either in the presence of several sub – optimal solutions close each other or if the search space is large and discrete. In the first case gradient – based algorithms, for instance, are likely to yield a sub – optimal solution if the starting point is close to this sub – optimum. In the second case, derivatives are not defined and gradient – based methods do not apply. However, strategies such as re – starting may avoid a gradient – based algorithm to be trapped in a local optimum and, on the other hand, other meta – heuristics may yield as equally good performance than evolutionary algorithms in discrete search spaces. Evolutionary computing theory may serve to give some insight into long run convergence of evolutionary algorithm. But rate of convergence is an issue that deserves further research. In fact it may well be the case that an evolutionary algorithm needs for exact convergence a number of steps comparable with the number of all possible feasible solutions to the problem at hand. In practice the most useful guide that is available to decide if it is worth the while using an evolutionary algorithm is experience. The capability of evolutionary algorithms to handle problems in a particular class is demonstrated by either applications or documented simulations. Again we have to stress the key role that availability of ever more powerful and cheaper computers has been playing as regards developments of evolutionary computing (and for so many new techniques and methods). At present the impressive improvement of computer resources allows calculations to be done that were simply impossible only few years ago.

At the same time the data storage facilities allow less and less expensive and larger and larger data bases to be available with easy and fast access to information.

Not only high complex models may be built and made operational but development of new tools is encouraged by the simple fact that software for practical applications may easily run on computers owned by researchers and practitioners. Another interesting circumstance resides in that methods developed in the past, that have been abandoned because of computational difficulties, are now becoming of practical usage. For example, neural networks have been studied since long time, but renewed interest has been possible after computers powerful enough allowed the calculations involved to be performed for real world scale problems. Though several evolutionary algorithms have been developed for solving problems arising in statistics, evolutionary computing is not to be considered a widespread tool in this domain. Statistical model building is of great importance in many fields of applications and requires more and more expertise from various disciplines. Environmental investigations on seismic events, analysis of the interactions among macro – economic variables, data mining and web mining are some examples of relevant problems where statistical models are essential part of the procedure solution. Even if a phenomenon is well understood, yet an estimation step is almost always needed to set up properly a number of problem – dependent details. Some numerical measures are not known in advance and cannot be easily computed nor offered ready – made from past experience. Namely, we have parameters to be estimated. Statistical estimation techniques proceed by setting up a probabilistic model which is specified up to a certain number of unknown parameters. Proper values are searched in a feasible space of solutions. The search is driven by criteria that amount to maximization or minimization of suitable functions derived by the probabilistic model. Evolutionary computing may intervene in this respect, suggesting evolutionary algorithms to be used as function optimizers. Non parametric approach may use evolutionary computing in a similar manner. Evolutionary algorithms have to be designed according to the appropriate optimality criteria. Of course, researchers and practitioners are faced with the dilemma what is the best choice among several algorithms grounded on different framework. As usual, algorithms that proved to work well for a particular problem should be retained until some shortcoming become apparent. Then we may either resort to hybridization for improving the technique or turn to different approaches, including evolutionary computing.

Finally, a connection has been pointed out recently between evolutionary computation and random numbers generation according to a specified probability distribution. This issue is object of current research.

1.2 Topics Organization

The book is composed of two parts. The first one is devoted to introduce evolutionary computing and the special techniques that are commonly included under this label. To date, we may list evolutionary programming, genetic algorithms, evolution strategies, genetic programming, estimation of distribution algorithms, evolutionary behavior and differential evolution. Applications in statistics are concerned mostly with genetic algorithms, so we will briefly illustrate the theoretical back ground of genetic algorithms. Special consideration will be given to convergence issues and fine tuning of algorithm parameters. Then we will describe the applications of genetic algorithms that have been tried to date as regards statistical problems. This will give some hints if and when the evolutionary computing approach may be preferred to different competing techniques.

Chapter 2
Evolutionary Computation

Abstract The evolutionary computation methods are introduced by discussing their origin inside the artificial intelligence framework, and the contributions of Darwin's theory of natural evolution and Genetics. We attempt to highlight the main features of an evolutionary computation method, and describe briefly some of them: evolutionary programming, evolution strategies, genetic algorithm, estimation of distribution algorithms, differential evolution. The remainder of the chapter is devoted to a closer illustration of genetic algorithms and more recent advancements, to the problem of convergence and to the practical use of them. A final section on the relationship between genetic algorithms and random sampling techniques is included.

2.1 Introduction

2.1.1 Evolutionary Computation Between Artificial Intelligence and Natural Evolution

Drawing an history of evolutionary computation is not an easy task nor within the scope of this book. However, we shall spend some words to outline where and when the framework, which has later become that of evolutionary computation, originated.

The term "evolutionary" started to be associated with concepts linked to computing and algorithms towards the beginning of the sixties, in the scientific community concerned with developing and studying computing machines, and specifically in a field which has been known as *artificial intelligence*. An excellent discussion may be found in chapter 1 of Fogel (1998).

Though the term artificial intelligence (AI) is widely accepted for denoting a specific research field, the definition of AI is controversial; proposals range from manipulations of symbols for solving problems, to developing intelligent computer programs, to mechanization of the human thought process, or even the study of mental faculties by means of computational models.

The starting contribution may be considered Turing (1950), who addressed the question: can a machine think? An essential requirement is that the process of thinking may be exactly objectified and formalized, then one may try to transpose that process into a digital machine program. In order to perform such a complex

R. Baragona et al., *Evolutionary Statistical Procedures*, Statistics and Computing,
DOI 10.1007/978-3-642-16218-3_2, © Springer-Verlag Berlin Heidelberg 2011

abstraction, scientists had been faced with enormous logical difficulties, and therefore they tried to limit their efforts, at least initially, to a narrower and well defined field: therefore, they started to study simple situations generally linked to games.

Moreover, it was necessary to find games where the purpose be unambiguously defined, and the measurement of the degree of attainment of that purpose be possible and not too hard; and finally, it was required that chance had no role at all in the game, in order to make the analysis deterministic, therefore simpler. It is not surprising that soon many researchers focused on the chess game, and in subsequent years a great deal of effort was devoted by scientists both in academy and in computer research centers, to derive software and more and more powerful machines able to defeat a human chess top player (in 1997 IBM's Deep Blue defeated the world champion Garry Kasparov).

However, it was soon clear to many researchers that those computers exploited their ability to evaluate very rapidly an enormous database of information, and compare them to the specific instances when they have to decide a move, but no form of *learning* automatically is involved.

But how to define that last requirement? A possible answer is that *learning* means connecting together pieces of knowledge to create new knowledge. Such a (apparently) simple idea led to the development of the so-called expert systems. In this software, a set of entities (objects) are defined, and sets of relationships between pairs (or more) of entities are enunciated (the knowledge base). A set of logical rules (what is called the inference engine) allows to discover possible new relationships between two given entities by following chains of relations contained in the knowledge base. Compared to chess programs, expert systems are also based on a large information set, and exploit the computer ability of managing rapidly its elements, but also attempt to connect them to create new knowledge. However, in the expert systems also, the difficulty of making explicit all the knowledge related to but the simplest problems makes application to real problems extremely complex.

An alternative framework which was soon explored, also starting from the middle of twentieth century, is turning to a microscopic view rather than macroscopic, leading to the nowadays well established framework called (artificial) neural networks. In the same fashion as the fundamental brain activity is governed by electrical impulses that flow through the neural cells, a neural network is a set of entities (also named neurons) which are connected to each other by ordered links. Each (artificial) neuron receives from each of its antecedents some numerical information, and depending on the whole set of received signals transmits a numerical information to each of their successors. The information flow is oriented, thus a neural network has distinct input and output information. According to a given input the network produces a specific output depending on its structure. If, for a given input, a target output is defined, the network parameters may be tuned in order to achieve the required output, and in all cases but the simplest this has to be done by iterative approximation. This is known as the training activity of the network: a recursive process that brings an entity to approach progressively the attainment of its goal. Indeed, the distinctive feature of changing continuously the behavior in order to obtain benefits according to a given measure of satisfaction has been advocated as an essential characteristic of intelligence, and provides the link between artificial intelligence and evolutionary computation.

A similar link may be drawn in nature between intelligence and adaptation. In effect, it is doubtless that intelligence arises when an organism reacts to the external forces (say, the *environment*) and many reactions are possible, with different consequences. Intelligence may be thought of as related to choosing reactions that ensure best results and it in turn calls for a definition and a measure of reaching goals, or satisfaction. Thus, the concept of intelligence requires, on one hand, that different courses of action may be alternatively chosen, in other terms, is concerned with decision maker entities, and, on the other hand, requires that each possible action may be evaluated, in order that good and bad behaviors may be distinguished. But the outcome of each action depends generally on the environment, therefore intelligence requires that information from the environment may be recovered and analyzed. Fogel et al. (1966) state: "intelligence is the capability of a system to adapt its behavior to meet its goal in a range of environments". In a word, though extremizing: *intelligence is evolution*.

The last word, evolution, introduces the second framework which inspired the development of evolutionary computation methods, and from which they inherited the name itself, the terminology and the fundamental ideas: the theory of natural evolution, named after Charles Darwin.

The main results obtained by Darwin in the middle of the nineteenth century received confirmation later and further development from the progress of genetics, and now a systematic theory of natural evolution has been formulated and its validity recognized almost everywhere, known as *neo-Darwinism*.

Neo-Darwinism proposes to explain the dynamics of life through few interaction mechanisms among individuals, and between individuals and the environment. Each of such mechanisms is subject to random forces, and their outcome is stochastic.

The first process is reproduction, where each individual, or each pair if sexual reproduction is considered, bears new individuals that have some features of their parents, and can mix characters of their two parents in sexual reproduction. Mutation is the second process, which arises also in the transition from parents to children, and allows new characters to appear in the population. The competition mechanism implies that individuals in the same population, owing to finite resources, are antagonists and compete to ensure sufficient (or satisfying) benefits, and implies also that some individuals are successful while others are not and are, at various extent, eliminated from the population. Finally, the selection process dictates that not all individuals have the same reproduction ability, and such differences are related to the capacity of the individual to adapt to the environment and survive to the competitors and predators.

Given a population at a certain time (the initial generation), a new population (the new generation) is formed, after all such processes have acted on each individual of the initial population. Some individuals of the initial population survive to the new population, and some new individuals are born. Modifications are random but the essential feature is that individuals that are more adapted (fitted) to the environment tend to survive and reproduce to a larger extent than individuals that are less fitted, therefore favorable characteristics tend to spread into populations, generation after generation.

2.1.2 The Contribution of Genetics

The outstanding contribution of Charles Darwin, based on the principle of *survival of the fittest*, has led to the theory of natural evolution which enables to explain the biological history of species. Darwin's theory was essentially observational, because it was not possible at that time to explain and describe in detail how the physical modifications of individuals take place, and which biological processes lead to recombination and mutation. This is the subject of genetics and it was developed only later: reason is, on one hand, that substantial progress in knowledge of biochemical processes was needed, and, on the other hand, that the mechanisms involved are extremely complex.

Modern genetics allow to describe the evolution process at different levels of detail, but a rather general description is sufficient for a mathematical formalization.

Living beings are constituted by cells with specialized tasks, but each cell contains a fixed number of chromosomes (number varies according to the species) which carry the genetic information of the whole individual. Each chromosome in turn contains several information, each piece of elementary information is called a gene. A gene may be conceptually thought of as a binary code, that may assume two different states (for genes the words expressed and unexpressed are used). The whole of information carried by genes of all chromosomes (the genotype) determines all characters of an individual (the phenotype). Chromosomes are ordered in pairs, and when sexual reproduction takes place, children receive, for each pair, one chromosome from each of their parents.

Reproduction is a complex process during which two phenomena may occur (among others) which modify the overall information transmitted from parents to children: mutation and recombination. Mutation happens when the single piece of information carried by a single gene changes: this modification may arise due to several complicated biochemical reasons, and may be assumed as a random event, generally a rare event. Recombination involves a couple of different chromosomes, and produces an exchange of genetic material so that part of the information carried by one chromosome is exchanged with the corresponding information of the other one. Recombination is also a random event, though more frequent in nature than mutation.

Once the physical and chemical processes involved in natural evolution had been discovered, it became possible to formalize them into a mathematical algorithm, but obviously this may be done only through many simplifying assumptions, because such processes are too complex.

The description of genetical evolution given above is very approximate and imprecise and does not approach in any detail the physical and chemical processes involved: really, we have not mentioned DNA at all. However, it is rich enough to be suitable for most purposes, and indeed the best mathematical metaphor of the evolution process, the genetic algorithm, is based on an even more simplified scheme.

In a genetic algorithm, each individual is assigned only one chromosome which characterizes all its features (possibly including several distinct fragments), and most often the information carried by each gene is simply binary. Moreover, there is no sex distinction, thus any individual may mate with any other to bear an offspring; finally, no growing up or ageing exist, and the fitness of each individual is constant in time. In spite of its simplicity, the genetic algorithm proved a formidable, all purposes optimizing tool; its simplicity explains also why an overwhelming number of variants and generalizations have been proposed in the literature.

Genetic algorithms originate from the work of John Holland in the sixties, and were developed by him and his students at the University of Michigan during several years. The fundamental reference, where genetic algorithms are formally introduced and thoroughly explored, is Holland's book *Adaptation in Natural and Artificial Systems* printed in 1975. As is clear from the title, Holland's idea was to formalize and describe a quantitative framework for studying the process of adaptation and evolution of a biological population, and to learn from them rules and principles which could allow artificial systems, in a similar fashion, to evolve. The latter are often related to optimization problems, thus employing the genetic algorithm environment for solving optimization problems has obvious advantages.

Each individual of the population is associated to a possible solution of the problem, and the function to be optimized assumes the meaning of fitness. Therefore, the fittest individual in each generation represents the best solution reached thus far, and evolution allows to discover a solution that gets better, as the generations evolve. In this way, running a genetic algorithm allows to produce a sequence of solutions (the best fitted individuals at each generation) which approach the optimum.

There has been considerable discussion on the role of genetic algorithms as function optimizers (see De Jong, 1993): it is clear that trying to optimize a function by means of a genetic algorithm means following only the best fitted individual at each generation, therefore focusing only on a particular aspect of the algorithm behavior; we return to this topic at the end of the present chapter.

Genetic algorithms have been successfully employed for solving optimization problems in many fields. Several are related with the design of complex systems and their optimal control. Among them, we can cite filters in communications and acoustics; neural networks; communication systems; wireless networks; computer networks; and even nuclear reactors. Genetic algorithms proved their validity in many classical operations research problems, such as the travelling salesman, scheduling and task planning. Finally, notable applications of genetic algorithms are found in several difficult applied problems, such as speech recognition and medical diagnosis. An especially suitable field where genetic algorithms find increasing applications is protein engineering. Hundredth of references may be found in any good genetic algorithms textbook (to cite just a few: Goldberg, 1989a; Davis, 1991; Man et al., 1999; Michalewicz, 1996a; Mitchell, 1996), and a review is beyond the scope of this book.

What all these problems have in common is complexity. In effect, there is no point in trying to solve by means of a genetic algorithm a problem whose solution may be found by means of analytical methods (such as equating derivatives to zero), or simple and well-behaved problems where classical numerical techniques such as Newton's method are generally adequate. Therefore genetic algorithms are employed in problems for which, essentially, no method for determining the optimum is known better than enumerating all the possible solutions. Such problems are known in the computational complexity theory as NP-complete problems, as discussed in the next section.

The last 30 years have seen an enormous development of the theory originated by John Holland, bridges have been built between the several similar attempts linked to the idea of evolution, and now a generally accepted framework called *evolutionary computation* has been established; however, genetic algorithms still appear the most general and flexible tool for evolutionary computation, and often evolutionary computing and genetic algorithms are used as synonymous.

2.2 Evolutionary Computation Methods

2.2.1 Essential Properties

Though we have observed that evolutionary computation is not only optimization, most applications in Statistics are concerned, at least at present, with optimization problems.

Schematically, an optimization problem may be defined as a pair (f, Ω) where f is a function from Ω to the set of real numbers $\mathbb{R}$, and Ω is the set of possible solutions. If Ω is a subset of $\mathbb{R}^n$ but is not a subset of $\mathbb{R}^{n-1}$, then n is the dimension of the problem. The aim may be to maximize or minimize the value of the objective function f. Solving the problem means finding the element(s) of Ω for which f attains its maximum (minimum) value, if they exist.

In many lucky (or simplified) cases, f is a well-behaved mathematical function of n real arguments, and Ω is a sufficiently regular subset of $\mathbb{R}^n$ so that the solution is found simply by equating to zero the derivatives of f. But in the great majority of cases this is not possible, the most relevant instance in Statistics is when Ω is a discrete, though very large, set. In that case we speak of combinatorial optimization problems.

Optimum problems may be classified according to their computational complexity, as measured by the number of elementary operations (generally specified as computer elementary arithmetical or logical instructions) needed to solve them. Problems for which an algorithm requiring a number of operations of order equal to a polynomial in n is known, are called P problems, while problems for which only algorithms exist whose number of required operations grows faster with n than a polynomial are called NP problems. Whether a given problem for which a polynomial algorithm is not known, is P or NP, cannot generally be shown, and the question if a NP problem actually exists is still essentially formally open. However, a class of problems may be defined, which are (at present) NP, but it may be shown that if for one of them a polynomial algorithm may be found, then a polynomial algorithm exists for any NP problem. Problems in that class are called NP-complete. Though one cannot exclude that for a NP-complete problem an algorithm in polynomial time will be discovered, this is most unlikely, and in this case it would be possible to solve with the same complexity level all NP problems: it would essentially mean that the class of P problems and that of NP problems coincide.

Therefore, in practice a NP-complete problem can be exactly solved only enumerating, and evaluating, all possible solutions (all elements of the set Ω) and this becomes rapidly impossible as n increases. Thus, we have to be satisfied with approximate solution methods, trying to build algorithms which enable to obtain "sufficiently good" solutions in a reasonable time: such methods are called *heuristic* algorithms.

An exact and widely shared definition of heuristic algorithm does not exist, but a generally accepted idea is that a heuristic method searches for best solutions of a problem at a reasonable computational cost, without ensuring to reach optimality, and consists in an iterative sequence of moves inside the solution space towards better points, trying to avoid evident errors. From a computational complexity point of view, a heuristic is an approximate algorithm which provides nearly optimal solutions to a NP problem in polynomial time.

Most heuristic methods are based on local search algorithms, in the sense that they wander inside the solution space, and each move is determined by evaluating neighboring candidates, and entering those which are considered more promising according to pre-specified given criteria.

Since heuristics may profit of the particular and specific features of each single problem, it is likely that ad-hoc techniques be suitable, and that a heuristic that performs well on a kind of problem does not work so good in another. A series of theorems (called *no free lunch theorems*) originated by the work of D. H. Wolpert and W. G. Macready (1997) state, essentially, that, if averaged on sufficiently broad classes of problems, any pair of heuristic algorithm give equivalent results. Therefore, heuristic methods are often tailored to the specific problems they have to solve.

There are, however, some all-purposes stochastic search methods which rely on basic ideas useful for any optimization problem, and for this reason are called *meta-heuristic*.

A heuristic optimization algorithm may be essentially described as an iterative method which defines a sequence of elements in the solution space, with the aim of progressively improving the values of the objective function. It is based at least on the following items:

(a) A set of possible solutions Ω
(b) A function $f(\cdot)$ defined on Ω and taking values on the set of real numbers (or some subset), called the objective (or target, or score) function, and a scope: maximization or minimization

(c) A set of neighborhoods defined for each element of Ω, or a rule for describing the neighboring elements of each point $\omega \in \Omega$, say $\{N(\omega), \omega \in \Omega\}$.
(d) A set of moving rules, which determine, for each $\omega \in \Omega$, which element in the neighborhood $N(\omega)$ is chosen as the next solution to be evaluated. Rules are often random, in that case they specify a probability distribution on the elements of the neighborhood $N(\omega)$.
(e) A starting point $\omega_0 \in \Omega$
(f) A stopping rule for deciding when the iterative process should be terminated, and the best-so-far found solution to be declared the result of optimization.

The heuristic is iterative: starting from ω_0, it computes its neighborhood $N(\omega_0)$ according to (c), chooses a point $\omega_1 \in N(\omega_0)$ according to (d), and turns from ω_0 to ω_1; then the elements of $N(\omega_1)$ are examined and one of them, ω_2, is selected; then $N(\omega_2)$ is computed and a new element ω_3 in it is selected and so on. If the stopping rule is met at iteration n, then ω_n is assumed as the solution and $f(\omega_n)$ as the optimized value of the objective function.

If the decisions concerning items (c), (d), (e) and (f) do not depend on the particular behavior of the objective function $f(\cdot)$, but are specified in terms of mathematical procedures defined on the formal objects $f(\cdot)$ and Ω, and may therefore applied to any particularization of them, the algorithm is called a *meta-heuristic*.

Many different heuristic methods have been proposed and are employed in various fields, their differences are essentially in the way the neighborhoods, and, more important, the moving rules, are selected, the most relevant alternatives being between deterministic and stochastic procedures, and between monotonic – $f(\omega_{k+1})$ always better than $f(\omega_k)$ – or non-monotonic rules.

Relevant examples of meta-heuristic methods are the descent methods, threshold accepting, simulated annealing, tabu search.

Evolutionary computation methods share the common features of meta-heuristics, but in addition have specific characteristics:

1. Evolutionary computation methods are population-based algorithms. It means that they consider at each stage an entire subset of possible solutions as the individuals of a population, and at each iteration (in this framework called *generation*) each member of the population changes (or only some of them); furthermore, the number of individuals may also change iteration by iteration. The essential feature, however, is that evolution originates from reciprocal interactions among individuals, in other terms the choice of which individual will become part of the population at generation n depends on the whole set of individuals in generation $n-1$.
2. The moving rules are stochastic. Therefore, at each step, each individual is assigned a neighborhood and a probability distribution on that, and the individual is changed to a new one inside the neighborhood according to a random trial on that probability distribution.

In summary, and reconciling the naturally inspired terminology of Sect. 2.1.1 with the more mathematical style of this Section, an evolutionary computation method may be described as follows:

(a) The algorithm motivation is to search for the maximum value of a given function $f : \Omega \rightarrow \mathbb{R}$. Each element of the set Ω is called an individual, and the value of $f(\cdot)$ measures the success of that individual in its environment, therefore f is called the fitness function and the aim is to maximize it.
(b) The algorithm is iterative and at each stage n (called a generation) produces a subset of Ω, called the population at generation n. A rule for choosing the population at the initial stage (generation 0 population) is therefore needed, and also a stopping rule for determining at which generation the iterations should terminate, has to be selected.
(c) The composition of population at generation n is determined by the population of the previous generation according to a stochastic procedure, which is inspired by the natural evolution theory, and tries to translate into formal mathematical operations the biological processes of reproduction, mutation, recombination. Members of generation $n - 1$ are seen as parents, and those of generation n as children. The number of individuals in the population may increase or decrease at each iteration (according to the different evolutionary computation algorithms), therefore the neighborhood usually includes the null element, and a jump to that means the elimination of the individual.

The essential innovation of population based methods is that the "destiny" of each individual at generation n depends on the whole set of individuals in the population at that time; this means that for each individual $\omega \in \Omega$ its neighborhood, defining what it will become in the next generation, depends on the other individuals of the contemporary population. Furthermore, different individuals in the same generations may have different types of neighborhood. Thus, the most common way of analyzing and following the evolution across generations does not refer to neighborhoods of each individual, but rather focuses on offsprings arising at each generation from the population as a whole.

Since the transition from a generation to the next one has a complicate mechanism, it may be generally decomposed into different successive phases. The first one consists in selecting, from the individuals of the population at the current generation, a set of candidates for bearing new offsprings (a stage often referred to as selection); then, each of them (or more frequently each pair) undergoes a process consisting in the successive application of some modification rules (the evolutionary "operators", frequently inspired by analogies with nature), ending up in the creation of one (or sometimes two) new individual (the child). Finally, children may replace their parents (totally or partly or not at all according to different replacement schemes), and constitute the population for the next generation.

A classification of evolutionary computation method is not simple, and many different criteria have been proposed. However, at least on an historical ground, there is a general agreement that three methods: evolutionary programming, evolution strategies and genetic algorithms, originated the family of evolutionary computation algorithms. We describe briefly these three frameworks in the next sections. More recently, many new methods have been proposed and explored. Among them, we shall address only a few methods which appear more suitable for applications in Statistics: the estimation of distribution algorithm, the differential evolution and some evolutionary behavior algorithms.

2.2.2 Evolutionary Programming

Evolutionary programming is the first methodology which relies on evolutionary concepts and was invented by Lawrence Fogel at the beginning of the sixties. He was concerned with artificial intelligence and developed the original idea that intelligence is intimately related with the ability of predicting a dynamic environment, in order to be able to increase self adaptation. In order to formalize such process, he considered *finite state machines*.

A finite state machine is a black box system which transforms a sequence of inputs in a sequence of outputs, given a finite alphabet of input and a finite alphabet of output. The finite state machine may be in a (also finite) number of different states, and the response depends on the state. The behavior of a machine is dynamical: it starts in an initial state, and receives the first input symbol; according to this, it outputs a symbol among the allowed alphabet, and changes state. Now, the second input is received and analyzed, and according to the current state an output symbol is chosen, and so on: each received input symbol produces an output and a state transition.

The output symbol of a state machine has the meaning of an attempt to predict the next input symbol (or some feature of it). Therefore an evaluation function (called the payoff) on the pairs {output symbol, next input symbol} is defined. At each stage of evolution, the entire sequence of input symbols is compared with the sequence of outputs, and the fitness of the machine is evaluated by taking the sum of the payoff values at each time.

As a very simple example, consider an average weekly forecast exercise. At each stage (say on Monday) the average temperature of the last week is received in input, while the current system state denotes the season: spring, summer, autumn or winter. According to the input temperature, the state is updated, and the related average seasonal temperature is output. This simple procedure may be formalized through a four–state finite machine: states are denoted by Spring, sUmmer, Autumn, Winter, input symbols may be $f$rozen, $c$old, $m$ild, $w$arm, $h$ot, and output symbols t_S, t_U, t_A, t_W, the four average seasonal temperature.

A possible behavior of this finite state machine is sketched in Table 2.1. If the input temperature is more suitable for the next (in time) season rather than the current one, the state is changed to the next, otherwise the state remains unchanged. For example, if the current state is Winter and the input temperature is too high, the state is changed to Spring. The transition table associates each pair (current state, input)

Table 2.1 State transition of the finite state machine in the example

input / state	f	c	m	w	h
Spring	(S, t_S)	(S, t_S)	(S, t_S)	(U, t_U)	(U, t_U)
sUmmer	(A, t_A)	(A, t_A)	(A, t_A)	(U, t_U)	(U, t_U)
Autumn	(W, t_W)	(W, t_W)	(A, t_A)	(A, t_A)	(A, t_A)
Winter	(W, t_W)	(W, t_W)	(S, t_S)	(S, t_S)	(S, t_S)

to the resulting pair (new state, output). The payoff values may be evaluated through the absolute difference between the temperature in output and the input temperature of the next week.

Evolutionary programming is a population based algorithm (and it was essentially the first population based method in literature). An initial population of finite state machines is generated at random, and exposed for a certain time to the environment (receiving a sequence of input symbols), then a next generation is produced by mutation. Each parent finite state machine produces an offspring by randomly changing one of the following characteristics: initial state, number of states, a response to an input symbol, or a transition from a state to the following. Also, the number of mutations undergone by a single offspring may be selected at random. Once each finite state machine has produced an offspring, they are evaluated by means of the payoff-based fitness. Then, on considering the whole set of parents and children, only half of the machines, those which provide the largest fitness, are retained and constitute the next generation population.

The brief account above refers to evolutionary programming as was originally introduced by Lawrence Fogel and is formalized in the book *Artificial Intelligence through Simulated Evolution* by Fogel et al. (1966). However, the procedure is of a general nature and may be adapted to many different problems, since the representation of each individual as a finite state machine is very flexible. Indeed, evolutionary programming has received a great deal of generalization and implementations in different fields, specially in the last decade, where increasing similarities with evolution strategies were enlightened. Most relevant extensions to the original scheme include:

- definitions of individuals by means of data structures such as real vectors or matrices
- the use of recombination operators which allow offsprings to be generated, that inherit features of more than one individual
- choice of the method for selecting the best individuals to be retained in the generation by stochastic rather than deterministic rules
- parameters which drive reproduction may be evolved together with the individuals

Evolutionary programming (as well as genetic algorithms) was also proposed as a basis for evolving computer software, and it led to a new emerging discipline known as *genetic programming* which is now developing rapidly, but lies beyond the scope of the present book (for an account, see Koza, 1992).

2.2.3 Evolution Strategies

A different approach which is also based on the idea of evolution was proposed in the sixties by I. Rechenberg and H. P. Schwefel at Berlin Technical University. Here the motivation comes from a process control problem in an engineering framework, and was soon extended to optimization of general functions of multiple variables. A detailed account may be found in Back (1996), and a more concise and recent introduction in Beyer and Schwefel (2002).

Like evolutionary programming, evolution strategies have been extended and widened in several directions, and at present these two evolutionary frameworks are becoming more and more similar and integrating.

In its original formulation, an evolution strategies is an algorithm for optimizing a real valued function of M real variables: $f : \mathbb{R}^M \to \mathbb{R}$. Evolution strategies also are based on populations of individuals, which evolve through successive generations. An individual is a possible solution to the problem, and therefore is identified by a vector in $\mathbb{R}^M$. The fitness evaluation is obviously made through the function to be optimized f (thus proportional to f if the maximum is needed, and to $-f$, or inversely proportional, if the minimum is required).

The algorithm is iterative and the population at the beginning is composed by individuals chosen at random, uniformly, in the whole space of solutions. At each generation, offsprings are generated by selecting a parent and perturbing it by simply adding a random realization of a $M-$variate gaussian variable with zero mean and a given (diagonal) dispersion matrix. Formally, from the individual $x = (x_1, x_2, \ldots, x_M)'$ the offspring $y = (y_1, y_2, \ldots, y_M)'$ is obtained from

$$y_i = x_i + z_i\sigma_i \quad i = 1, 2, \ldots, M \tag{2.1}$$

where $(z_1, z_2, \ldots, z_M)$ are independent realizations of a gaussian N(0,1) variable, and $(\sigma_1, \sigma_2, \ldots, \sigma_M)$ are pre-specified values.

Once all offspring are created, the population for the next generation is formed by selecting only the fittest individuals, according to different strategies, called $(\mu + \lambda)$ or (μ, λ), where μ is the (constant) number of individuals in the population, and λ is the number of offsprings at each generation:

$(\mu + \lambda)$–ES μ parents are employed for creating λ children, then all $(\mu + \lambda)$ individuals are ranked and the best μ are chosen to constitute the next generation population

(μ, λ)–ES λ offsprings are generated by μ parents, $\lambda > \mu$, and only the μ best fitted out of the λ offsprings are returned for the next generation population: therefore each individual disappears at the next generation.

A number of important extensions and generalizations were introduced in later years, so that the actual evolution strategies employed in recent applications are much more elaborated. Main evolutions of the original strategy concern *self-adaptation* and *recombination*.

Self-adaptation means that the parameters governing mutation are also evolved together with individuals. Therefore each member of the population is characterized not only by its numerical vector related to the solution, but also by the vector of the standard errors of the perturbations: an individual is coded by $(y_1, \ldots, y_M, \sigma_1, \ldots, \sigma_m)$. The standard deviation parameters σ_i are also inherited by the offsprings, and are subject to mutation too. The mutation operator for σ is often described by:

$$\sigma_{\text{new}} = \sigma_{\text{old}} \exp\{\tau z\}$$

where z is a realization of a gaussian standard variable and τ is a fixed constant (called the learning parameter).

Recombination was proposed in order to get offspring that share characteristics of more than one parent solution. The corresponding evolution strategies, indicated with $(\mu/\rho, \lambda)$–ES or $(\mu/\rho+\lambda)$–ES, rely on a fixed number ρ chosen in advance and called the mixing number ($\rho < \mu$) which defines the number of parents involved in an offspring. For each offspring to be born, ρ parents are selected at random from the population, let $x_i(k), i = 1, \ldots, M; k = 1, \ldots, \rho$ be the solution coordinates of the selected parents: then each coordinate y_i of the offspring depends on the set of the corresponding coordinates of its parents $\{x_i(k), k = 1, \ldots, \rho\}$, and two alternative recombination operators may be adopted:

- discrete (or dominant) recombination: y_i is selected at random with equal probabilities out of $\{x_i(1), x_i(2), \ldots, x_i(\rho)\}$, for each $(i = 1, 2, \ldots, M)$.
- intermediate recombination: y_i is chosen equal to the arithmetic mean of the parents coordinates:

$$y_i = \frac{1}{\rho} \sum_{k=1}^{\rho} x_i(k)$$

Even more elaborated strategies have been proposed more recently. One of the most interesting is *covariance matrix adaptation* ES, where the solution vectors are mutated by perturbing through correlated gaussian variables, or equivalently (2.1) is substituted by

$$y = x + \sigma Q z$$

where $z = (z_1, z_2, \ldots, z_M)'$ is a vector of random observation of m independent standard gaussian variates, and $V = QQ'$ is the covariance matrix of the mutation step. When self-adaptation is used, the parameter σ and the entries of the matrix Q are evolved together with individuals.

Evolution strategies are more naturally employed when the space of the solutions is $\mathbb{R}^M$ or at least a compact subset, but they have to be modified and generalized to cope also with discrete spaces or even with mixed, or constrained spaces, though it may impose several restrictions on the mutation and recombination operators.

2.2.4 Genetic Algorithms

Among the evolutionary computation methods, genetic algorithms are those which most rely on biological inspiration and try to develop farther a metaphor of the natural evolution of biological populations. The terminology itself bears many analogies with genetics and biology.

A genetic algorithm is an iterative procedure that follows the evolution of a population of individuals through successive generations . The features of each individual are formalized in a vector of symbols from a given alphabet (usually a binary or decimal digit) called the *chromosome*. Each entry of this vector is called a *gene*. Not only the value of each gene, but also its position (the *locus*) in the chromosome is relevant in defining the characteristics of the individual. The whole set of characteristics of each individual determines its ability to survive and reproduce in the environment, and this is supposed to be measurable by means of a single valued real (often positive) number, called the fitness of the individual. Thus, a real-valued function may be defined on the set of chromosomes, which measures the fitness and is called the fitness function.

We shall denote by g the index of the generation, by i the index of the individual in the population ($i = 1, 2, \ldots, N$) and by j the index of the gene in the chromosome ($j = 1, 2, \ldots, M$). Therefore the individual i at generation g is associated to the following chromosome :

$$x_i^{(g)} = (x_{i,1}^{(g)}, x_{i,2}^{(g)}, \ldots, x_{i,M}^{(g)})'$$

and $f[x_i^{(g)}]$ will denote its fitness value.

Transition from a generation to the next consists in a reproduction process, of a stochastic nature, articulated in the three stages of selection, recombination and mutation.

The selection step results in choosing which individuals of the current population are going to reproduce. Owing to the natural population similarity, we want that most fitted individuals reproduce more frequently than less fitted ones, therefore, we set up a random procedure where the probability of being selected for reproduction is an increasing function of the fitness value. Most popular rules (or selection operators) are the *roulette wheel*, the *stochastic universal sampling*, and the *tournament selection*.

The roulette wheel method simply selects an individual with probability proportional to its fitness. Therefore, each choice of a candidate to reproduction is made by a random trial with possible results $\{x_i^{(g)}, i = 1, \ldots, N\}$ and associated probability

$$P\left[x_i^{(g)}\right] = f\left[x_i^{(g)}\right] \Big/ \sum_{k=1}^{N} f\left[x_k^{(g)}\right].$$

The roulette wheel rule may be also seen in terms of the fitness empirical distribution function $F_g(y) = \text{Freq}\ \{\text{individuals with fitness} < y \text{ at generation } g\}$, and amounts simply to choosing independently N times a number r uniformly distributed between 0 and 1, and selecting the corresponding r-quantile of F_g (i.e., the individual that has the largest value of F_g less than r).

Stochastic universal sampling, on the contrary, is obtained by generating uniformly at random only one number ℓ in $(0, 1/N)$, and choosing the individuals corresponding to quantiles $\ell, \ell + 1/N, \ell + 2/N, \ldots, \ell + (N-1)/N$ of F_g.

Tournament selection is a method which tries to exploit further similarities with natural populations, and is based on comparisons of individuals (a tournament) where the best fitted wins. For each candidate to reproduction to be selected, a group of individuals is chosen at random (but with different modalities according to variants of this method), they are compared and the one with the largest fitness is selected. The replacement actually takes place with probability p_s (*selection pressure*).

Once the selection stage has produced candidates for reproduction, the recombination stage considers randomly chosen pairs of individuals. They mate and produce a pair of offsprings that may share genes of both parents. This process, also called *cross-over*, is applied with a fixed probability (usually large than 0.5 but smaller than one) to each pair. Several different types of cross-over are common, the simplest is called one point cross-over. It consists in pairing the chromosomes of the two individuals and choosing at random one locus: the genes which appear before that locus remain unchanged, while the genes appearing after the cross-over point are exchanged together. The process produces, from two parents, two children, each of which inherits part of the gene sequence from one parent, and the remaining part from the other parent. If cross-over does not take place, the two children remain identical to their parents. A more elaborated cross-over type is called uniform cross-over: each gene of the offspring is selected at random, from the corresponding genes of the two parents, with equal probability. Note that in this way the number of offsprings from a pair may be chosen to be one, two or even more.

Once offsprings are generated, they are subject to the mutation operator. Mutation is needed to introduce innovation into the population (since selection and cross-over only mix the existing genes), but is generally considered a rare event (like it is in nature). Therefore, a small probability p_m is selected, and each gene of each individual's chromosome is subject to mutation with that probability, independently of all other genes. If the gene coding is binary, a mutation simply changes a 0 to a 1 or vice versa, while if the alphabet for a gene is richer, a mutation rule has to be defined. Often a uniform random choice among all possible symbols (different from that to be mutated) is preferred if the alphabet is finite, or a perturbation based on a gaussian variable if the genes are coded as real numbers.

A final important topic is the way new offsprings replace their parents, also called reproduction (sometimes replacement) strategy. We assume that the number of individuals in the population for each generation remains equal and fixed to N; the simplest rule is generating N offsprings and replacing entirely the population at each generation. However, this way may eliminate the best fitted individual with non zero probability, therefore a common modification is as follows: if the best fitted offspring is worse than the best fitted parent, this last is retained in the next generation population, usually replacing the least fitted offspring. It is called the *elitist* strategy. More generally, we may decide to replace at each generation only a fraction (called the *generation gap*) of the population, or even to replace just one individual (usually the worst) at each generation (a procedure called *steady state* or *incremental rule*).

Many modifications of the genetic algorithm have been proposed in literature, and several types of different procedures concerning mutation, recombination and replacement have been introduced. Furthermore, some new operators have been considered, for example *inversion* (which consists in reversing the order of the genes in a chromosome) that are employed less frequently: some of them will be used for specific purposes in later chapters.

Genetic algorithms start from an initial population (generation 0) whose individuals are usually selected at random uniformly in the solution space, or, sometimes, are chosen in a deterministic fashion in order to represent different subsets of that space. As generations proceed, new individuals appear: owing to the selection mechanism, their fitness is on the average larger than their parents; moreover, the cross-over operator allows appearance of new individuals that may enjoy favorable characteristics of both parents. Thus, it is likely that after many generations the best chromosome that may be obtained by combining the genes of the initial population is discovered and starts to replicate itself; however, this process would be unable to experiment new genetic material. In other words, in case that all individuals at generation 0 have say a gene code equal to 1 in the first locus of their chromosome, this would be true for any offspring, indefinitely, and if the maximum fitness corresponds to a chromosome whose first gene equals 0, this would never be discovered. The solution to this drawback is obviously mutation: such operator ensures that all possible gene sequences may be obtained in the chromosome of the offspring, and therefore, in principle, we may be confident that running a genetic algorithm for a sufficiently large number of generations the space of solutions is thoroughly explored, and the best individual found. We shall return to this topic (the algorithm convergence) in the next section.

2.2.5 *Estimation of Distribution Algorithms*

These algorithms are best explained, and were originally derived, in the case that the chromosomes are real vectors $x = (x_1, x_2, \ldots, x_M)'$, though they have been extended to more general settings. In the real vector case, the problem may be formulated as that of maximizing a fitness function $f(x)$ where x is a real vector $x \in \mathbb{R}^M$.

The proposal originates from the attempt of explicitly taking into account the correlation between genes of different loci (components of the vector x), that may be seen in good solutions, assuming that such correlation structure could be different from that of the less fitted individuals. The key idea is to deliver an explicit probability model and associate to each population (or a subset of it) a multivariate probability distribution.

An initial version of the estimation of distribution algorithm was originally proposed by Muhlenbein and Paas (1996), and then many further contributions developed, generalized and improved the implementation. A thorough account may be found in Larrañaga and Lozano (2002) and in a second more recent book (Lozano et al., 2006).

The estimation of distribution algorithm is a regular stochastic population based evolutionary method, and therefore evolves populations through generations. The typical evolution process from one generation to the next may be described as follows:

1. Generate an initial population $P^{(0)} = \{x_i^{(0)}, i = 1, \ldots, N\}\ ; c = 0$.
2. If $P^{(c)}$ denotes the current population, select a subset of $P^{(c)}$: $\{x_j^{(c)}, j \in S^{(c)}\}$ with $|S^{(c)}| = n < N$ individuals, according to a selection operator.
3. Consider the subset $\{x_j^{(c)}, j \in S^{(c)}\}$ as a random sample from a multivariate random variable with absolutely continuous distribution and probability density $p^{(c)}(x)$, and estimate $p^{(c)}(x)$ from the sample.
4. Generate a random sample of N individuals from $p^{(c)}(x)$: this is the population at generation $c + 1$, $P^{(c+1)}$.
5. If a stopping rule is met, stop; otherwise $c + 1 \to c$ and return to 2.

The originally proposed selection operator was the truncation selection, in other words only the n individuals with the largest fitness out of the N members of the population are selected. Later, it was proposed that other common selection mechanism such as the roulette wheel (proportional selection) or the tournament selection (choice of the best fitted inside a group of k individuals chosen at random) can be adopted.

Note that the most critical and difficult step is the third one: the aim is to summarize the properties of the most fitted part of the population through a probability distribution, and then to employ that distribution to generate new offsprings. Many papers concentrated on the problem of "estimating" the distribution, meaning to derive, from the finite set of individuals $\{x_j^{(c)}, j \in S^{(c)}\}$, the probability density function $p^{(c)}(x)$. It can be observed that this is not an uncommon problem in Statistics, and many proposals (frequently based on non parametric density estimation) appear in the statistics literature. However, the estimation of distribution algorithms were proposed and developed in a different field, and methods for deriving $p^{(c)}(x)$ were proposed which are somewhat unusual in Statistics.

The simplest way is called Univariate Marginal Distribution Algorithm (UMDA) and assumes that $p^{(c)}(x)$ is a multivariate normal with independent components, therefore its parameters (means and variances) are obtained by the usual estimators on the marginal distributions of each gene in the subset $S^{(c)}$. Obviously, this is in principle a very inefficient choice, which also contradicts the basic assumption of exploiting correlations among genes, though it has been reported that in some cases it leads to successful algorithms.

A more elaborated solution takes into account the dependence between genes, but to this aim a simplifying assumption is formulated, and is known as Factorial Distribution Algorithm (FDA). The key assumption is that the fitness function may be additively decomposed in terms, each depending only on a subset of genes. In other words, if $s_1, s_2, \ldots, s_k$ all are subsets of $\{1, 2, \ldots, M\}$, it is assumed that there exist k functions $f_1, f_2, \ldots, f_k$, each of which depends on x only through the coordinates corresponding to the subset s_j, and the fitness $f(x)$ may be written as follows:

$$f(x) = \sum_{j=1}^{k} f_j[x(s_j)]$$

where $x(s_j) = \{x_i, i \in s_j\}$. If it is true, the multivariate probability distribution $p^{(c)}(x)$ is factorized as a product of conditional distributions on smaller subsets, and this simpler factorization helps to estimate the whole distribution. The choice of the subsets may be done also using graphical models. To be more specific, let us define, basing on the s_j, the following sequences of subsets d_i (histories), b_i (residuals), c_i (separators):

$$d_0 = \emptyset\,;\; d_i = s_1 \cup s_2 \cup \ldots \cup s_i\,;\; b_i = s_i \cap \overline{d_{i-1}}\,;\; c_i = s_i \cap d_{i-1}\,,\; i = 1, 2, \ldots, k.$$

Then, if no b_i is empty, and each c_i is a subset of at least one s_j with $j < i$, the multivariate density may be written as a product of conditional distributions:

$$p(x) = \prod_{i=1}^{k} p[x(b_i)|x(c_i)].$$

Therefore the problem is reduced to estimating lower order distributions. In addition, to simplify the problem a gaussian form is often assumed.

More complicated ways of estimating the multivariate distribution have also been proposed, based on Bayesian Networks.

As should be clear, the accent in estimation of distribution algorithms is essentially on extracting the typical features of best fitted individuals, and reproducing them in the next generation. Since the use of the complete multivariate probability distributions accounts for relationships between genes, no recombination tool (cross-over operator) is contemplated. Neither mutation operator are used: new individuals (carrying never experienced gene values) may be generated by random sampling the estimated multivariate probability distribution. In fact, since $p^{(c)}(x)$ is a density, sampling may result in elements not belonging to $S^{(c)}$.

Finally, it may be observed that, strictly from the point of view of probability theory, estimation of distribution algorithms are based on a very unusual and non standard framework, because the critical step (step 3 in our pseudo-code) from a subset of individuals $S^{(c)}$ to a multivariate distribution $p^{(c)}(x)$ would need assumptions on the properties of $S^{(c)}$ as a random sample drawn from $p^{(c)}(x)$, and these have not been precisely specified (and, regrettably, they cannot be easily formulated).

2.2.6 Differential Evolution

Differential evolution is an algorithm arising in a pure optimization framework, and is best explained by referring to a real function f of M real variables: $f : \mathbb{R}^M \to \mathbb{R}$ to be optimized. Though differential evolution papers refer generally to minimization, we shall continue our biological populations similitude and consider f as a fitness function to be maximized.

Differential evolution is a recent method, which was first proposed by Storn and Price in the middle of nineties. A complete account may be found in Price et al. (2005).

Differential evolution is also a population based method, and evolves populations of solutions through successive generations. Each individual represents a possible solution, and is codified by a real vector $x = (x_1, x_2, \ldots, x_M)' \in \mathbb{R}^M$. Though not frequently used in the present framework, we continue to denote x by the word chromosome, and their components by the word gene.

The transition from one generation to the next is obtained by treating each individual separately, and producing an offspring which replaces it in the next generation. This makes differential evolution particularly suitable for a parallel implementation.

The evolution mechanism is based on *difference vectors* (the difference between two randomly selected chromosomes of the current population) which is the basic perturbation type allowing new features to appear in the population. The word vector is usually preferred to chromosome, because differential evolution has a convenient geometrical interpretation, and individuals may be advantageously seen as points (or vectors) in $\mathbb{R}^M$.

The number of individuals in the population is held fixed throughout generations; the initial population has a special importance, and the authors stress that good performances of the differential evolution algorithms are critically influenced by the initial population : "in order for differential evolution to work, the initial population must be distributed throughout the problem space" (Price et al., 2005, p. 53). This happens, as it will be soon clear, because the offsprings always lie in the convex closure of the set of the points representing parents population. Therefore, the population at generation 0 should contain points which are as much as possible different with each other, and anyway it should be reasonably ensured that the best solution vector is a linear combination of the vectors forming the initial population. The initial individuals are selected at random by defining a probability distribution on the solutions space, the chosen distribution is usually uniform but different families of distributions are obviously possible.

At each generation, each individual is subject to the process of *differential evolution*, which may be explained as follows. Let x denote the individual to be evolved.

A completely different individual is formed as follows: select at random a vector in the population, different from x, and called the *base vector* v_0; also, select at random two more individuals in the population, different both from x and v_0, and different each other: v_1 and v_2. Scale the difference between these two last vectors by a factor F (the *scale factor*) obtaining $F(v_1 - v_2)$, and add this difference to the base vector, to obtain a new individual u called the *mutant*:

$$u = v_0 + F(v_1 - v_2)\,.$$

The scale factor F has a fixed value chosen by the implementer, usually between 0 and 1. The mutant vector u is then recombined with the initial individual vector x to produce an offspring by means of uniform cross-over. It means that each gene of the offspring will be selected at random to be equal to the corresponding gene of the mutant u with a fixed probability p_c, or equal to the original gene of the individual x with probability $(1 - p_c)$. This random selection is performed independently on all genes. Formally, if $y = (y_1, y_2, \ldots, y_M)'$ denotes the offspring vector, then

$$y_i = \delta_i u_i + (1 - \delta_i)x_i\,, \quad i = 1, \ldots, M$$

where $\{\delta_i, i = 1, \ldots, M\}$ are independent Bernoulli random variables with equal parameter p_c. The number of genes inherited from the mutant has therefore a binomial distribution.

Finally, a replacement step is performed: the original individual x and the offspring y are compared, and only that with the best fitness is retained and entered in the next generation population. The process of differential evolution is repeated for each individual in the population.

It is apparent that the process induced by differential evolution is logically simple; though the evolution of each member takes place separately, it depends on the whole population because the mutant which may contribute to generate the offspring is obtained by a linear combination of three other individuals selected at random.

A number of different variants and modifications are possible, in various directions:

- The initial population may be selected according to particular probability distributions on the solution space, or taking advantage of possible natural bounds on the values of each gene.
- The choice of the base vector may be performed at random uniformly, or using a selection rule based on the fitness.
- Decision about which base vector to assign to each individual may be based on different rules, deterministic or random.
- The choice of the individuals originating the difference vector, v_1 and v_2, is subject to various decision rules.
- The scale factor F may be chosen a fixed constant: smaller values are related to local search, while larger values of F correspond to a global search. The scale factor F may also be selected at random (gaussian, lognormal or uniform

distributions have been proposed); furthermore, one can use a different scale factor for each gene (i.e., for each coordinate of the vector).

- A cross-over operator different from uniform may be used for recombining the individual and the mutant.
- Finally, the survivor between parent and offspring may be chosen not by pure fitness but according to different criteria.

Like all other evolutionary computation methods, differential evolution is iterative and the best individual in the population approaches the optimum as the generations flow; therefore, a stopping rule has to be selected. Owing to the geometrical interpretation, it would appear natural to stop generations when the points representing all members of the population appear nearly undistinguishable, however this problem is not specific to differential evolution, but has similar characteristics for all evolutionary computation algorithms, and any stopping rule (which we discuss briefly in a next section) is plausible.

2.2.7 Evolutionary Behavior Algorithms

Many more optimization algorithms inspired by nature have been proposed in recent years. Among them, some methods are particularly interesting, also population based, but suggested by analogies with the social behavior of the individuals rather than biological reproduction features. Rather than concentrating on the evolution of a population through generations, these methods consider each individual as an agent searching iteratively for the solution of a given problem (equal for all of them). At each stage, each individual proposes a solution, and the stages are iterated until a stopping criterion is met. The crucial point is that the solution proposed at each stage by each individual depends on the goodness score (or fitness) of the solutions proposed in the previous stage by all (or some) other individuals in the population. Therefore the solution proposed by each individual depends on the best results reached by the community. These methods try to idealize and reproduce the social behavior features of living communities, thus we have called them *evolutionary behavior* algorithms.

The main contribution in this field are the *ant colony optimization* and the *particle swarm optimization*.

Ant colony optimization was introduced by Dorigo in his ph. d. thesis in 1992 (Dorigo, 1992) and was developed by himself and his co-workers in the last 15 years (e.g., Dorigo and Gambardella, 1997; Dorigo and Stützle, 2004). The method is inspired by the way ants search for food. Each ant initially wanders searching for food, but upon finding it, the ant returns to its colony laying down, in the way back, a substance called *pheromone*. Later on, ants tend to follow pheromone trails rather than wander at random, therefore advantageous paths are characterized by a large amount of pheromone, and are more attractive. However, pheromone evaporates in time, so that paths to places where food has been exhausted lose their attractiveness and are soon neglected.

Ant colony optimization's most natural application is to problems where any possible solution may be described by a path on a graph, like in the traveling salesman problem, and it will described here in that framework, though these methods have been applied also to different environments.

Let us consider a graph with n vertices denoted by $1, 2, \ldots, n$ and edges $(i, j) \in E$, and suppose that any possible solution is associated to a path, possibly with some constraints. Each edge has a known cost c_{ij} (often proportional to its length if applicable) and a pheromone loading τ_{ij} (initially set to zero). We consider a population of m ants, and the algorithm is iterative: at each stage each ant proposes a solution, by building an admissible path on the graph. Each ant starts from a randomly selected vertex and chooses which vertex to reach by means of a probabilistic rule: if the ant is in vertex i, it will select vertex j with probability proportional to $\tau_{ij}^{\alpha} c_{ij}^{-\beta}$, where α and β are positive constants. Depending on the nature of the problem, constraints on the edge set E and on the single solution components, and a rule for deciding when a solution is complete, have to be fulfilled (e.g., in the traveling salesman problem each vertex has to be visited once and no more than once).

When each ant k has completed its proposed solution s_k $(k = 1, 2, \ldots, m)$, these are evaluated by means of a fitness function $F(s)$, and the pheromone values of each edge are updated:

$$\tau_{ij} \quad \leftarrow \quad (1 - \rho)\tau_{ij} + \rho \sum_{s \in S*} F(s)$$

where ρ, between 0 and 1, controls the evaporation rate, and the sum over s is extended to all solutions including the edge (i, j) contained in a subset of solutions S^* ; in the simplest implementation S^* is the set of the solutions proposed by each ant in the current stage, as in ant systems (Dorigo, 1992). Other ant colony optimization algorithms differ essentially for the way S^* is built, therefore the differences are in the pheromone updating rule: one may add to S^* the best so far found solution, or on the contrary S^* may contain only the best solution found so far, or just in the current stage, or S^* may contain only the solutions found by the most successful ant at each stage. Finally, the pheromone values may be limited by a priori chosen minimum and maximum values (max-min ant systems, Stützle and Hoos, 2000). The fitness $F(s)$ may also be chosen in various ways, the most common seems an inverse proportionality to the sum of the costs of all edges in the solution.

Particle swarm optimization is a more recent set of algorithms which tend to reproduce a sort of social optimization induced by interactions among individuals with a common problem to solve, also known as *swarm intelligence*. Particle swarm optimization was introduced by Kennedy and Eberhart (1995, 2001). In its simplest form, a swarm is composed by many particles moving in a multidimensional continuous space, and the particle behavior is recorded at discrete times or stages. At each stage, each particle has a position and a velocity. Suppose that there are m particles moving in $\mathbb{R}^n$, denote by $x_i \in \mathbb{R}^n$ the position of the particle i, and by $v_i \in \mathbb{R}^n$ its velocity: then at the next stage the particle will move to $x_i + v_i$. Each point of the space may be evaluated, according to the problem, by means of a fitness function $F(x)$ defined on $\mathbb{R}^n$. After each stage the particle velocities are updated, allowing the particles change directions, and this is done by exploiting knowledge of the best solution found so far by the particle (local best lb_i), the best solution found so far by all particles (global best gb), and (possibly) the best solution found by a set of neighboring particles (neighborhood best nb_i). In any case, particles tend to be attracted towards the promising points found by the neighbors or the community. The velocity updating equations are linear and of the following type:

$$v_i \quad \leftarrow \quad \omega v_i + c_1 r_1 (lb_i - x_i) + c_2 r_2 (gb - x_i) + c_3 r_3 (nb_i - x_i)$$

where ω is an inertial constant usually slightly less than 1, c_1, c_2, c_3 are constants representing the relative strength of personal, community and neighborhood influence, and r_1, r_2, r_3 are random vectors, introducing a probabilistic perturbation.

Though especially suitable for optimization in $\mathbb{R}^n$, discretized versions for searching over discrete spaces have also been proposed.

Ant colony and particle swarm optimization methods have been rarely employed in statistical analysis applications, but given their increasing development it is likely that they will be soon found useful and appropriate for statistical problems too.

2.2.8 A Simple Example of Evolutionary Computation

It is now time to present a worked example of evolutionary computation. It relates to time series modeling and it is a simplified version of the problems which will be addressed in Chap. 4, and a genetic algorithm will be employed. First, only a full iteration of a simple GA with selection, crossover and mutation will be analyzed, then we shall outline what happens in successive generations.

We consider a time series, that is a stretch of observations taken at equally spaced time intervals simulated from the random process

$$y_t - \phi y_{t-1} = a_t - \theta a_{t-1}, \tag{2.2}$$

where $\phi = 0.9$ and $\theta = -0.5$, and the sequence $\{a_t\}$ is a zero mean unit variance ($\sigma_a^2 = 1.0$) normal white noise, that is a sequence of independent identically normally distributed random variables. Model (2.2) is known as a ARMA(1,1) random process. The usual requirements of stationarity and invertibility are fulfilled provided that $-1 < \phi < 1$ and $-1 < \theta < 1$ respectively.

By using a normal random number generation routine we generated 1100 artificial observations from the random process (2.2). The first 1000 observations have been discarded to eliminate the influence of the starting values so that a time series of $n = 100$ observations is available. As it is often the case, time series observations are affected by abnormally large or small observations that do not fit the overall time series behavior. So we contaminate the artificial time series $y = (y_1, y_2, \ldots, y_n)'$ by adding 3.5 to the observation at time $t = 17$ and -3.5 to the observation at time

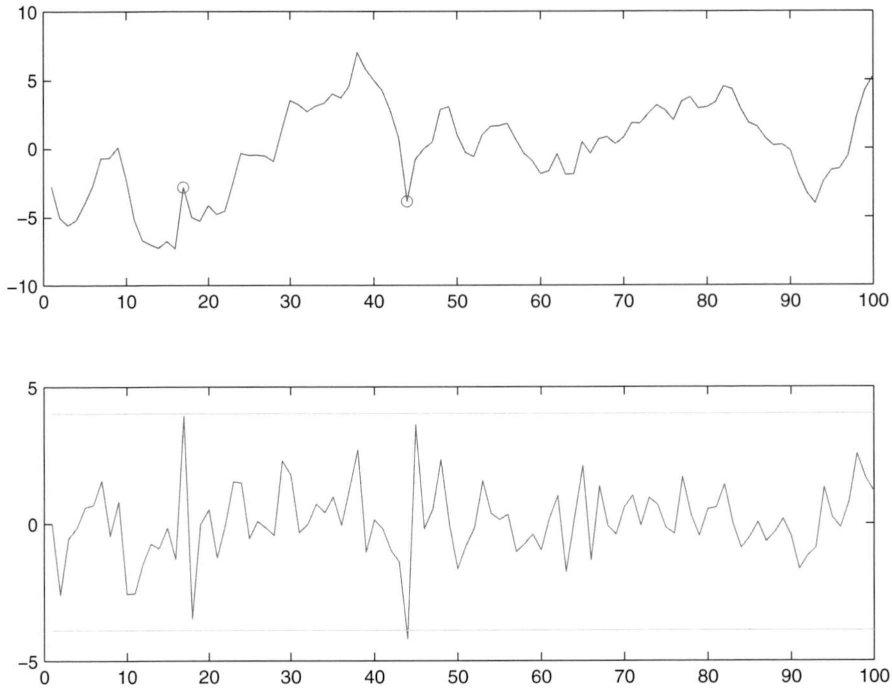

Fig. 2.1 Artificial time series generated by a ARMA(1,1) random process ($n = 100$ observations). *Top panel*: time series values (*solid line*) with outliers marked by circles. *Bottom panel*: Residuals computed by ordinary least square model estimate and lower and upper thresholds for outlier identification

$t = 44$. It results the artificial time series y plotted in Fig. 2.1. The top panel displays the artificial observations as a line where the outliers at $t = 17, 44$ are marked with circles. The bottom panel displays the residuals computed by estimating the model (2.2) parameters ϕ and θ by ordinary least squares. The straight lines represent the thresholds $3\hat{\sigma}_a$ and $-3\hat{\sigma}_a$ for outlier identification. The outliers at $t = 17, 44$ are clearly outlined.

The residual variance $\hat{\sigma}_a^2$ has been computed

$$\hat{\sigma}_a^2 = \frac{1}{n} \sum_{t=1}^{n} \hat{a}_t^2, \tag{2.3}$$

where the residuals $\{\hat{a}_t\}$ have been calculated recursively from model (2.2) by replacing the parameters ϕ and θ with their ordinary least squares estimates $\hat{\phi} = 0.8820$ and $\hat{\theta} = -0.2401$. The estimate $\hat{\sigma}_a^2 = 1.7319$ has been computed.

The ordinary least squares estimation method actually ignores the presence of the outliers. As a result the parameter estimates are often severely biased toward zero and the residual variance is larger than the white noise variance. We may proceed in two ways to take the presence of the outliers into account properly. We may identify the outliers, estimate their size and remove them before performing the model parameters estimation. Alternatively if we do not want to perform such preliminary step we may resort to a outlier resistant estimation method. We want to implement this latter course of action and we shall use a version of the median of absolute deviation (MAD) criterion as the objective function to minimize in order to obtain the model parameter estimates. Let

$$\tilde{a}_t(\phi, \theta) = y_t - \phi y_{t-1} + \theta a_{t-1},$$

where we search for the values $\tilde{\phi}$ and $\tilde{\theta}$ such that

$$\mu_a = \text{median}\,(|\tilde{a}_1|, |\tilde{a}_2|, \ldots, |\tilde{a}_n|) \tag{2.4}$$

is minimized. It is apparent that using the MAD criterion we avoid abnormally large or small residuals to influence model (2.2) parameter estimates. A problem arises, however, that is the objective function (2.4) is not differentiable and does not share with the objective function of the ordinary least squares method any good mathematical properties. As an illustration, Fig. 2.2 displays the likelihood function computed for the time series y varying the model parameters ϕ and θ in the set of admissible values, that is the square with vertices $(\pm 1, \pm 1)$. The variance has been computed as a function of each and every pair (ϕ, θ) by using formula (2.3). The surface is smooth and searching for the maximum of such function is rather easy for gradient-based methods as there is only a global maximum and no local maxima are present. Figure 2.3 displays the likelihood function of y where the variance is estimated by the squared MAD given by (2.4). In this case the likelihood surface is not smooth and searching for the global maximum is rather difficult because of the presence of several local maxima. If we want to use gradient-based methods we have to resort to numerical derivatives because actually analytical derivatives do not exist everywhere and good results are not to be expected. Also, heuristics such as the grid search may easily get into trouble because the grid cannot be too much detailed to avoid the need for lengthy computations and, as a consequence, the pair that yields the global maximum may not be possibly included in the grid.

We shall use this maximization problem to describe in detail an iteration of the GA. The necessary preliminary step consists in defining the solution space and the code to represent each and every admissible solution. We have two real parameters to estimate and we want to use the binary code. So our first choice will be how to represent real numbers in the interval $(-1, 1)$ by means of a binary string. Let x be such binary string and let us choose its length equal to ℓ. Choosing, for instance, $\ell = 8$ means that we have a byte available to represent a real number between -1 and 1. Let m be the positive integer that represents the value of the binary string by using the ordinary binary code. For instance, the 8-bit string 11110000 stands for the integer 240. In general for a binary string of length ℓ the integer m encodes the real number r given by

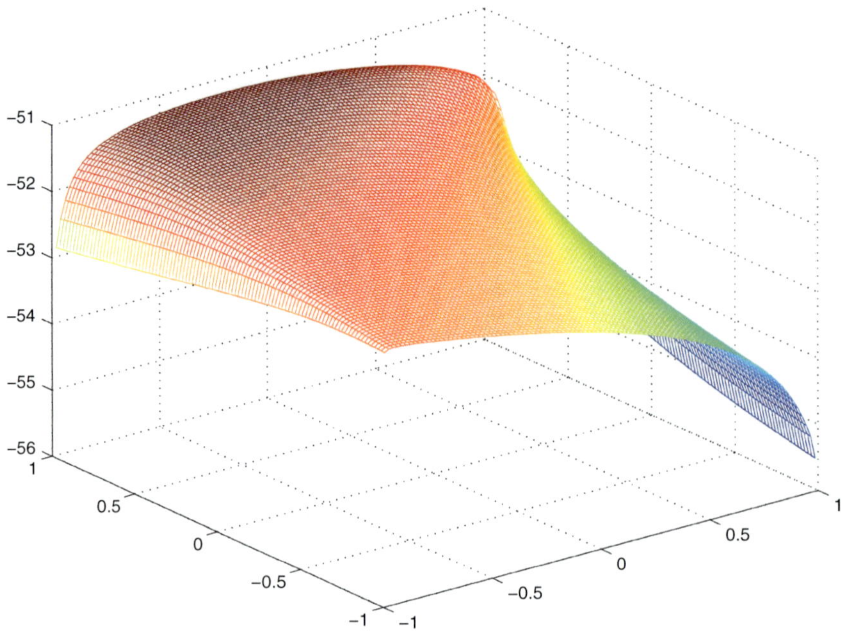

Fig. 2.2 Likelihood function of the observed time series y by assuming a ARMA(1,1) model with parameters varying in the interval $(-1, 1)$. The residual variance is estimated by the residual sum of squares divided by the number of observations n

$$r = -1 + 2\frac{m}{2^{\ell} - 1}. \tag{2.5}$$

For instance, according to (3.1) and for given $\ell = 8$, $m = 240$ means the real number $r = 0.8824$. As a solution is a pair of real numbers we may concatenate two strings of length ℓ_1 and ℓ_2 respectively to obtain a complete solution as a binary string of length $\ell = \ell_1 + \ell_2$. Let, for example, $x = 0000100111110000$ and let $\ell_1 = \ell_2 = 8$ so that $\ell = 16$. Decoding x yields the integer pair $(9, 240)$ and, using (2.5), the real pair $(-0.9294, 0.8824)$ that is the solution $\phi = -0.9294$ and $\theta = 0.8824$. This mapping operates the other way round as well, that is for any given pair (ϕ, θ) a binary string x may be computed. In this case, however, depending on the given precision and due to rounding approximations, different pairs, if close enough, may lead to the same binary string. Precision is as larger as greater the binary string length ℓ.

Another important preliminary choice is concerned with the fitness function. The solution space for the problem of model (2.2) parameters estimation is $\mathcal{X} = (-1, 1) \times (-1, 1)$. Searching $\mathcal{X}$ aims at minimizing the criterion (2.4). The fitness function has to be positive and has to be as larger as closer to the global optimum. So we have to define the fitness function as a suitable transform of (2.4). The most natural choice consists in assuming as objective function to be maximized the likelihood function where the residual variance is replaced by the MAD as given by (2.4).

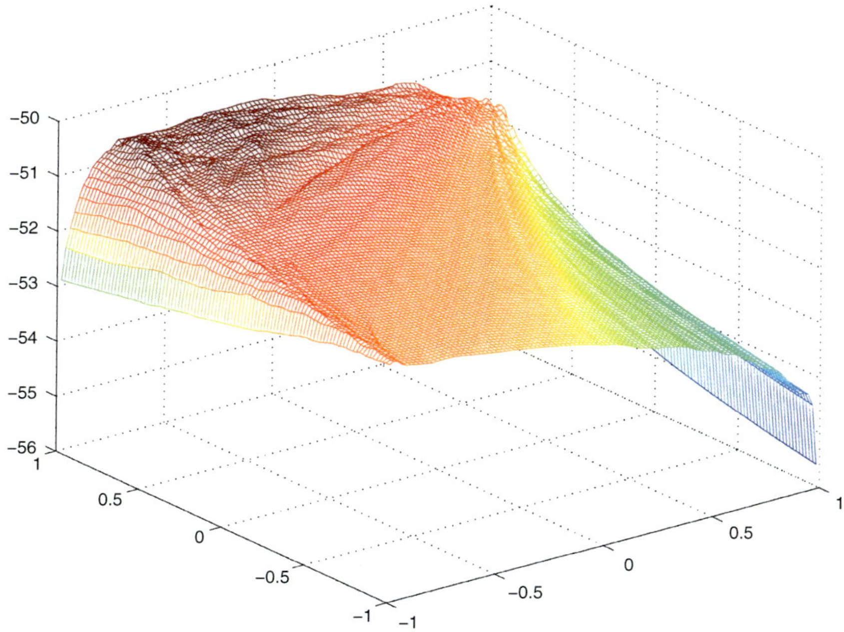

Fig. 2.3 Likelihood function of the observed time series y by assuming a ARMA(1,1) model with parameters varying in the interval $(-1, 1)$. The residual variance is estimated by the squared median of the absolute values of the residuals

Once we assume that σ_a^2 is estimated by μ_a^2, it may be shown that approximately the logarithm of the likelihood L may be written

$$\log L = -\frac{n}{2}\log(2\pi) - n\log(\mu_a) - \frac{n}{2}.$$

However, we obtain values too small that may cause underflows and are difficult to deal with. So let us define the fitness function

$$f(x) = \exp\left(\frac{\log L}{n}\right) = \exp\left\{-\frac{1}{2}(\log(2\pi) + 1)\right\}(\mu_a)^{-1}, \tag{2.6}$$

where x is a binary string of length ℓ that may be decoded to yield the model parameters.

We are now in the position of initializing a GA for searching for the binary string x which encodes the pair $(\tilde{\phi}, \tilde{\theta})$ in the solution space $\mathcal{X}$ that maximizes the fitness function f given by (2.6). For illustration purpose let us define a small population size $s = 5$ and randomly generate the binary strings $\{x^{(1)}, x^{(2)}, x^{(3)}, x^{(4)}, x^{(5)}\}$ displayed in Table 2.2. For clarity of exposition in each line, after the binary string, the integer values, the real parameters, the MAD index μ_a and the fitness function value are displayed. The random number generation routine produces only the binary strings, each bit may take the values 0 or 1 with equal probability. At this point we may recall the GAs terminology and each binary string is a chromosome which is included in the initial population.

Now we are ready for starting the GA. For illustration we shall consider only one iteration and the usual three steps selection, crossover and mutation.

2.2.8.1 Selection

For selection we choose the roulette wheel rule with the replacement of the entire population. The fitness function values in the rightmost column of Table 2.2 may be normalized to yield the sequence

$$0.3620 \ 0.2424 \ 0.1843 \ 0.1204 \ 0.0909$$

that represents the probabilities that the chromosomes in the initial population be chosen to enter the population at the next iteration of the GA. Then we may compute the cumulated normalized fitness function, that is the sequence

$$0.3620 \ 0.6044 \ 0.7887 \ 0.9091 \ 1.0000.$$

According to the roulette wheel rule we draw for 5 times a number between 0 and 1 and we select the chromosome 1 if such number is between 0 and 0.3620, the chromosome 2 if it is between 0.3620 and 0.6044, the 3-rd one if the random number belongs to the interval $(0.6044, 0.7887)$, the 4th if it is in $(0.7887, 0.9091)$ and the 5th if it is in $(0.9091, 1.0000)$. This procedure may be illustrated by drawing a circle as in Fig. 2.4 and dividing it in spikes proportional to the fitness function values. Then the selection by the roulette wheel rule may be performed by pointing at random at the circle and selecting the chromosome associated to the spike which has been hit.

We draw the following random number sequence in (0, 1)

$$0.0576 \ 0.3676 \ 0.6315 \ 0.7176 \ 0.6027$$

and, as a consequence, chromosomes 1, 2 and three copies of chromosome 3 are selected for the next iterations. The population after selection is displayed in Table 2.3. The average fitness function increases from 0.1456 to 0.1685. Note that unlike selection, that always yields an increase of the average function, both crossover and mutation may cause the fitness function to decrease.

Table 2.2 GA example: initial population

Chromosome	x		Integer values		Real values		MAD	$f(x)$
$x^{(1)}$	11110001	10011001	241	153	0.8902	0.2000	0.9178	0.2636
$x^{(2)}$	10011110	01100000	158	96	0.2392	−0.2471	1.3710	0.1765
$x^{(3)}$	01110010	01000111	114	71	−0.1059	−0.4431	1.8033	0.1342
$x^{(4)}$	00000111	00110111	7	55	−0.9451	−0.5686	2.7605	0.0877
$x^{(5)}$	10010110	11000100	150	96	0.1765	0.5373	3.6539	0.0662

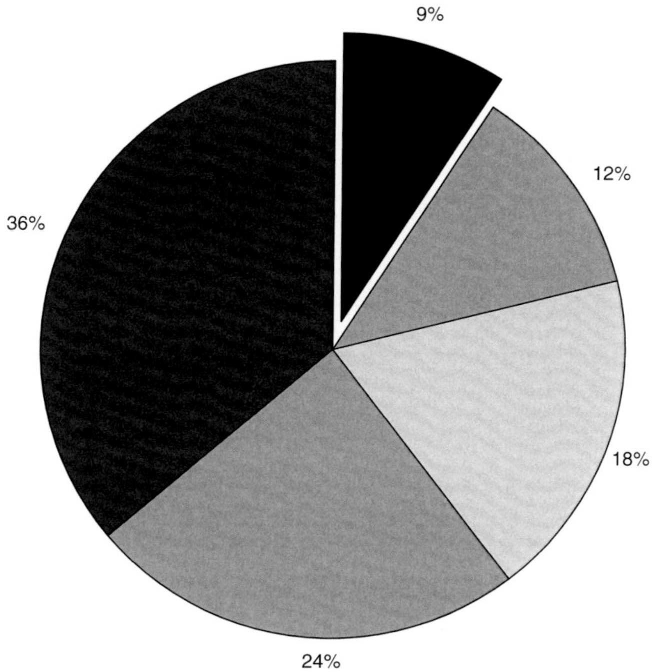

Fig. 2.4 Roulette wheel: each spike is proportional to the probability that the associated chromosome be selected for the next iteration of the GA

Table 2.3 GA example: current population after selection

Chromosome	x		Integer values		Real values		MAD	$f(x)$
$x^{(1)}$	11110001	10011001	241	153	0.8902	0.2000	0.9178	0.2636
$x^{(2)}$	10011110	01100000	158	96	0.2392	−0.2471	1.3710	0.1765
$x^{(3)}$	01110010	01000111	114	71	−0.1059	−0.4431	1.8033	0.1342
$x^{(4)}$	01110010	01000111	114	71	−0.1059	−0.4431	1.8033	0.1342
$x^{(5)}$	01110010	01000111	114	71	−0.1059	−0.4431	1.8033	0.1342

2.2.8.2 Crossover

For crossover we have to choose in the current population chromosome pairs that exchange bits according to some pre-specified rule. We adopt the simplest one, that is the one-point crossover. Let the chromosome pair be $(x^{(1)}, x^{(2)})$ and let a random number c be generated in the interval $(1, \ell - 1)$. Such number c is called the cutting point. Then the chromosomes $x^{(1)}$ and $x^{(2)}$ exchange the bits from location $c + 1$ to location ℓ to produce two new chromosomes that replace the old ones in the current population. Crossover takes place with a given probability p_c. We choose $p_c = 0.9$ and let the chromosome pairs selected for crossover be $(x^{(1)}, x^{(4)})$ and $(x^{(2)}, x^{(3)})$. Chromosome 5 is not selected and remains in the current population unchanged. Let us consider now the crossover for the pair $(x^{(1)}, x^{(4)})$ and assume that the randomly generated cutting point is $c = 1$. We may write the two chromosomes on the following two lines and mark the cutting point with a vertical bar

1| 1110001 10011001

0|1110010 01000111

The exchange produces the two new chromosomes

1| 1110010 01000111

0| 1110001 10011001

where the first bit is unchanged but is followed by the bits from the other chromosome. Likewise, the pair $(x^{(2)}, x^{(3)})$ may be displayed, by assuming that $c = 7$ is the randomly generated cutting point,

1001111| 0 01100000

0111001| 0 01000111

The exchange produces the two new chromosomes

1001111| 0 01000111

0111001| 0 01100000

where the first 7 bits are unchanged but are followed by the bits from the other chromosome.

The result of the crossover may be summarized in Table 2.4. The average fitness function is equal to 0.1726 (greater than the previous average fitness function 0.1685).

Table 2.4 GA example: current population after crossover

Chromosome	x		Integer values		Real values		$f(x)$
$x^{(1)}$	11110010	01000111	242	71	0.8980	−0.4431	0.3260
$x^{(2)}$	01110001	10011001	113	153	−0.1137	0.2000	0.0838
$x^{(3)}$	10011110	01000111	158	71	0.2392	−0.4431	0.2046
$x^{(4)}$	01110010	01100000	114	96	−0.1059	−0.2471	0.1142
$x^{(5)}$	01110010	01000111	114	71	−0.1059	−0.4431	0.1342

2.2.8.3 Mutation

Let p_m be the probability of mutation and let $p_m = 0.1$. As each and every bit is allowed to mutate with probability p_m this choice means that 10% on the average of the bits that form the chromosomes in the population may change its value from zero to one or vice versa. As $\ell = 16$ and $s = 5$ the total number of bits in the current population is equal to 80 and 8 are expected to mutate. In the present case the randomly generated numbers make mutation to operate on 9 bits. The mutation outcome is the population displayed in Table 2.5. The bits that have been changed are reported in boldface. Except chromosome 2 all chromosomes have been changed by mutation. The average fitness function still increases from 0.1726 to 0.1776. However in the current population there is a chromosome that has fitness function less than the original chromosome in the population yielded by crossover. At the end of the iteration the solution to be assumed is the pair (0.9608, −0.4431) which corresponds to the largest fitness function 0.3281. This solution is an apparent

Table 2.5 GA example: current population after crossover

Chromosome	x		Integer values		Real values		$f(x)$
$x^{(1)}$	11111010	01000111	250	71	0.9608	−0.4431	0.3281
$x^{(2)}$	01110001	10011001	113	153	−0.1137	0.2000	0.0838
$x^{(3)}$	10111010	01000110	186	70	0.4588	−0.4510	0.2552
$x^{(4)}$	01100010	01000000	98	64	−0.2314	−0.4980	0.1221
$x^{(5)}$	01100010	01100110	98	102	−0.2314	−0.2000	0.0989

improvement with respect to the solution found in the initial population, that is the pair (0.8902, 0.2000) with fitness function equal to 0.2636. In this latter case the estimate of the parameter θ is severely biased while after one iteration of the GA we have an estimate of θ with rather small bias.

2.2.8.4 Outcomes from Some Complete GA Runs

Estimating the parameters of model (2.2) by means of GAs-based methods requires a large population to evolve for several iterations. We performed a small simulation experiment to illustrate the performance of GAs in comparison with a grid search heuristic and a gradient-based method. The variability of the estimates has been taken into account by running each method (excepted the grid search which is an exhaustive deterministic search) 10 times and computing the average and the standard deviation of the estimates. The first simulation experiment uses the square root of the residual variance $\hat{\sigma}_a^2$, i.e. the root mean square error (RMSE), as objective function to be minimized, and fitness function

$$f(x) = \exp\left\{-\frac{1}{2}(\log(2\pi) + 1)\right\}(\hat{\sigma}_a^2)^{-1/2}.$$

We adopt the GA with binary encoding that has been described in detail but the population size has been $s = 30$ and the number of iterations is 100. In addition a version of the GA which uses a floating-point encoding has been tried. The grid search has been performed on a 100×100 lattice. Then a gradient-based method has been used with a stopping rule that causes the algorithm to end as soon as the change between the values of the objective function computed in two consecutive iterations is less than 0.0001. The number of iterations does not exceed 100 anyway. In comparison, the GAs perform 3000 fitness function evaluations and the grid search performs 10000 objective function evaluations. The results are displayed in Table 2.6. The estimates are all biased towards zero due to the presence of the outliers in $t = 17, 44$. The results yielded by the different methods are comparable and close each other.

Let us perform the same simulation experiment but let us use as objective function the residuals MAD. The results are displayed in Table 2.7. The GAs yield less biased estimates as we expect by using a outlier resistant objective function. The other methods fail to take advantage by this circumstance because the optimization problem has become more difficult and the two methods are not efficient in the

Table 2.6 Estimates and standard errors by GAs, grid search and gradient methods with the RMSE as objective function

Method	$\hat{\phi}^a$	$\hat{\theta}^a$	RMSE[a]
Grid search	0.8800	−0.2400	1.3160
Gradient	0.8820	−0.2403	1.3160
	(0.0001)	(0.0003)	(0.0000)
GA binary	0.8823	−0.2399	1.3160
	(0.0008)	(0.0008)	(0.0000)
GA floating-point	0.8843	−0.2379	1.3162
	(0.0046)	(0.0152)	(0.0003)

[a] Standard errors are enclosed in parentheses

presence of many local optima. This motivates using the GAs for solving this class of optimization problems.

Table 2.7 Estimates and standard errors by GAs, grid search and gradient methods with the MAD as objective function

Method	$\hat{\phi}^a$	$\hat{\theta}^a$	MAD[a]
Grid search	0.8600	−0.7200	0.6556
Gradient	0.8631	−0.3145	0.7016
	(0.1524)	(0.1855)	(0.0415)
GA binary	0.8837	−0.4727	0.6494
	(0.0131)	(0.2035)	(0.0008)
GA floating-point	0.8983	−0.3932	0.6509
	(0.0238)	(0.1658)	(0.0044)

[a] Standard errors are enclosed in parentheses

2.3 Properties of Genetic Algorithms

2.3.1 Genetic Algorithms as a Paradigm of Evolutionary Computation

The essential features of a genetic algorithm are typical in any evolutionary computation method. Its main elements: coding, selection, mutation, recombination, replacement, may be found to various extents, in all evolutionary algorithms, therefore by extending the meaning and the rules of those elements we may obtain a sufficiently wide framework where most evolutionary methods may find their place.

For this reason, the remainder of this book will be devoted essentially to genetic algorithms, but we shall address with the words genetic algorithm a somewhat wider concept allowing for many variations of coding and of the selection, mutation, cross-over and replacement mechanisms, so that they may describe a large variety of optimization methods. On passing, we note that most heuristic and meta heuristic algorithms may be seen as (degenerate) genetic algorithms, where the number of individuals in the population is set to one, and/or the stochastic nature of the operators vanishes by setting the variance to zero; recombination is not used (or equivalently the cross-over probability p_c is taken to be zero) and the mutation operator is somewhat specialized (e.g., for simulated annealing the mutation probability is changed in accordance to the ratio between the fitness value and the current temperature).

Interpreting many evolutionary computation methods as genetic algorithms requires allowing a complete freedom in redefining and extending the main steps across generations, concerning coding, selection, mutation, recombination, replacement: but this has been done implicitly, to a large extent, in the literature starting from the seventies onward, when proposing adaptation of genetic algorithms to an increasingly wide range of applied problems. We review some of these proposals briefly.

Coding is probably the most difficult and uncertain element of genetic algorithms, especially when they are employed for an optimization problem and each individual corresponds to a possible solution. Though it is unanimously recognized that the way a phenotype is coded into a genotype is crucially relevant to the result, and may exert a striking influence on the success of the optimization process, theoretical support for helping the choice of coding schemes is very limited. There are some problems whose solutions may be coded naturally in a binary string (for example, arranging objects of a set in two alternative categories), and in these cases binary is generally recognized as the best coding. However, for most problems it is not sufficient: if we want our coding to have an intuitive and appealing immediate meaning, each solution is generally associated to a string composed of integer or real numbers. In this case a chromosome can be a vector where each gene is not binary but an integer or real number. Obviously this requires that a range of admissible values is defined. However, the assumption of continuously varying real values is untenable, as usual, if computer arithmetics is employed, since the computer representation of a real number is based on a finite though large number of different states: therefore, distinction between integer and real genes is inessential.

Two possibilities arise. The first one is assuming the string of integer numbers as the chromosome representation: this forces to redefine mutation rules for taking into account the richer gene coding, and possibly also to reconsider cross-over and other operators rules. The second alternative is substituting to any integer number its binary representation, and obtaining this way a binary chromosome to which the simple genetic algorithm may be directly applied. This second way appears much simpler, but it has some drawbacks. First of all, the natural binary representation of integer numbers (the ordered coefficients of the expansions in power of 2) does not preserve topology: two similar integer numbers may correspond to binary representations which are very different (for example, number 15 and 16 have natural binary representations 01111 and 10000). This concept needs to be made precise by defining a distance on each of the two spaces: if we consider the arithmetic difference in modulus for the set of integers, and the Hamming distance (number of different correspondent digits) in the set of binary representations, one may control that two different integers with minimal distance (therefore consecutive numbers) may be mapped to binary codings whose distance is not minimal.

Table 2.8 Binary and Gray coding for integer numbers

Integer	Natural binary	Gray code
0	0000	0000
1	0001	0001
2	0010	0011
3	0011	0010
4	0100	0110
5	0101	0111
6	0110	0101
7	0111	0100
8	1000	1100
9	1001	1101
10	1010	1111
11	1011	1110
12	1100	1010
13	1101	1011
14	1110	1001
15	1111	1000

The property of maintaining such a distance ordering may however be obtained through a different binary encoding, called Gray code (after Frank Gray, a researcher in Bell Laboratories who first introduced it in 1947 calling it *reflected binary code*). This method ensures that consecutive numbers have binary representations with Hamming distance equal to one (see Table 2.8). There are, however, at least two drawbacks: Gray coding is cyclical, therefore Gray code procedures are not unique; and, further, the appealing interpretation of each digit as the coefficient of a power of 2 is no longer valid for Gray codes.

The second disadvantage of a gene coding obtained by representing integer numbers in base two is concerned with the effect of genetic operators. Since each gene has a different significance, the mutation of a single gene may produce very different impact on the integer that chromosome encodes; mutating the leftmost gene produces a very large change, while mutation of the rightmost gene modifies the integer only a little. In the same fashion, cross-over when applied with one randomly selected point, will rarely involve leftmost digits, thus changes induced on chromosomes will rarely be conspicuous. In summary, a natural binary encoding may induce a reduced efficiency of genetic operators (and new, more complicated, encoding rules have been proposed to avoid this effect).

Only few general principles may be given to help building a good encoding: apart from the obvious precept of a one to one correspondence between individuals and chromosomes, one should try to avoid redundancy (possible chromosome values are more than possible individuals) and choose the coding with the smallest alphabet (number of different symbols). It is certainly much simpler if each gene, independently of its locus, may assume the same values, so that the search space is a cartesian product: but this poses problems of legitimacy (some values in some genes may produce a chromosome which does not correspond to any solution) and admissibility (a chromosome may correspond to a solution that violates some constraints of the problem). Such problems arise often in statistical applications, and in the next chapters it will be discussed how to solve them.

Since few guidelines are available concerning encoding, any one-to-one mapping from the space of solutions to a numerical vector space is reasonable in principle, and comparison between different methods has often to be left to experience. Furthermore, relatively simple problems sometimes advocate surprisingly complicate or long encodings. In this case it has been found that simpler and intuitively more appealing encodings may be obtained if we allow the length of the chromosome itself (number of genes) be different from solution to solution. An example of such variable-length chromosome encoding will be given when dealing with cluster analysis. In this case, when the number of clusters is left free, one of the proposed methods consists in coding the centroids of each cluster, therefore each gene denotes one point in the space of observations, and the number of genes equals the number of groups to be formed.

It should be stressed that when non binary codings are employed the mutation operator has to be redefined, and sometimes the cross-over mechanism also needs modification. Moreover, when variable-length chromosomes are adopted, sometimes cross-over (and possibly mutation) results in offsprings that are not meaningful as individuals (violating legitimacy or length constraints), therefore a validation stage has to be added to the reproduction process.

Mutation is extended to non-binary genes in a natural way, like adopted in evolution strategies. Besides deciding the frequency of mutation, here the substantial amount of mutation has to be selected; usually mutation consists in an additive perturbation by means of a random trial from an assigned probability distribution, which is applied to all genes, therefore $p_m = 1$, and the features of the distribution control the mutation effects. For genes encoding real numbers, bell-shaped symmetric zero-mean distributions are often used, denoting a zero-drift mutation type where negligible changes are most likely; the variance may be considered as an index of overall mutation amount, and the kurtosis (being linked to the modal density peak) may be interpreted as an index of frequency of significant mutations.

Cross-over involves no additional difficulty in non-binary coding if fixed-length chromosomes are employed, but variable-length or some more specialized coding require a corresponding more careful definition of cross-over (for example the PMX crossover, see Falkenauer, 1998).

The mutation and cross-over rates themselves may be subject to evolution rather than being held fixed throughout generations: a possibility is encoding them directly in the chromosome, and evaluating them in connection with the fitness results (we have seen that this is done in evolution strategies and differential evolution, for a treatment in the context of genetic algorithms see e.g. Davis, 1991).

Many extensions to the procedures used for selection have also been proposed, in addition to those mentioned in the preceding sections; we consider briefly some of the most relevant to our scopes: *stochastic tournament* and *rank selection*.

Stochastic tournament is an elaboration on the tournament selection method: each individual is compared with a group of competitors, but it has a chance to be selected even if it is not superior to each of them. If the tournament is lost, because a competitor has a largest fitness, however the individual is discarded only with probability p_R, and maintained in the population with probability $1 - p_R$.

Rank selection consists in organizing selection not according to the actual fitness value of each individual, but according only to the position it occupies in the increasing ranking induced by fitness. In other words, the individuals are ordered according to their fitness in increasing value, and let $\phi(x_i)$ denote the rank of the i-th individual, thus ϕ has integer values between 1 and N. The function $\phi(\cdot)$ replaces the fitness $f(\cdot)$ in the selection mechanism (this is sometimes called *ordered fitness*). For example, if roulette wheel is used, the probability of selecting individual x_j is computed as $\phi(x_j)/\{\phi(x_1) + \phi(x_2) + \cdots + \phi(x_N)\}$. This has obvious advantages if the range of the fitness function is not bounded, but with ranking selection we lose any information concerning the fitness difference between pairs of individuals, and this may be an advantage if we are not sure about the correctness of the fitness measurement, but a drawback when meaningful information is discarded.

More in general, the probability of reproduction may be based, rather than directly on the fitness function, on a transformation of the fitness, whose aim is to distort the scale, and therefore the relative selection probabilities of the individuals in the population, while maintaining their fitness ranking unchanged. This behavior is known as *fitness scaling* and consists in choosing the probabilities of selecting each individual as proportional to a scaled fitness $s(x_j) = \psi[f(x_j)]$ where ψ is monotone increasing, and often linear. Since this choice has a relevant impact on algorithm performance, we examine it in more detail in the section devoted to implementation. A related topic is *penalized fitness*, devised as a way of taking into account problems of legitimacy and admissibility without the need of a validation stage where each chromosome has to be examined. In fact, validation should be repeated at each new generation and may therefore prove computationally expensive. A measure of admissibility (or legitimacy) of each chromosome is incorporated into its fitness value, by subtracting a penalty term. The penalized fitness is therefore of the following type:

$$f^*(x) = f(x) - c\,v(x)$$

where $c > 0$ and $v(x)$ is a validity score for chromosome x, usually simply $v(x) = 0$ if x is admissible and $v(x) = 1$ if it is not. The penalized fitness approach works implicitly, since bad individuals receive a very small fitness and therefore they are much likely to disappear in the next generation. However, tuning the constant c appropriately requires a knowledge, at least approximate, on bounds of the fitness values in the solution space to avoid negative fitness and, on the other side, ineffective penalization. The penalization term may be made smoother by substituting the impulse function $v(x)$ with a more elaborate behavior, and a similar idea will be in effect used in statistical application of genetic algorithms, specially in model selection problems, where the penalized fitness approach has a stressing analogy with automatic identification criteria.

A relevant extension is evaluating possible solutions by means of several contemporaneous criteria, using a vector-valued fitness function. This involves completely new additional problems, and evolutionary computation methods for solving multi-objective optimization problems have been recently proposed (*evolutionary multi-objective optimization*); they will be addressed shortly in the chapter concerning cluster analysis.

Finally, replacement strategies have also been extended and specialized. When genes are not only binary, but encode a richer alphabet, replacement may be based not only on fitness increase, but also on differences of the single genes of the offspring compared to the corresponding gene of its parents, or a subset of the current population. A related technique is *crowding* (De Jong, 1975) which was originally proposed for helping to maintain population diversity and for avoiding that sets of very similar individuals are found in the same generation. Crowding works as follows: for each new offspring, a set of randomly selected individuals in the current population is considered, and the offspring replaces the individual which is most similar according to the Hamming distance (crowding was proposed for binary coding).

2.3.2 Evolution of Genetic Algorithms

The original structure of the genetic algorithm was enriched in 30 years by a large number of extensions and modifications concerning all of its particular aspects. Some of those proposals are particularly important and suited for statistical applications, and we concentrate here on two extensions which are critical for the use we are going to do of genetic algorithms as a means of optimally solving statistical problems: locus-dependent encoding and hybridization.

With locus-dependent encoding we mean simply that each gene may have its own encoding method, therefore in a chromosome some genes may be binary, others decimal integers, and still other genes may be encoded by letters of a different alphabet. In this way, each locus may be associated with a particular feature of the problem, and complicated optimization applications may be translated into relatively intuitively appealing chromosomes, so that both the fitness definition, and the immediate comprehension, are facilitated.

In principle, any alphabet may be used, and if a locus encodes a dimension of the problem where k different modalities are possible, one can employ an alphabet with k different symbols. It is true that the dilemma remains, when evolving the population, if to translate all genes into binary coding and apply the standard genetic operators, or to maintain the locus-dependent coding, and having to redefine mutation and cross-over operators that have different effects on different loci. This last choice seems to be often preferred in the literature, since it is believed that, in spite of its harder difficulty, employing genetic operators that are exactly tailored to their operands may ensure a better ability of finding optima, and a higher speed in the search.

Locus-dependent coding is especially useful in some statistical applications where the solution depends on many variables whose measurement scales are different (numerical, or ordinal, or categorical), or the solution space may be naturally partitioned into a finite number of disjoint sets. A relevant example is model selection in regression. Part of the model building decision concerns which variables to use as independent, and this part could be easily associated to a binary set of genes, each denoting the presence or absence of a given variable. To complete the definition of the model, we have to choose the regression parameters values, and the most natural encoding is a real value (within a specified interval). A locus-dependent encoding leading to chromosomes where, say, the first k genes are binary and define what variables are active as independent, and the remaining part composed of real numbers representing the regression parameters values, seems to provide the simplest and most easily understandable way of describing a multiple regression problem.

This example enlightens a further feature of such an enlarged concept of coding: since the number of regression parameters depends on the number of regressors, the second part of the chromosome may have a variable length, determined by how many ones are there in the first part.

Variable length chromosomes are often used in many applications and nearly always the length is encoded, implicitly or explicitly, in the chromosome itself. The variable length can involve difficulties in recombination operators, which are often defined in a more accurate or complicated way. Sometimes it is possible to ignore variable length, fixing the number of genes to the maximum allowable number, and filling meaningless genes in excess with a neutral code ("don't care"), but this rarely avoids legitimacy problems, and a validation stage is generally required.

Hybridization means integrating a genetic algorithm with other optimization methods, both heuristic or meta-heuristic, and analytical when possible. The resulting methods are called *hybrid genetic algorithms* or, more recently *memetic algorithms*.

An integration between the genetic process and other optimization methods is generally dependent on the specific problems and may occur at two levels: genetic operators and fitness function. Mutation (sometimes also cross-over) may be hybridized with meta-heuristic one point search methods such as simulated annealing, threshold accepting, or tabu search, by adopting specialized mutation mechanisms that change a gene (sometimes a group of them) in the direction suggested by the meta-heuristic search. Let us consider one specific chromosome, and suppose for example that we are going to mutate the first gene: on considering the set of chromosomes that have different codes at the first locus and the other genes equal, we obtain a neighborhood of the starting point, inside which a search for a new candidate may be performed in a typical simulated annealing way. Let x denote the initial chromosome (to be subject to mutation) and y denote a chromosome selected at random in the neighborhood of x specified above; then mutation is accepted surely if the fitness of y is larger than $f(x)$, while if y is less fitted than x, the mutation is accepted with probability $\exp\{-[f(x)-f(y)]/T\}$, where T is a parameter (temperature) generation dependent, which is decreased as long as the algorithm proceeds.

Hybridization of the fitness function, on the contrary, relies generally on analytical optimization methods, basing on exact methods (such as equating derivatives of some function to zero) or approximate numerical techniques (that are employed for obtaining optima of complicated but well-behaved functions to an arbitrary assigned precision). This type of hybrid algorithm is usually possible when the problem to be solved admits a hierarchical decomposition, and at the lowest level the conditional fitness has a relatively simple and well-behaved form, that may be optimized by classical methods. A relevant example concerning Statistics (where, happily, fitness hybridization is often possible) is again the variable selection problem in regression.

Given a dependent variable and a set of possible independent variables, we have to build a linear regression equation by first selecting which variables appear in the equation, and then by determining the appropriate regression coefficients. Without specifying exactly the fitness function, assume that it has a part depending on the number of parameters, and a part inversely proportional to the sum of squared regression errors. Then, once the decision concerning which independent variables are selected (the identification of the regression model, corresponding to choosing the gene values of the first part of the chromosome in our example above) is taken, the values of the regression parameters (second part of the chromosome) yielding the best solution may be obtained analytically by least squares. The result of the optimizing action of the external method may be either incorporated in the chromosome as in our example, where the second part genes encode the estimates of the parameters, or remain implicit in the fitness, which could in our example be redefined as "the best fitness for a regression with given independent variables", and in that case the chromosome could be limited to encode only the choice of the independent variables, therefore shorter.

Hybridization was proposed initially to improve the typical ability of the simple genetic algorithm to provide good solutions in complicate problems, but without getting rapidly to the best solution in absolute, a behavior that was noted early, starting from Holland, and became common sense. The first idea was to employ local search methods, which could enable to refine the large-scale search performed by the genetic algorithm. However, later implementation used many various optimization techniques and hybridization proposals are now problem specific. In fact, though bearing in mind the caveats of no free lunch theorems, if a genetic algorithm is hybridized with the best known optimization method for a given problem, it should perform no worse than that method, therefore hybridization, though more computationally expensive, would provide an advantage anyway (see e.g. Davis, 1991).

Hybridizing a genetic algorithm has also an interesting interpretation in terms of natural evolution, since the modifications induced on the chromosome by the effects of the external optimization method may be assimilated to learning. Incorporating the effect of hybridization into the chromosome corresponds to admitting that an individual may transmit genetically its learned behavior to offsprings, and is known as *Lamarckian hypothesis* (after the naturalist Jean Baptiste Lamarck, who hypothesized, well before Darwin, that favorable characters, such as the long neck of giraffe, once acquired may be transmitted to descendants). Though the Lamarckian hypothesis has been refused on a biological basis, it is commonsense that some kind of favorable behavior may spread, in time, into animal populations: it is called the *Baldwin effect*, and may be explained by noting that the positive behavior may increase natural fitness and ability to reproduce themselves.

There has been a large debate on hybridization. Whitley wrote in 1994: "Experimental researchers and theoreticians are particularly divided on the issue of hybridization", the main criticism being that hybridization introduces in the chromosome some modifications that cannot be explained nor controlled in terms of genetic operators, therefore the typical features and the long run behavior of a genetic algorithm would not apply to a hybrid. However, Whitley adds: "despite the theoretical objections, hybrid genetic algorithms typically do well at optimization tasks".

In the last years, the application of the genetic algorithm framework to an increasing range of applied problems has been uniformly successful partly because of hybridizing with problem oriented strategies and optimization methods, and in Statistics also hybrid genetic algorithms are nearly always preferred.

2.3.3 Convergence of Genetic Algorithms

The issue of characterizing the behavior of a genetic algorithm as the generations flow is obviously an important one and has been addressed under various points of view since the original proposal by Holland. A genetic algorithm is a stochastic procedure, therefore in the long run the population could reach an equilibrium behavior where each possible individual has a limiting probability to be present. Moreover, if the genetic algorithm is employed as an optimization method, the question if the best solution found so far approaches, or reaches, the optimum value arises. If $x_{\text{best}}^{(g)}$ is the chromosome of the fittest individual found at generation g, then $\{f[x_{\text{best}}^{(g)}], g = 1, 2, \ldots\}$ defines a sequence of random variables whose convergence properties have to be studied.

The early approach by Holland (1975) is based on the concept of *schema*. In perfect coherence with the current knowledge of Genetics, we may assume that relevant features influencing the adaptation of an individual to the environment are determined not only by the value assumed by a single gene, but rather by the combination of the values presented by several genes simultaneously. Therefore we may think that a well fitted individual corresponds to a chromosome where several subsets of genes are found that have the "right" sequence of values. This is called the *building blocks* hypothesis. This point of view was formalized by Holland through the notion of schema. A schema may be defined as a subset of the chromosomes space, composed of all chromosomes that have a given code at each of some specified loci.

Our discussion will be limited to binary encoding, as it was originally developed by Holland (1975). A schema may be denoted by a sequence of digits of the same length of the chromosome, but with a ternary alphabet: 0, 1, and $*$. A 0 means that we are selecting chromosomes that have value 0 in that locus, a 1 has a similar meaning, and a $*$ means that chromosomes belong to the schema regardless the value assumed at that locus. For example, if the chromosome length is 5 say, the subset of all chromosomes with the first gene value equal to one is a schema, denoted by the string $1 * * **$ while the subset of all chromosomes that assume value zero in genes located at loci 2 and 4 is a schema indicated by $*0 * 0*$, and so on.

A schema has fixed (or *defined*) loci, those filled by a 0 or 1, and free (or undefined) loci, those filled with an asterisk. The *order* of a schema is the number of fixed loci, while the *defining length* is the distance between the first and the last defined position. For example, $0 * *00$ has order 3 and defining length 4, while $1 * *0*$ has order 2 and defining length 3. A chromosome belonging to a schema is said an *instance* of that schema. A schema may be evaluated by means of the average fitness of its instances.

At a given generation, the current population (formed by N individuals) contains instances of many schemas. In fact, any given chromosome composed of M genes is an instance of all schemas that have, at each locus, the actual value of its gene or an asterisk, their number being therefore 2^M. Thus, any population of N individuals contains instances of a large number of schemas, between 2^M and $N\,2^M$, and possibly several instances of the same schema. The point made by Holland is that the genetic algorithm, while evaluating explicitly the fitness of N chromosomes, at the same time evaluates implicitly, by an estimate of the average fitness, also the schemas which are represented by instances in the population. This is called *implicit parallelism*, and is motivated by an attempt to evaluate the evolution of the number of instances of a given schema through generations, which leads to the so called *schema theorem*.

Let us consider a given schema H (the letter H is nearly always used for schemas, since they are geometrically interpreted as hyperplanes in the solution space) and denote by $m_H(g)$ the number of instances of schema H in the population at generation g. What we are trying to derive is a characterization of $m_H(g)$ based on a recursive equation in g: however, $m_H(g)$ is obviously a random variable which depends on the population at the previous generation $g - 1$, and on the stochastic result of the genetic operators. Therefore it is not possible to connect directly $m_H(g)$ to $m_H(g-1)$, while the probability distribution of $m_H(g)$ is completely defined by the population at generation $g - 1$ and the genetic algorithm mechanism. Thus, we can hope to derive some properties of that distribution: Holland addressed the behavior of its mean, by considering separately the effect of selection, mutation and cross-over.

Let us first take into account the effect of selection, assuming that we use proportional selection (roulette wheel rule). We denote by $\{x_i^{(g)}, i = 1, 2, \ldots, N\}$ the population at generation g, by $\overline{f}_g$ the average fitness:

$$\overline{f}_g = \frac{1}{N} \sum_{i=1}^{N} f[x_i^{(g)}]$$

and by $\overline{f}_{H,g}$ the average fitness of the instances of schema H contained in the same population, that is the average fitness of the $m_H(g)$ chromosomes that belong to schema H:

$$\overline{f}_{H,g} = \frac{1}{m_H(g)} \sum_{x_j^{(g)} \in H} f[x_j^{(g)}]$$

Since the probability of a chromosome $x_i^{(g)}$ being selected is $f[x_i^{(g)}]/\{N\overline{f}_g\}$, the probability of selecting a chromosome belonging to schema H is

$$\sum_{x_i^{(g)} \in H} f[x_i^{(g)}]/\{N\overline{f}_g\}$$

and the average number of instances of H in generation $g + 1$ is N times that probability:

$$E\{m_H(g+1)\} = \sum_{x_i^{(g)} \in H} f[x_i^{(g)}]/\overline{f}_g = \frac{\overline{f}_{H,g}}{\overline{f}_g} m_H(g) . \tag{2.7}$$

It follows that the ratio between the expected frequency of H in generation $g + 1$ and the frequency in generation g equals the ratio between the average fitness of the schema H and that of the whole population at generation g. This result may be interpreted in the sense that schemas enjoying a large fitness on the average tend to be increasingly more frequent in the population as generations flow.

We must now consider the effects of both mutation and recombination, since these operators may create, or eliminate, instances of H. The only process easy to describe is disruption of a schema, thus we shall try to follow only these events, deriving a lower bound to the probability that a given instance of schema H survives to mutation. A schema is preserved after mutation if only loci that are free mutate, while if mutation occurs in loci whose values are defined (fixed) then the resulting chromosome is not an instance of H any more. Recall that the number of defined loci is called the defining order, $o(H)$. Then if the mutation probability is p_m, and it is applied independently to each gene of each chromosome, the probability that a mutation does not change any of the $o(H)$ defined gene values is simply $(1 - p_m)^{o(H)}$. Therefore, we may modify (2.7) as follows:

$$E\{m_H(g+1)\} \geq \frac{\overline{f}_{H,g}}{\overline{f}_g} m_H(g)\,(1 - p_M)^{o(H)} . \tag{2.8}$$

Let us now turn to cross-over. In this case also, we can easily address only the probability that a schema H is eliminated by cross-over, we take into account the simple one-point cross-over. Moreover, only a bound can be easily derived: cross-over will destroy the schema if the chromosome part to be swapped contains at least one defined position. For example, if an instance of the schema $1 * 0 * 1 * *$ undergoes a cross-over with cutting point two, say, the resulting chromosome may have a bit 0 in the fifth locus, and therefore the schema may be destroyed. Vice versa, if the cutting point is 5 or 6, the exchanged segment relates only to free loci, and the schema survives. It is not difficult to realize that what is important is that the cutting point falls within the defining length of the schema H, $d(H)$ (the distance between the first and the last defined position). Since the cutting point is chosen uniformly at random among the $M - 1$ possible choices, the probability that it falls within the defining length may be computed simply as $d(H)/(M - 1)$, and multiplying by the cross-over probability p_c, we get: the probability that an instance of schema H is destroyed by cross-over is no more than $p_c\, d(H)/(M - 1)$ (no more because when cross-over takes place, the inherited genes could also be luckily equal to the defined values, so that the schema survives). Thus, we may finally correct formula (2.8) multiplying by the probability that the schema is not eliminated by cross-over:

$$E\{m_H(g+1)\} \geq \frac{\overline{f}_{H,g}}{\overline{f}_g}\, m_H(g)\,(1 - p_M)^{o(H)} \left\{1 - p_c \frac{d(H)}{M - 1}\right\}. \tag{2.9}$$

The interpretation of (2.9) is not simple, and sometimes incorrect convergence properties have been deduced from it. The terms related to mutation and cross-over are always less than one, therefore they reduce the right hand side. The reduction effect is increased by increasing p_m, $o(H)$ and $d(H)$, therefore for schemas whose defining length and order are small (short, low-order schemas) the effect of the third and fourth factors of (2.9) may be negligible. The first term, as seen before, is the ratio between an estimate of the average fitness of schema H and the average population fitness. Thus, the schema theorem is usually interpreted as follows: short, low-order schemas with average fitness above the mean tend to exponentially increase the number of their instances in the population. There are some immediate objections to that assertion:

- Formula (2.9) is an inequality, and does not take into account the probability that instances of H are created by mutation or cross-over.
- The fitness ratio $\overline{f}_{H,g}/\overline{f}_g$ depends on an estimate of the average schema fitness, computed only on the individuals in the population at generation g, therefore it may be a seriously biased estimate.
- The value of $m_H(G)$ is bounded by N and cannot really increase exponentially with g.
- Suppose that H is a very favorable schema with average fitness well above the mean, then after several generations many individuals will belong to H, and $\overline{f}_g$ will be about equal to $\overline{f}_{H,g}$, in that case the right hand side of (2.9) becomes less than $m_H(g)$.

But probably the most serious objection is that the schema theorem is based on a conditional argument, therefore it relates the actual number of instances in generation g, $m_H(g)$, to the average number of instances in generation $g + 1$, $E\{m_H(g + 1)\}$, but an evaluation of the variance of the distribution of $m_H(g + 1)$ is not possible. The schema theorem cannot be interpreted to involve the ratio of the number of instances of H in two successive generations: $m_H(g+1)/m_H(g)$, nor the mean of that ratio, nor the ratio of the means $E\{m_H(g+1)\}/E\{m_H(g)\}$. Despite this, the work on schemas by Holland and later researchers was important as an attempt to investigate the long run behavior of genetic algorithms, and contributed to stimulate a great deal of study concerning the limiting properties of genetic algorithms considered as stochastic processes.

It is by now generally acknowledged in the literature that the schema theorem cannot contribute to a formal convergence analysis of a genetic algorithm. Only at the beginning of the nineties rigorous results were obtained on this subject, by adopting exact mathematical models of the genetic algorithm, and exploiting results in probability and algebra. A comprehensive account may be found in Reeves and Rowe (2003).

The key observation is that the population at generation $g+1$ is created according to a stochastic mechanism whose probability distribution is completely determined by the population at generation g, therefore the sequence of populations indexed by generations may be seen as a Markov process. Then a genetic algorithm may be thought of as a stochastic process in discrete time, $g = 1, 2, \ldots$, whose realization at each generation g is a population, coded by a set of N chromosomes, or N points in the solution space; thus, the univariate marginal distributions have support equal to the Nth cartesian product of the solution space.

This poses some representation problems, and two different approaches have been proposed: following the population as a whole, or the frequencies of different individuals. We suppose that coding is binary, that each chromosome has M genes and the population is composed by N individuals. Thus, on taking the individuals in a given order, any possible population is associated to a string of MN binary digits, with 2^{MN} different possible states. However, not all states correspond to different populations, since the same population correspond to all states obtained by permutating the order of the M-digits sequences inside the MN digit string: the actually different populations are $\binom{N+2^M-1}{N}$ (combinations with repetition of the 2^M possible different individuals in sets of cardinality N). Anyway, the number of states of the process is finite, and it may be considered a finite Markov chain. Given an arbitrary ordering of states, the transition probabilities form the matrix P and the state probabilities at generation g will be denoted by w_g, while w_0 denotes a vector with all entries equal to zero except that indicating the initial population, which is set to 1. From Markov chains theory,

$$w_g = P w_{g-1} \;\; ; \;\; w_g = P^g w_0 \,.$$

The transition matrix would be very large, and difficult to derive. An alternative representation, proposed by Vose (1999) with the aim of facilitating the study of transition, consists in considering the frequency in the current population of each of the possible 2^M individuals. A state is identified by a vector of 2^M rational numbers $p_g = \{p_g(1), p_g(2), \ldots, p_g(2^M)\}'$ where $p_g(i)$ denotes the relative frequency of individual i in the population at generation g. Obviously $p_g(i) \geq 0$ and $p_g(1)+p_g(2)+\cdots+p_g(2^M) = 1$. This achieves a great reduction in the dimension of the representation because the states are in a one-to-one correspondence with the possible populations; also, the transition mechanism is no more described by a matrix but a single vector is sufficient, which specifies the probability that a given offspring will be generated at generation $g+1: s_g = \{s_g(1), s_g(2), \ldots, s_g(2^M)\}'$ where $s_g(i) \geq 0$ represents the probability that individual i is generated by the population at time g, and $s_g(1) + s_g(2) + \cdots + s_g(2^M) = 1$. Each new offspring is generated independently, and with a probability distribution which is multinomial with parameters s_g ; then, the transition mechanism may be entirely described in terms of the probabilities s_g by means of a transition operator $G(\cdot)$:

$$s_{g+1} = G(s_g)$$

where $G(\cdot)$ incorporates all features of the algorithm. The link between s_g and p_g may be expressed through distribution, since $p_g(i)$ is the relative frequency of a realized event with probability $s_g(i)$, then

$$E\{p_{g+1}\} = s_g .$$

Therefore, conditional on the population at generation g, p_g, we may write $E\{p_{g+1}\} = G(p_g)$. This suggests a way of studying the limiting behavior of the population: admitting that the number of individuals N tends to infinity, the variance of the distribution tends to zero and we get $p_{g+1} = G(p_g)$. The limiting behavior of this recursive equation may be analyzed, concluding that as $g \to \infty$, p_g tends to the fixed point(s) of $G(\cdot)$ (Vose, 1999).

The difficult task is to compute the transition matrix P or operator G, in order to derive the limiting properties of the Markov chain.

We shall not address such a problem here, but just quote some relevant results. First, if the genetic algorithm has a mutation probability greater than zero, then any population may be generated from any preceding one at each generation, therefore the chain is ergodic. The limiting distribution w_∞ has been characterized by Davis and Principe (1993). If we denote by P the transition matrix, and by P_j the matrix obtained from P by replacing the jth column with zeroes, then the kth element of the limiting probability vector w_∞ is

$$w_\infty(k) = |P_k - I| / \sum_j |P_j - I| .$$

On the contrary if mutation is not allowed, using only selection and recombination induces closed sets of states in the chain. Moreover, from the point of view of optimization, when the chain is ergodic each state has a strictly positive limiting probability, therefore convergence to the optimum is not ensured with probability one. An exception is when we employ the elitist strategy (the best-so-far found chromosome is automatically copied to the next generation). In that case, suppose that there is only an optimal individual, coded by chromosome y. Let j denote the state corresponding to the population composed of all individuals equal to y : the transition matrix P has a 1 in the diagonal at position j, it is an absorbing state and convergence is certain. More precisely, it may be shown (Rudolph, 1997) that, on denoting as before by $x_{\text{best}}^{(g)}$ the best fitted chromosome at generation g, then the sequence $\Delta_g = f(y) - f[x_{\text{best}}^{(g)}]$ is a non-negative supermartingale converging to zero almost surely.

More elaborated results have been derived: essentially, if the elitist strategy is not employed, it may be shown that the chain spends most of the time in the state (or states) with maximum fitness. If, on the contrary mutation is not allowed, the set of the optimal states is closed (therefore once entered it will never be abandoned), therefore convergence depends essentially on the starting state, i.e., the initial population. In fact, with no mutation, if we start for example with an initial population where all chromosomes have the gene in the first locus equal to one, all subsequent offsprings will also have a one in the first position. Similarly, the set of populations having a given digit at a specified locus form a closed set, and the further steps will only improve the fitness by increasing the proportion of best fitted individuals inside the closed set, driving in the limit to a uniform population composed of copies of the best fitted individual compatible with that closed set (a formal proof may be found in Schmitt et al., 1998). A similar behavior is usually exhibited, at least for an initial time, also by a genetic algorithm with very small mutation probability, and was called *premature convergence*.

In his book, Rudolph (1997) presents also a study of the properties of the random variables "number of generations to reach the optimum". Essentially, it is seen that in reasonably simple problems the mean number is bounded by a polynomial function of the chromosome length, but such a bound does not hold in general for any optimization problem.

A different approach, inspired by statistical mechanics, was proposed by Shapiro, Prügel-Bennett, Rattray and Rogers (see, e.g., Shapiro, 2001). They consider a genetic algorithm as a complex system described, at each generation, by the statistical distribution of a given variable measured on each individual, and propose to follow the behavior through generations of some distribution summary like the cumulants. The chosen variable is the fitness value. Thus, at generation g the statistical distribution $\{f[x_1^{(g)}], f[x_2^{(g)}], \ldots, f[x_N^{(g)}]\}$ is considered and its cumulants computed. It is possible to evaluate the effect of selection, mutation and cross-over on the cumulants, and thus to follow their behavior in successive generations. Interesting results have been obtained for binary chromosomes and the *onemax* fitness (the number of genes equal to 1 in the chromosome), but an extension to more general fitness functions is very complicate.

A final additional observation concerns the case of genetic algorithms in statistical applications. Most often the genetic algorithm will be run operating on a sample with the aim of estimating parameters of the distribution, and the result will depend on two sources of variability, that due to sampling and that due to the stochastic nature of the algorithm. Suppose that a sample x is drawn from a distribution belonging to the family $\{F_\theta(\cdot), \theta \in \Theta\}$ and we want to make an inference on θ by optimizing some function of x (a likelihood, for example); denote by $\theta^*(x)$

the best theoretical value. We run a genetic algorithm and obtain an estimate $\hat{\theta}(x)$, therefore the bias is:

$$\hat{\theta}(x) - \theta = \{\theta^*(x) - \theta\} + \{\hat{\theta}(x) - \theta^*(x)\}$$

where the first term is due to the sampling variability and the possible bias implied by the estimation method, which is controlled and studied by classical statistical inference, while the second term is typical of the genetic algorithm and is what we addressed in the present analysis of convergence. However, a statistician would probably like that $\hat{\theta}(x) - \theta$ converges to zero, implying that both terms on the right hand side must degenerate,[1] and this requires attention since the second term also depends on the sample x. Such a problem is typical of statistical applications and still needs to be addressed in literature.

2.3.4 Issues in the Implementation of Genetic Algorithms

When a genetic algorithm has to be employed in practice for solving a specific problem, a number of decisions have to be taken. Suppose we have chosen the encoding type already, and the fitness function has also been defined. At least the following points need to be clarified:

1. Choice of the number of individuals in the population.
2. Choice of the selection mechanism.
3. Choice of the mutation type and its probability.
4. Choice of cross-over operator and its probability.
5. Definition of the initial population at generation 0.
6. Decision on how many generations to reproduce, and when the algorithm should stop.

Though the last question may also be deferred to a later time, when the genetic algorithm is being run, the first five topics have to be addressed before we can start the procedure. Few theoretical guidelines are available for this, and experience with practical applications of the genetic algorithm is offered by a vast literature. The most instructing conclusion is that (as one could expect) there is no uniformly best choice of the parameters, but any particular problem may require different values, as the no-free-lunch theorems suggest.

A preliminary step is however to make explicit what objectives we have in mind. A distinction in this respect was proposed by De Jong (1975), whose work is one of the main contributions in the literature on the present subject. De Jong proposes

[1] Formally, convergence to zero could also arise from $\hat{\theta}(x) - \theta^*(x)$ tending to assume the same values of $\theta - \theta^*(x)$, but this seems very artificial and unreasonable, thus we shall not admit this possibility

to distinguish between on-line and off-line applications. In the first ones, we want that the genetic algorithms drive rapidly to a good solution, without pretending to arrive to the optimum, while in off-line applications we are prepared to wait for many generations, but we want to get as close as possible to the best solution. In the first case, speed is more important than precision, while the contrary is true in the second approach, and one can expect that a different parameter choice is needed. De Jong, and later Grefenstette (1986), who tried to evolve the decision itself by means of a genetic algorithm, experimented a large number of parameter combinations on many typical fitness functions. De Jong's indications are towards small values of the mutation probability, around 0.001, and rather high cross-over probability, around 0.6, with a population of around 50 individuals. Grefenstette noted that according to the on-line or off-line points of view the parameters give different results: if off-line is more relevant, lower cross-over rates and larger population sizes produce better results, while the contrary is true if on-line arguments are more important; he also suggested a somewhat larger mutation probability, about 0.01.

As far as the population size is concerned, it is clear that it should be large enough to enable a multiple search inside the solution space, but not too large for avoiding heavy computational effort. Empirical studies indicate that values around 50 (or even 30) are usually satisfying, while Alander (1992) suggested values between M and $2M$, where M is the chromosome length (number of genes). On the theoretical ground, the choice of the population size has been addressed by several authors. Notably, Goldberg (1989c) suggested an exponential function of the chromosome length, and later studies by himself and co-authors (e.g. Goldberg et al., 1992), on considering favorable building blocks and adopting sampling size strategies, suggested rather a linear dependence. Recently, Gao (2003) derived a lower bound for the population size, depending on the mutation probability, the effect on fitness of each single gene, and the natural logarithm of the chromosome length.

In all cases, there is evidence that the performance of a genetic algorithm is a non linear function of its parameter values.

As a consequence, one may conclude that a good choice may be obtained only by experimenting a range of possible values on the same problem. Mutation is necessary for exploring the solution space thoroughly, but a too large mutation rate would drive the genetic algorithm towards a purely random search, with worse results. On the contrary, cross-over has the positive effect of combining schemas and makes the search for the optimum easier, therefore a substantial probability is always suggested, though not too close to one for avoiding nearly certain disruption of high order schemas. In fact, we already noted that schemas with a long defining length are likely to be destroyed by cross-over, which preferentially preserves short schemas; moreover, not all loci have the same chance to be involved in cross-over, since the last genes of the chromosomes (end points) are always exchanged, while the preceding genes are not (this is called *positional bias*). To avoid these features, two-point cross-over is sometimes used: two cutting points are selected at random between 1 and $M - 1$, and the internal segment is exchanged. Along the same line, uniform cross-over has been proposed, where each gene of the chromosome of the offspring is selected at random, with equal probability, between the two correspondent genes of the parents. Syswerda (1989) found that uniform cross-over was definitely better than two-point cross-over (which in turn was found better than one-point): it certainly avoids positional bias and end-point effects, but some authors consider that it may be highly disruptive of any schema (Mitchell, 1996, p. 196).

Let us now turn to consider the selection mechanism. Holland introduced the dichotomy between *exploration* and *exploitation* in describing adaptation of systems: exploration means searching for new and useful characteristics, and is obtained by genetic operators (mutation and cross-over), while exploitation means propagation of the favorable characters found so far, and relates to selection. A balance is needed for enhancing adaptation, therefore, given the genetic operators probabilities, selection should not be too strong (for maintaining sufficient diversity and allowing new phenotypes to appear) nor too weak (which would slow the evolution). If we use fitness- proportionate selection, the probability of selecting an individual is given by the ratio of its fitness to the sum of the fitness values of all individuals in the population, and if this sum is large it may decrease the difference between the selection probabilities of the different chromosomes. In other words, at the initial generations the individuals are likely to be very different, and their selection probabilities will also be largely different, but in later generations the average fitness will increase, and this implies generally that the fitness variability decreases, therefore all individuals tend to receive selection probabilities with similar values. Mitchell (1996) observes: "the rate of evolution depends on the variance of the fitnesses in the population". A simple method for avoiding this is standardizing the fitness distribution at each generation, dividing by its standard deviation: this is called *sigma scaling*. Let

$$\sigma_g^2 = \frac{1}{N} \sum_i \left\{ f[x_i^{(g)}] - \overline{f}_g \right\}^2$$

denote the fitness variance at generation g, then we may consider the following possible transformations of the fitness:

$$\alpha_g(x_j) = f(x_j)/\sigma_g$$
$$\beta_g(x_j) = \{f(x_j) - \min_i f(x_i)\}/\sigma_g$$
$$\gamma_g(x_j) = \text{const} + \{f(x_j) - \overline{f}_g\}/\sigma_g\,.$$

Some authors propose that selection should not be uniform, starting with a less selective reproduction and later increasing pressure as generations flow, suggesting an approach similar to simulated annealing by defining a sequence of temperatures T_g,varying with generations and gradually decreasing to zero. A consistent choice of the transformed fitness would be:

$$s_g(x_j) = \exp\{f(x_j)/T_g\} / \sum_i \exp\{f(x_i)/T_g\}$$

and is called the *Boltzman selection*. Obviously this leaves the problem of how to select the initial temperature and the rate of its decrease. Finally, rank selection also enables to avoid the selection pressure problem, since it is independent of the fitness variance. Rank selection is usually successful in preserving diversity, though it sometimes slows convergence, and it has always to be considered that with rank selection all information concerning the absolute fitness differences between individuals is discarded. The elitist strategy (maintaining in the next generation the best fitted individual) is considered advantageous by most authors, and is generally unanimously employed, in view also of the aforementioned theoretical results. The best individual is added to the new population in case it did not survive, and is usually substituted to the individual with the least fitness value, or to one selected at random.

A few words are also opportune concerning the choice of the initial population. The most popular choice is selecting the initial individuals completely and uniformly at random inside the solution space: each individual is selected independently of the others, and usually also each gene value is selected independently of the other genes. The method depends on the coding; for binary and k-ary alphabets equal probabilities are assigned, while when a real encoding is employed, without any bound, often a gaussian distribution is adopted. We have already noted that if mutation is not used, all individuals will belong indefinitely to the convex closure of the set of the initial population; thus, if the mutation probability is very small, it may be a good idea starting from an initial population that is not selected (or not entirely) at random, but contains the extremal or "corner" points of the solution space, in order to ensure that a large part of that space may be reached also by cross-over and not relying only on mutation. Moreover, any a priori information may be included in the initial population, for example individuals which are known to be well-fitted or with promising features.

A relevant problem when using genetic algorithms for optimization is the stopping rule: how many generations should we wait before taking the best-so-far found chromosome as the optimum solution? The best obtained fitness value can be monitored against generations, and a typical behavior is a fast increase in the first generations, which later stabilizes with a decreasing rate of occasional improving, as in Fig. 2.5.

Sometimes we know what is the optimum value of the fitness, therefore we may safely decide when to stop, but it rarely happens in statistical applications. The simplest solution is deciding in advance how many generations to evolve, but this is possible only when preceding experience with similar problems may suggest suitable values. An alternative is stopping the process when a sufficiently large number of generations have passed without any improvement in the best fitness value, or when a population statistics reaches a pre-defined bound. Several indices have been proposed, such as the variance or the range of the fitness distribution, or else some diversity measures relating to the chromosomes rather than the fitness. An example, with binary encoding is the maximum Hamming distance between two chromosomes: evolution may be stopped when the maximum Hamming distance is less than $\alpha M/100$ (where M is the number of genes), which means that no more than α percent genes are different in any pair of individuals.

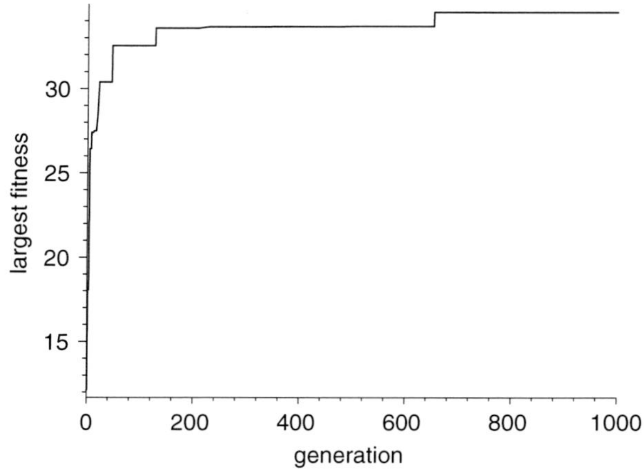

Fig. 2.5 An example of the best fitness value behavior against generations

Finally, it should be remembered that genetic algorithms are stochastic procedures: thus, also starting from the same initial population and evolving the same number of generations, repeating the process may lead to different solutions. Thus, it is customary, and recommended, to repeat the genetic algorithm application for several runs. This may be done choosing each time a different initial population at random, or starting always from the same initial population (when there are reasons to select a particular initial set of individuals) and proceeding with different random numbers streams. Running a genetic algorithm several times on the same data allows to control the variability of the results, which is implicitly a measure of their reliability. A too large variability may suggest the need to increase the number of generations to be evolved.

At the end of this section a concluding remark may be drawn, concerning the computational complexity of the problems to be addressed by means of genetic algorithms. Since in statistical applications the most hard computations are usually found in calculating the fitness, an overall measure of the effort may be obtained through the number of times the fitness is evaluated. On this respect, a substantial advantage is attained by the simple device of storing the fitness values together with each chromosome, as an additional artificial gene. Therefore, in a genetic algorithm with a population of N individuals, at each new generation we must evaluate the fitness only for the new offsprings, whose average number is approximately $MNp_m + Np_c$, where p_m is the mutation, and p_c the cross-over, probability. Therefore in G generations an average number of $(MNp_m + Np_c)G$ fitness evaluations are necessary. This number should be compared with the effort needed for a complete enumeration of all possible individuals, and their fitness. With binary encoding, and a cartesian product solution space, the different individuals are 2^M. Therefore, employing a genetic algorithm is plausible only if $(MNp_m + Np_c)G$ is of a considerably smaller order of magnitude than 2^M, otherwise complete enumeration, which obviously solves the optimization problem with certainty, is the best strategy. For example, with $p_m = 0.001$, $p_c = 0.6$, $N = 50$, 100 generations and a chromosome with $M = 40$ genes, we have $(MNp_m + Np_c)G = 3200$ while 2^M is as large as 10^{12}. The main point is the number of genes, since with the same parameter choice but taking $M = 20$ the average number of fitness evaluations for the genetic algorithm is about the same (3100), while 2^{20} is only about one million. We can conclude that the progress in computer speed will probably enable us to solve exactly by enumeration problems which are now addressed by evolutionary computation; on the other hand, such progress will make it possible to solve by genetic algorithms increasingly hard problems.

2.3.5 Genetic Algorithms and Random Sampling from a Probability Distribution

We discuss now some connections between evolutionary computation and methods for generating random samples according to a given multivariate probability distribution. Though we are dealing in effect with pseudo-random sampling, since we are not drawing real samples, but using numbers generated by algorithms running on a computer, we shall discard the prefix pseudo as usual in the statistical literature.

The problem of generating samples from an assigned distribution is an old one in Statistics, but received a great deal of attention, essentially for the multivariate case, in more recent years, when Bayesian researchers started addressing increasingly complicated problems, where the posterior probabilities do not belong to standard families, and the posterior mean – or other indices – are given by integrals whose primitive is not known. These studies led to the MCMC (Markov Chain Monte Carlo) methods, which have been a major research subject in Statistics in the last 20 years.

A detailed illustration of MCMC methods is beyond the scope of this book (and may be found e.g. in Gilks et al., 1996). Let $\pi(x)$, $x \in \mathbb{R}^p$ denote a multivariate probability distribution whose direct simulation by standard random number generators is difficult. The MCMC techniques generate a vector sequence $\{x_t\}$ in $\mathbb{R}^p$ that may be considered a random realization of a Markov chain with equilibrium distribution equal to $\pi(\cdot)$. To this aim, a proposal distribution $q : \mathbb{R}^p \times \mathbb{R}^p \to [0, 1]$ is defined from which random numbers may easily be generated. At time t, given the state x_t, a random realization y from the distribution $q(\cdot|x_t)$ is generated. The move is accepted, i.e., x_{t+1} is set equal to y, with probability given by

$$\alpha(x_t, y) = \min\left\{1, \frac{\pi(y)q(x_t|y)}{\pi(x_t)q(y|x_t)}\right\}. \tag{2.10}$$

If the move is not accepted, then $x_{t+1} = x_t$. It may be shown that the chain generated this way is ergodic, and its equilibrium distribution is $\pi(\cdot)$. As a consequence, after an initial "burning-in" period, the generated data are recorded and assumed as a random sample from $\pi(\cdot)$, even though they, strictly speaking, are not obviously a sequence of independent realizations.

This method (known as Metropolis-Hastings) has the main advantage that random numbers generation is needed only from the proposal distribution $q(y|x)$, which may be chosen in such a way that generation is conveniently easy. Even if the large dimensionality makes this task difficult, a dimensional reduction is possible by using a scalar form of the algorithm, by considering the components of the vector x_t one at a time. Let $x_{t,i}$ denote the components of the vector $(i = 1, 2, \ldots, p)$ and let $x_t(-i)$ denote the vector with all components except the ith. Then, the components are sequentially updated by using different proposal densities $q_i[x_{t+1,i}|x_t(-i)]$ combined with the conditional distributions induced by $\pi(\cdot)$, in a similar way as (2.10). In this way each step of the procedure requires that random numbers be generated from univariate probability distributions. Different choices of the proposal distribution q lead to different techniques: if $q(y|x) = q(x|y)$, then q disappears in (2.10), yielding the Metropolis algorithm. If $q(y|x) = q(y)$ the algorithm is called independence sampler, if $q(y|x) = q(y-x)$ it is known as random walk Metropolis algorithm. A relevant case is the scalar procedure where the proposal densities are chosen equal to the univariate conditional distributions induced by $\pi(\cdot)$, and is called the Gibbs sampler. In this case the probability $\alpha(x_t, y)$ is always equal to one, and the moves are always accepted.

It was noted that if $\pi(\cdot)$ is multimodal and with strongly correlated components, the sequence generated by the chain may be easily get trapped in a local maximum, and many modifications were proposed to avoid such a drawback. A popular idea is to use many chains in parallel. Several proposals in the literature are aimed at improving the "mixing" ability of the algorithm, i.e., its capability of generating chains which are able to visit exhaustively the whole support (for example, the Metropolis Coupled MCMC of Geyer, 1991, or the Simulated Tempering of Marinari and Parisi, 1992). As soon as the practice of using N parallel chains became popular (these algorithms were sometimes called Population Based MCMC), the idea of exploiting interactions between the different chains arose, and some authors proposed to use techniques similar to the genetic operators mutation and cross-over to evolve the N contemporaneous states of the chains as they would be a population. An important difference here is that one has to use operators that do not destroy the convergence of the chains to the equilibrium distribution π. To this aim the operator has to satisfy the property of *reversibility*. Reversibility may be described as follows: for an operator ω which changes x to y with probability $p_\omega(y|x)$, ω is reversible with respect to $\pi(\cdot)$ if $\pi(x)p_\omega(y|x) = \pi(y)p_\omega(x|y)$ for any x, y in $\mathbb{R}^p$. For operators that change pairs of states into pairs of states (as in cross-over), the reversibility property may easily be modified: if ω changes (x_i, x_j) into (y_i, y_j) with probability $p_\omega(y_i, y_j|x_i, x_j)$ then ω is reversible w. r. to π if $\pi(x_i)\pi(x_j)p_\omega(y_i, y_j|x_i, x_j) = \pi(y_i)\pi(y_j)p_\omega(x_i, x_j|y_i, y_j)$ for any x_i, x_j, y_i, y_j in $\mathbb{R}^p$.

A MCMC procedure exploiting genetic operators, called Parallel Adaptive Metropolis Sampler, was proposed by Holmes and Mallick (1998). Liang and Wong (2000, 2001) introduced the Evolutionary Monte Carlo methods, combining also concepts from simulated annealing, and several other papers appeared in the literature, a review may be found in Drugan and Thierens (2004).

As far as the mutation operator is concerned, since coding is usually real, generally a small modification by adding a random normally distributed noise with zero mean and moderate variance is adopted (like in evolution strategies). The probability of mutation, however, is not constant at p_m as before, but is determined by a Metropolis acceptance rule: if x_t is the parent and $x_t^* = x_t + \varepsilon$ is the candidate offspring (the mutant), then the mutation is accepted with probability

$$\min\left\{1, \frac{\pi(x_t^*)}{\pi(x_t)}\right\}.$$

This ensures reversibility so that mutation does not destroy the chain ergodicity. Note however that with this mechanism the mutation probability is usually rather large compared with the small values of p_m generally adopted in evolutionary computation.

Cross-over operations may be realized through different operators, but always considering that the ergodic character of the chain should be preserved, therefore the cross-over results should leave the equilibrium distribution unchanged. In fact, if two states x_i and x_j are generated according to $\pi(\cdot)$, the results of a standard cross-over operation between x_i and x_j are not in general distributed exactly according to $\pi(\cdot)$. Two solution have been proposed: one is subordinating cross-over results to an acceptance rule of Metropolis-Hastings type, the other consists in modifying the cross-over mechanism itself.

Let us consider the first solution. Suppose that two independently randomly chosen states x_i and x_j are subject to a cross-over operator ω which generates offsprings y_i and y_j with probability $\phi(y_i, y_j|x_i, x_j)$. We accept the new pair of states y_i, y_j, substituting them to x_i and x_j, with probability

$$\alpha(x_i, x_j, y_i, y_j) = \min\left\{1, \frac{\pi(y_i)\pi(y_j)\phi(x_i, x_j|y_i, y_j)}{\pi(x_i)\pi(x_j)\phi(y_i, y_j|x_i, x_j)}\right\}.$$

Then, the probability distribution $p_\omega(y_i, y_j|x_i, x_j)$ of the accepted changes (therefore of the cross-over results) may be easily computed as follows:

$$\begin{aligned} p_\omega(y_i, y_j|x_i, x_j) &= \alpha(x_i, x_j, y_i, y_j)\phi(y_i, y_j|x_i, x_j) \\ &\quad + I(x_i = y_i, x_j = y_j)\left\{1 - \int\int \phi(z, w|x_i, x_j)\alpha(x_i, x_j, z, w)dzdw\right\} \end{aligned}$$

where $I(\cdot)$ is the indicator function. Now, α satisfies the detailed balance equation:

$$\begin{aligned} &\alpha(x_i, x_j, y_i, y_j)\pi(x_i)\pi(x_j)\phi(y_i, y_j|x_i, x_j) \\ &\qquad = \alpha(y_i, y_j, x_i, x_j)\pi(y_i)\pi(y_j)\phi(x_i, x_j|y_i, y_j) \end{aligned}$$

from which we obtain:

$$\pi(x_i)\pi(x_j)p_\omega(y_i, y_j|x_i, x_j) = \pi(y_i)\pi(y_j)p_\omega(x_i, x_j|y_i, y_j) .$$

Therefore this mechanism satisfies the reversibility property. It follows that if x_i and x_j are independently distributed according to $\pi(\cdot)$, then the results of cross-over y_i and y_j are also independent and distributed according to $\pi(\cdot)$. The only difficult task could be determining the exchange distribution $\phi(y_i, y_j|x_i, x_j)$. However, for most common cross-over forms, such as fixed one-point and uniform, the distribution satisfies

$$\phi(y_i, y_j|x_i, x_j) = \phi(x_i, x_j|y_i, y_j)$$

thus it disappears in the acceptance probability, which is simply computed as:

$$\min\left\{1, \frac{\pi(y_i)\pi(y_j)}{\pi(x_i)\pi(x_j)}\right\} .$$

The alternative way of proceeding is taking as offsprings not directly y_i and y_j, but a suitable transformation which enables maintaining ergodicity. The most common solution of this type is called *snooker cross-over* (being inspired by the snooker algorithm proposed by Roberts and Gilks (1994), in the MCMC framework). Let, as before, x_i and x_j denote the parents, and y_i and y_j the results of a one-point cross-over operator. The offsprings from x_i, x_j are selected as two new points belonging to the lines joining x_i to y_i and x_j to y_j respectively. They are determined by random trials from the conditional distributions induced by $\pi(\cdot)$ along the lines. Thus, if x_i^c and x_j^c denote the results of the snooker cross-over, then

$$x_i^c = x_i + r_1(y_i - x_i) \quad ; \quad x_j^c = x_j + r_2(y_j - x_j)$$

where r_1 and r_2 are generated at random from the probability distributions $g_1(\cdot)$ and $g_2(\cdot)$ defined as follows:

$$g_1(r) \propto \pi[x_i+r(y_i-x_i)]|1-r|^{M-1} \quad ; \quad g_2(r) \propto \pi[x_j+r(y_j-x_j)]|1-r|^{M-1} , \ r \in \mathbb{R}$$

the proof that the chain remains ergodic in this case is more difficult and will not be given here (see, e.g., Goswami and Liu, 2007).

What precedes suggests a close relationship between MCMC methods and genetic algorithms, and one may expect that the issue of random sample generation according to a given distribution might be developed in a complete genetic algorithms framework. A proposal in this direction is in Battaglia (2001), where a genetic algorithm is introduced for drawing random samples from a given multivariate probability distribution.

The main difficulty seems to be that in MCMC procedures the selection operator is completely missing. The behavior of the individuals does not depend on their adaptation to the environment, since a fitness function is not explicitly defined. Evolution here has the aim of obtaining a population that represents adequately the probability distribution $\pi(\cdot)$, so it would be natural to evaluate the adaptation to the environment of the population as a whole, for example considering an index of similarity between $\pi(\cdot)$ and the empirical distribution of the population. However, such kind of fitness measurement, evaluating at each generation the population as a whole, could not be employed for driving selection, because for defining the selection probabilities each chromosome has to be assigned its own adaptation value. To overcome such difficulties, Battaglia (2001) proposes to consider a partition $\{P_j, j = 1, \ldots, n\}$ of the support of $\pi(\cdot)$, and adopt the procedure introduced by Smith et al. (1993) in modelling the immune systems. Let

$$\pi_j = \int_{P_j} \pi(x)dx \quad , \; j = 1, \ldots, n$$

denote the probability of the set P_j, and $s_j^{(g)}$ the absolute frequency of the chromosomes belonging to P_j in generation g. Obviously, $\pi_1 + \cdots + \pi_n = 1$, $s_1^{(g)} + \cdots + s_n^{(g)} = N$ (the number of individuals in the population), and the scope of the genetic algorithm is generating a vector $\{s_1^{(g)}, s_2^{(g)}, \ldots, s_n^{(g)}\}$ converging to $\{N\pi_1, N\pi_2, \ldots, N\pi_n\}$.

In the work by Smith, Forrest and Perelson a finite number of different antigens are considered, each of which having at least one specialized antibody. Each different chromosome corresponds to a different antibody, and its genes encode what antigens it is able to contrast; the aim is to defend against all antigens, maintaining diversity within the population. In order to define an individual adaptation score, an effectiveness measure of each antibody on each antigen is first defined. Then, an antigen is chosen at random with a given probability distribution, and a block of r antibodies is selected at random too. The antibodies are examined to check the effectiveness of each of them against the given antigen, and the most effective antibody is assigned a positive score. By repeating such a procedure several times, and taking the average results, each chromosome receives an adaptation score.

For the present case, the antigens are identified with the partitions P_j, the antibodies with the chromosomes $x_i^{(g)}$. The effectiveness of $x_i^{(g)}$ on the antigen P_j is set to unity if $x_i^{(g)} \in P_j$ and zero otherwise. By selecting antigens at random with the equilibrium probabilities π_j of the associated partitions, the mean adaptation score of $x_i^{(g)}$ may be computed as (Battaglia, 2001):

$$\varphi_r(x_i^{(g)}) = N \frac{\pi_j}{s_j^{(g)}} \left\{ 1 - \frac{\binom{N - s_j^{(g)}}{r}}{\binom{N}{r}} \right\}$$

where j is the partition to which $x_i^{(g)}$ belongs. These fitness scores depend on the group width r adopted in the random assignment, larger values of r yield more cooperative procedures, and for $r = N$ we obtain:

$$\varphi(x_i^{(g)}) = N \frac{\pi_j}{s_j^{(g)}} \quad , \; x_i^{(g)} \in P_j \, .$$

If a fitness proportionate selection is used, the selection probability of a single chromosome $x_i^{(g)}$ is

$$p(x_i^{(g)}) = \frac{\pi_j}{s_j^{(g)}} \left\{ \sum_{k \in J_g} \pi_k \right\}^{-1} \quad , \; x_i^{(g)} \in P_j$$

where the summation extends over the indices of partitions which are actually represented in generation g: $J_g = \{j : s_j^{(g)} > 0\}$. If in the population there is at least one chromosome belonging to each partition, then the selection probabilities are in accordance to the target distribution π_j. The task of ensuring that each partition is represented in the population is left to mutation and cross-over, as described above.

The procedure relies on the selected partition $\{P_j, j = 1, \ldots, n\}$ of the support, and the computation of the probabilities π_j of each set of the partition. An appropriate choice of the partition may be crucial for ensuring good mixing properties, but no simple guidelines are available, though for some problems symmetry properties may suggest an intuitive partition in equal probability subsets. When the probabilities π_j are not exactly known, Battaglia (2001) proposes to start with approximate values and use an adaptive procedure for updating them through generations:

$$\pi_j^{(g)} = \beta s_j^{(g)} / N + (1 - \beta) \pi_j^{(g-1)} \, .$$

Chapter 3
Evolving Regression Models

Abstract Regression models are well established tools in statistical analysis which date back early to the eighteenth century. Nonetheless, problems involved in their implementation and application in a wide number of fields are still the object of active research. Preliminary to the regression model estimation there is an identification step which has to be performed for selecting the variables of interest, detecting the relationships of interest among them, distinguishing dependent and independent variables. On the other hand, generalized regression models often have nonlinear and non convex log-likelihood, therefore maximum likelihood estimation requires optimization of complicated functions. In this chapter evolutionary computation methods are presented that have been developed to either support or surrogate analytic tools if the problem size and complexity limit their efficiency.

3.1 Introduction

The first and most natural topic where genetic algorithms may find an useful application is the analysis of multivariate random samples. When analyzing dependence among variables in a multivariate data set, two essential features may be distinguished: the functional form of the dependence, and the measurement of its strength. In order to build a statistical dependence model among many variables, one has therefore to make explicit both the mathematical form of the function, and the values of its parameters. We shall refer to these two tasks as *identification* and *estimation*.

Genetic algorithms have been proposed for both tasks: in identification they are useful for selection of variables, which is usually difficult because a choice has to be done inside a very large discrete space of solutions. In estimation, genetic algorithms are employed when the function to be optimized, often the likelihood, is highly nonlinear, non convex and the optimum cannot be found using derivatives.

We shall review separately evolutionary computation proposals in identification and estimation. For model identification, most relevant applications are found in linear regression, generalized linear models and principal component and canonical analysis. Parameter estimation by evolutionary computation has been proposed for regression models and independent component analysis. Contributions concerning mixture models will be considered in the chapter on cluster analysis.

R. Baragona et al., *Evolutionary Statistical Procedures*, Statistics and Computing,
DOI 10.1007/978-3-642-16218-3_3,

3.2 Identification

The choice of the independent variables to be entered in a regression model, when many variables are available, is a difficult task that should balance accuracy and parsimony. The popular methods of sequential selection: forward, backward or stepwise, do not always ensure the optimal choice, therefore evolutionary computation methods are a natural candidate, and have been proposed in literature for several types of linear and generalized linear models.

3.2.1 Linear Regression

A typical issue in linear model identification is variable selection. A linear relationship is postulated between a dependent variable y and a set of independent variables $\{x_1, x_2, \dots, x_p\}$. Let n observations be available so that we may write the usual linear regression model

$$y_i = \beta_0 + \beta_1 x_{1i} + \beta_2 x_{2i} + \dots + \beta_p x_{pi} + u_i, \qquad i = 1, \dots, n,$$

where $\beta = (\beta_0, \beta_1, \dots, \beta_p)'$ is the parameter vector and $u = (u_1, \dots, u_n)'$ is a sequence of independent and identically distributed random variables with zero mean and unknown variance σ_u^2. Let $y = (y_1, \dots, y_n)'$ and $X = [1, x_1, x_2, \dots, x_p]$ where 1 denotes a column vector of ones. The linear regression model may be written in matrix form

$$y = X\beta + u.$$

For the sake of simplicity let us assume that the matrix X is non random and has full rank. Then the best linear unbiased estimates may be written

$$\hat{\beta} = (X'X)^{-1}X'y, \qquad \hat{\sigma}_u^2 = \hat{u}'\hat{u}/(n - p - 1),$$

where $\hat{u} = y - X\hat{\beta}$. The variance-covariance matrix of the parameter estimates $\hat{\beta}$ may be computed $\hat{\sigma}_u^2(X'X)^{-1}$. With the further assumption that u is normally distributed these are also the maximum likelihood estimates.

If p is large it is desirable to reduce the number of independent variables to the set that includes only the variables really important to explain the variability of y (Miller, 1990). Common available methods are the iterative forward, backward and stepwise methods. The goodness-of-fit of each model is usually evaluated computing the sum of squares of residuals and using the two statistics R^2 and F defined by:

$$R^2 = 1 - \hat{u}'\hat{u}/y'y, \qquad F = \frac{R^2/p}{(1 - R^2)/(n - p - 1)}.$$

We would be more confident about the final result if we could compare several alternative subsets simultaneously, since we want to select the variables that really matter in a linear regression.

The GAs are an easy-to-use tool for performing this comparison exactly: the encoding is straightforward as it suffices to define a mapping from a binary string of length p and the parameter sequence $\beta_1, \ldots, \beta_p$. If the kth gene is 0, then the parameter β_k is constrained to zero. The constant term β_0 is always included in the regression.

Let us illustrate a GAs-based procedure for subset regression on an example of $n = 100$ artificial data and a set of $p = 15$ variables. The independent variables are sampled from a standard unit normal distribution. The y are generated by a model with parameters

$$\beta = (0.01, 0.7, -0.8, 0.5, .01, .01, .01, -0.7, 0.6, 0.8, 0.01, 0.01, 0.01, 0.01, 0.01, 0.01)'$$

and $\sigma_u^2 = 2.25$. It is apparent that only the variables 1–3 and 7–9 impact y significantly. This is shown by the plot in Fig. 3.1 where the confidence intervals of the parameters $\hat{\beta}$ at the 5% significance level are displayed. Only the intervals that correspond to the variables 1–3 and 7–9 do not include zero.

A GA has been employed to search for this best subset model. The fitness function has been the F statistic. The chromosome is a binary string of length 15, for instance

$$000110000011100$$

is decoded to a regression model that includes only the variables 4, 5, 11, 12, 13 as independent variables to explain y. The GA parameters have been chosen

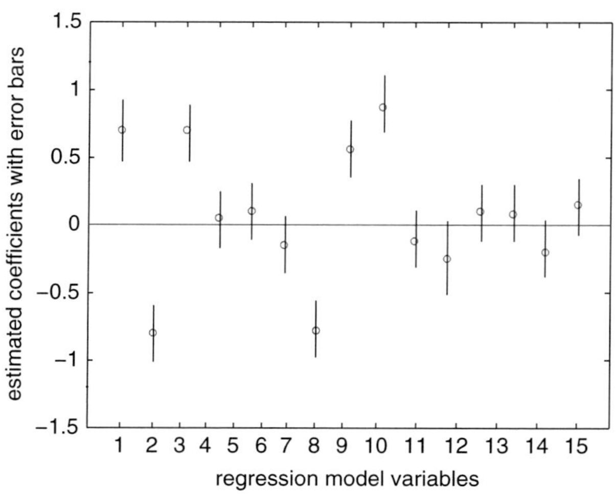

Fig. 3.1 Confidence intervals of 15 parameters in a linear regression model

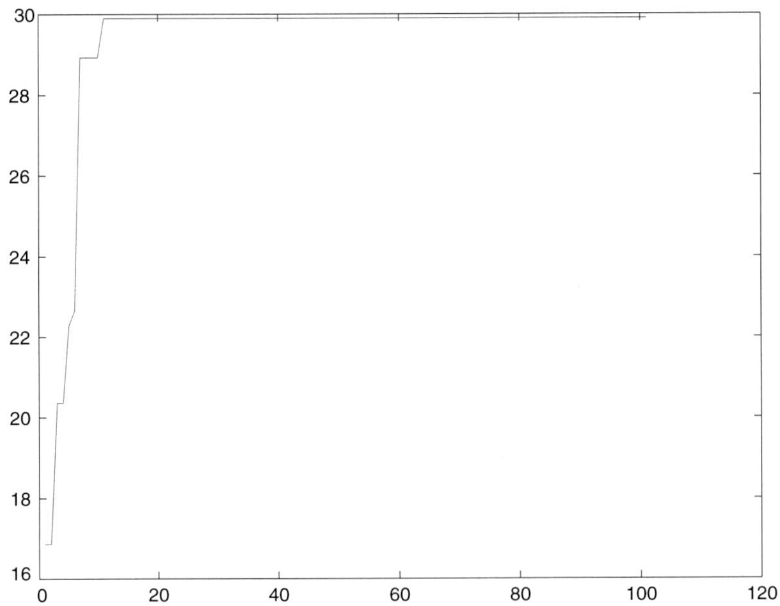

Fig. 3.2 Fitness function in the subset regression problem versus the number of iterations

NIND = 30 the number of chromosomes in the population (i.e. the population size), MAXGEN = 100 the maximum number of generations, GAP = 0.9 the generation gap (how many new chromosomes are created out of NIND), $p_c = 0.7$ and $p_m = 1/15$. Roulette wheel rule for selection, single cutting point crossover, binary mutation and the elitist strategy are employed. The fitness function evolution is displayed in Fig. 3.2. This is the typical fitness function behavior in the presence of elitist strategy. While fitness function improves quickly in the first iterations, then no better solutions are found and the elitist strategy prevents the best obtained fitness from decreasing. The GA finds the best solution corresponding to $F = 29.8941$ and variables $1-3$ and $7-9$ ($R^2 = 0.6945$ and RMSE $= 1.423$).

The use of genetic algorithms for variable selection in regression was first suggested by Chatterjee et al. (1996) who also noted that GA might also be used for symbolic regression models, where, together with the variables, the mathematical form of the regression function may be selected in a set of allowable functions. Further contributions are by Minerva and Paterlini (2002) and by Balcombe (2005), who discusses extension to the study of bivariate Granger causality and to detection of seasonal unit roots. Recently Kapetanios (2007) has considered employing simulated annealing and genetic algorithms for variable selection in regression. He compared, in an econometric framework, the evolutionary computation algorithms with a method based on sequential selection, and a different technique related to Bayesian model averaging, obtaining very promising results.

An interesting contribution in this field is the omitted variable search by Sessions and Stevans (2006). They assume that an indicator (0/1) variable is omitted in a regression equation, and search in the space of all possible indicator variables defined on the observations, by means of a GA, in order to maximize the coefficient of determination R^2. This choice is motivated by some real world instances, but their simulations suggest that the method may also be useful for more general situations. The same formal addition of a binary indicator variable may also be interpreted as an outlier indicator, and employed for outlier detection in regression. Tolvi (2004) suggested to perform simultaneously both variable selection and outlier identification, on considering binary chromosomes with length $p + 1 + n$, where the first $p + 1$ bits indicate selection of the regressors (including intercept) and the last n digits indicate presence or absence of outlying observations.

3.2.2 *Generalized Linear Models*

When the linear model is inadequate, the wider class of generalized models may be considered (see, e.g., McCullagh and Nelder, 1989). They are characterized by two features:

1. What is explained as a linear function of the regressors is not the mean of the observation $\mathbb{E}(y)$ but a transformation $g[\mathbb{E}(y)]$, where the *link* function $g(\cdot)$ is invertible;
2. The probability distribution of the data belongs to the exponential family.

In this framework, genetic algorithm applications have been proposed for the identification of loglinear models and for mixed models in the analysis of variance.

Loglinear models are used for describing statistical dependence in a set of categorical variables, and are applied to contingency tables. If M categorical variables are observed, and the number $n_{i_1,i_2,\ldots,i_M}$ denotes the frequency of simultaneous occurrence of modality i_1 of the first categorical variable, modality i_2 of the second character, ..., modality i_M of the Mth character, then $\log n_{i_1,i_2,\ldots,i_M}$ is described as an additive analysis of variance model with main effects of the single variables, and interactions of order $2, 3, \ldots, M$. It is usual to restrict the model to dependence only among some variables, the most popular restricted models are called *hierarchical*: they describe independence in subset of characters in an effective way, and the maximum likelihood estimates are relatively easy to compute.

The selection of the independent and dependent variables subsets in a hierarchical loglinear model is not a simple task, Roverato and Poli (1998) proposed to employ a genetic algorithm. They consider loglinear graphical models (Lauritzen, 1996), exploiting the property that there is a one-to-one correspondence between them and the (undirected) graphs with M vertices. Thus, each chromosome is associated with an M-points graph, and codifies, through $\binom{M}{2}$ binary digits, the presence or absence of each of the possible edges.

The cross-over operator is rather specialized, and is based on exchanging the entire set of edges related to a randomly chosen subset of vertices, while the fitness is based on the Akaike's AIC criterion, and depends essentially on the model log-likelihood minus the number of edges (equal to the sum of the gene values). In a simulation study, the genetic algorithm provided better results than a stepwise procedure.

A further application of genetic algorithms to this framework was proposed by Bremer and Langevin (1993). They consider a 3-way mixed analysis of variance model with the first factor fixed and the others random. Here the effect of factors is described by a representation of the variance and covariance structure in terms of main effects and interactions. The chromosome is based on integer coding and describes which subsets of possible parameters are constrained to zero. This setting requires specialized cross-over and mutation operators, while the fitness is based on the Akaike's criterion.

3.2.3 Principal Component Analysis

A few papers consider the possible use of genetic algorithms in principal component analysis or other methods aimed at summarizing large multivariate data sets into few variables. To give an idea of the possible applications we review here a recent paper by Sabatier and Reynés (2008).

Sabatier and Reynés (2008) consider principal component analysis where the loading coefficients are restricted to assume only integer values. This feature is intended to help interpretation of the meaning of principal components. Instead of using as a criterion only the variance of the extracted components, they also consider the number of distinct integers in the loading coefficients vector, to be minimized. On the other hand, they do not impose strict uncorrelation of successive components, but only penalize correlation. The final criterion is a mixture of the three, and is used for the fitness:

$$\text{fitness} = F_{\text{variance}} + F_{\text{distinct}} + F_{\text{correl}} \; .$$

Each of the F terms is restricted to assume values between 0 and 1. F_{variance} is a linear transform of the extracted component variance, assuming value 1 for the (best) unrestricted first principal component solution, while $F_{\text{distinct}} = (M - d)/(M - 1)$, where d is the number of distinct loadings values, and M the number of variables. Finally, for the ith extracted component, the sum of the absolute correlation coefficients with the already extracted components, $r^* = |r_1| + |r_2| + \cdots + |r_{i-1}|$ is computed, and $F_{\text{correl}} = (i - 1 - r^*)/(i - 1)$.

The genes encode directly the integer loading coefficients, cross-over is standard and mutation takes place by adding or subtracting, at random with equal probability, a one to the gene. Rank selection and elitist strategy are adopted. Sabatier and Reynés experienced some applications, and conclude that genetic algorithms show a good accuracy in solving these problems. They also proposed a similar method for building a linear discriminant function with integer coefficients.

Several contributions concerning the application of genetic algorithms to multivariate analysis are also found in the chemometrics literature, e.g., Kemsley (1998, 2001) on canonical variate analysis, and Guo et al. (2002) on selection of subsets of variables via Procrustes analysis.

3.3 Parameter Estimation

Many models, even moderately complex, lead to a likelihood function which turns out to be very complicated, non differentiable or with a difficult domain, and in such cases evolutionary computation may be useful for determining the optimum value, and hence the maximum likelihood estimators of parameters. For instance, Vitrano and Baragona (2004) proposed a genetic algorithm for estimating the parameters of a class of exponential power function distributions. In order to evaluate the variability of the estimators obtained from genetic algorithms, and since the classical results based on the Fisher's information matrix will be difficult to apply, Chatterjee et al. (1996) proposed to evaluate the parameters estimators variance by means of bootstrap.

Another case where evolutionary computation may be useful is when the model is fitted by means of residuals-based criteria but different from least squares, that may require optimizing a non convex and non differentiable function.

3.3.1 Regression Models

In the classical linear regression models the parameter estimates are usually derived by least squares, but several different criteria have been proposed. In robustness, robust estimators are obtained by considering functions of the residuals different from the square. The simplest instance is the LAD (least absolute deviation) estimation where we minimize the sum of the absolute values of residuals. This makes the objective function non differentiable.

A still more complicated problem, that has been addressed by genetic algorithms, arises when the observed data are censored, as it often happens, for example, in lifetime studies. In a censored experiment each observation is registered exactly only if it does not exceed a given (and known) maximum, otherwise it assumes a value equal to that maximum. Thus, if the independent variable is y, we do not observe y_i values, but $\min\{y_i, T_i\}$. On assuming a linear regression for y: $y_i = x_i'\beta + u_i$, the fitted data may be written $\min\{x_i'\beta, T_i\}$ and the least absolute deviation function to be minimized with respect to β is:

$$\sum_i |\min\{y_i, T_i\} - \min\{x_i'\beta, T_i\}| .$$

Zhou and Wang (2005) studied the properties of this function and employed a genetic algorithm for finding the minimum. They use real-coded genes, mutation consists of adding, with random sign, a random quantity approaching to zero as the generations flow. The cross-over operator produces children genes that are convex linear combinations of the parents' genes, with random coefficients, in a similar way as snooker cross-over (see Sect. 2.3.5), and the fitness is simply the opposite of the function to be minimized. The generations cycle and selection are unusual: first cross-over and mutation are applied to the existing population, then the most fitted individuals, chosen from both parents and children (in a deterministic fashion) are selected to form the next generation's population.

Zhou and Wang (2005) obtained satisfying results in their simulations, where they also compared genetic algorithms with threshold accepting (see Fitzenberger and Winker, 1998) and found that GA required less computing time to get a similar performance.

3.3.2 The Logistic Regression Model

Applications of evolutionary computation to logistic regression have also been proposed. Logistic regression is a generalized linear model useful for analyzing dependence of binary data on other quantitative or categorical variables. The binary dependent variable is associated with the presence or absence of a given feature, and its probability distribution is Bernoulli, so that its mean equals the probability of finding that feature. The link function used in logistic regression is the logit function $\text{logit}(x) = \log\{x/(1-x)\}$. The regression parameters may be estimated by maximum likelihood, but the likelihood is not linear in the parameters, and the normal equations system cannot be solved directly, therefore evolutionary computation algorithms might be conveniently employed. Genetic algorithms were proposed by Chatterjee et al. (1996) and by Pasia et al. (2005), while Robles et al. (2008) addressed the same problem by means of estimation of distribution algorithm.

We illustrate their contributions through a worked example, comparing also with a more classical numerical optimization method.

Let y denote a binary dependent variable and $\{x_1, x_2, \ldots, x_p\}$ a set of independent variables. The logistic regression (Hosmer and Lemeshow, 1989) assumes a non linear relationship between y, called in this context the response variable, and the covariates $x_1, x_2, \ldots, x_p$. Let Y denote a binary random variable and assume that $y = (y_1, \ldots, y_n)'$ is a sample from Y. Let π be the probability $P(Y = 1|x_1, \ldots, x_p) = E(Y|x_1, \ldots, x_p)$. The logistic regression model is defined by using the logit transform

$$\text{logit}(\pi) = \log\frac{\pi}{1-\pi} = \beta_0 + \beta_1 x_1 + \beta_2 x_2 + \cdots + \beta_p x_p,$$

where $\beta_0, \beta_1, \ldots, \beta_p$ are the parameters that have to be estimated from the observed data y and $x_j = (x_{j1}, x_{j2}, \ldots, x_{jn})'$, $j = 1, \ldots, p$. It may be shown that the logarithm of the likelihood function may be written

$$L = \sum_{i=1}^{n} y_i(\beta_0 + \beta_1 x_{1i} + \cdots + \beta_p x_{pi}) - \sum_{i=1}^{n} \log\{1 + \exp(\beta_0 + \beta_1 x_{1i} + \cdots + \beta_p x_{pi})\}.$$

The vector estimate $\hat{\beta}$ has to be found that maximizes L. Equating the gradient of L to zero yields a system of non linear equation that has not an analytical solution. Usually iterative methods are employed either to solve this set of non linear equations or to directly deal with the maximization of L.

As an example, we fitted a logistic regression model to a real data set, namely the coronary heart disease (CHD) data from Hosmer and Lemeshow (1989). We used several algorithms to estimate the two parameters β_0 and β_1 of the logistic regression model

$$\text{logit}(\pi_i) = \beta_0 + \beta_1 x_i, \qquad i = 1, 2, \ldots, 100,$$

where $y_i = 1$ if insurgence of coronary heart disease in the ith patient has been recorded and $y_i = 0$ otherwise and x_i is the ith patient's age (years). The iterative re-weighted least squares (IRLS), the GAs and EDAs algorithms implemented for maximizing the logarithm of the likelihood

$$L = \sum_{i=1}^{n} y_i(\beta_0 + \beta_1 x_i) - \sum_{i=1}^{n} \log\{1 + \exp(\beta_0 + \beta_1 x_i)\}$$

are outlined as follows. Upper and lower bounds for the two parameters have been chosen $(-10, 10)$ for β_0 and $(-2, 2)$ for β_1. The input matrix is defined $X = [1, x]$ where 1 denotes a column vector of ones.

- *IRLS*. This iterative algorithm implements the Newton method applied to the problem of maximizing the likelihood of a response variable y given X. Let a preliminary guess of the model parameter $\hat{\beta}^{(0)}$ be available. Then the following steps describe the move from $\hat{\beta}^{(k)}$ to $\hat{\beta}^{(k+1)}$ at iteration k.

1. Set, for $i = 1, \ldots, n$,

$$\pi_i^{(k)} = \frac{\exp\left(\hat{\beta}_0^{(k)} + \hat{\beta}_1^{(k)} x_{1i} + \cdots + \hat{\beta}_p^{(k)} x_{pi}\right)}{1 + \exp\left(\hat{\beta}_0^{(k)} + \hat{\beta}_1^{(k)} x_{1i} + \cdots + \hat{\beta}_p^{(k)} x_{pi}\right)}.$$

2. Define the weights matrix $W^{(k)} = \text{diag}(w_1^{(k)}, \ldots, w_n^{(k)})$ where $w_i^{(k)} = \pi_i^{(k)}(1 - \pi_i^{(k)})$.
3. Compute $z^{(k)} = X\hat{\beta}^{(k)} + \left(W^{(k)}\right)^{-1}(y - \pi^{(k)})$.
4. Solve with respect to $\hat{\beta}^{(k+1)}$ the weighted linear regression problem

$$\left(X'W^{(k)}X\right)\hat{\beta}^{(k+1)} = X'W^{(k)}z^{(k)}$$

5. Replace $\hat{\beta}^{(k)}$ with $\hat{\beta}^{(k+1)}$ and repeat from step 1 until some termination condition is met.

- *GA-1* (binary encoding). The potential solutions to the maximization problem have been encoded as two binary strings of length 20 each. Let c denote a non negative integer coded as a binary number by using the Gray code. Then a real parameter x is encoded as a binary string of length ℓ as follows

$$x = a + c(b - a)/(2^{\ell} - 1). \tag{3.1}$$

As c ranges from 0, the null string, to $2^{\ell} - 1$, the all ones string, the formula may encode any real number in an interval (a, b) placed at equi-spaced intervals each of which has length

$$(b - a)/(2^{\ell} - 1).$$

Equation (3.1) has been used to obtain the value of each of the two parameters given the integer c encoded as a binary string. The population size has been taken equal to 30, the number of generations has been 300 and 30 bootstrap samples have been generated to compute the estimates as the average estimates and the standard errors. The stochastic universal sampling method has been used for selection, then the single point crossover with $p_c = 0.7$ and the binary mutation with $p_m = 1/20$ (see Sect. 2.2.4 for a definition of these evolutionary operators).
- *GA-2* (real encoding). The potential solutions to the maximization problem have been encoded as floating-point numbers. The population size has been taken equal to 30, the number of generations has been 300 and 30 bootstrap samples have been generated to compute the estimates as the average estimates and the standard errors. The stochastic universal sampling method has been used for selection, then the line recombination crossover with $p_c = 0.7$ and the floating-point mutation with $p_m = 1/20$. Line recombination is a special crossover operator that may be applied to real variables only. According to a real encoding, a pair of chromosomes c_1 and c_2 chosen at random are real vectors that we may assume for the sake of simplicity to have the same dimension. Then a new chromosome c_3 is generated by the rule $c_3 = c_1 + \alpha(c_2 - c_1)$ where α is a uniform real random number in a given interval (α_1, α_2). The interval bounds have to be chosen by the user and in principle no constraints are imposed on such choice. For instance negative values and values greater than one are both allowed. So line recombination may produce a new chromosome that is not constrained in the segment between c_1 and c_2. Likewise a real chromosome c_1 may use a special mutation operator called floating-point mutation. The entry $c_1^{(i)}$, i.e. the gene at locus i of a chromosome c_1, becomes $c_2^{(i)} = c_1^{(i)} \pm 2\delta c_1^{(i)}$ if $c_1^{(i)} \neq 0$ or $c_2^{(i)} = \pm 2\delta$ if $c_1^{(i)} = 0$. δ is a real number generated from a uniform distribution in the interval

(0, 1) and the + or − sign may occur with equal probability. More details on genetic operators designed for use in the presence of real encoding may be found in Mühlenbein and Schlierkamp-Voosen (1993).

- *GA-3* (Chatterjee et al., 1996). Equation (3.1) has been used to obtain the value of each of the two parameters given the integers c_0, c_1 encoded as binary strings. The chromosome is the binary string $c = [c_0, c_1]$. The population size has been taken rather large, 1000 chromosomes, and the number of generations has been chosen equal to 30. Tournament selection with $p_s = 0.7$, single point crossover with $p_c = 0.65$, and binary mutation with $p_m = 0.1$ have been used. An additional operation, the inversion (Mitchell, 1996), has been applied with probability $p_i = 0.75$ to each chromosome in each generation. Inversion consists in choosing two points ℓ_1 and ℓ_2 at random in the chromosome and taking the bits from ℓ_1 to ℓ_2 in reverse order. The standard errors of the parameter estimates are computed by applying the GA on 250 bootstrap samples of the data.
- *GA-4* (Pasia et al., 2005). The potential solutions to the maximization problem have been encoded as two pairs of numbers, a real number $r \in (0, 1)$ the first one and an integer in a given interval (N_a, N_b) the second one. The parameter estimates are obtained as $\hat{\beta}_0 = r_0 N_0$ and $\hat{\beta}_1 = r_1 N_1$. Binary encoding which uses the Gray code has been employed. The population size has been taken equal to 100, the number of generations has been 100 and 30 bootstrap samples have been generated to compute standard errors of the parameter estimates. The binary tournament has been used as selection process. Then special crossover (modified uniform crossover) and mutation are suggested. For crossover, the chromosomes are paired at random and the integer parts exchange. If the integer parts are equal, then the exchange takes place as regards the real part of the chromosome. Only the offspring with better fit is placed in the new generation. Mutation applies, with probability $p_m = 0.1$, only to the real parts of each chromosome. This part, r say, is multiplied by a random number between 0.8 and 1.2, namely r is multiplied by $0.8 + 0.4u$, where u is an uniform random number in (0, 1). If mutation yields a number greater than 1 the first component is set to 1.
- *EDA* (Robles et al., 2008). The potential solutions to the maximization problem are represented by s vectors of 2 real numbers, the parameters β_0 and β_1. The initial population is generated at random. Then the s chromosomes are evaluated according to the likelihood function and the better s^* are retained. Other than using the likelihood, also the *AUC* (Bradley, 1997) criterion is suggested as an alternative fitness function. This is recommended when the logistic regression model is used as a classifier and the *AUC* is the area under the receiver operating characteristic (ROC) curve, a graphical device to describe the predictive behavior of a classifier. The s^* best vectors found are used to estimate a bivariate probability density function. From this latter distribution s new chromosomes are generated and a new iteration starts. We adopted a bivariate normal distribution so that only the mean vector and the variance-covariance matrix are needed to estimate the distribution in each iteration. We assumed $s = 50$ and $s^* = 30$, 300 generations and 30 bootstrap samples.

Table 3.1 Parameter estimates for logistic regression fitted to the CHD data by using IRLS, 4 GAs and an EDA-based algorithms

	IRLS	GA-1	GA-2	GA-3	GA-4	EDA
$\hat{\beta}_0$	−5.3195	−5.1771	−6.0010	−5.4360	−5.0915	−5.4985
	(1.1337)	(1.3775)	(1.6355)	(1.2580)	(1.0066)	(1.5062)
$\hat{\beta}_1$	0.1109	0.1070	0.1248	0.1130	0.1056	0.1147
	(0.0241)	(0.0290)	(0.0331)	(0.0270)	(0.0208)	(0.0301)
L	−53.6774	−53.1873	−53.8577	−53.6886	−53.2021	−53.6907

The results are reported in Table 3.1 for the 6 algorithms. Estimates $\hat{\beta}_0$ and $\hat{\beta}_1$ are displayed with standard errors enclosed in parentheses. As a measure of adaptation the logarithm of the likelihood ℓ computed on the average estimates is reported.

According to the figures displayed in Table 3.1 the best algorithm is GA-1 as it shows the largest log-likelihood. The second best is the algorithm GA-4. This latter allows the smallest standard errors of the estimates to be attained. This result may be surprising because the encoding method splits each parameter in two parts so that an increase of the variability of the estimates would be expected. Moreover, the fitness function is not linked to the parameters as directly as the other algorithms as there is an intermediate step, i.e. the multiplication of the two parts of each parameter, that separates the chromosomes decoding from the fitness function evaluation. In spite of these considerations algorithm GA-4 takes advantage from the flexibility due to the separate treatment of the order of magnitude (the integers N_0, N_1) and the accurate definition of the decimal digits (the real numbers r_0, r_1). The other algorithms lead to slightly smaller values of the log-likelihood and yield results similar to the algorithms GA-1 and GA-4. The standard errors of the estimates $\hat{\beta}_0$ and $\hat{\beta}_1$ obtained by algorithms IRLS, GA-1 and GA-3 are slightly larger than those recorded for the algorithm GA-4. As an overall result it seems that binary encoding performs better than the real one for evolutionary computing algorithms. For instance, we tried to use in the algorithm GA-4 a real encoding by defining a chromosome as an array of real numbers and obtained rather poor results.

3.4 Independent Component Analysis

Let $\{y_1(t), \ldots, y_m(t)\}$ be an observed data set that we may assume originated by the linear combination of a set of unobservable variables $\{s_1(t), \ldots, s_h(t)\}$ that we may call sources. The link between the data and the sources is as follows

$$y_i(t) = a_{i1}s_1(t) + a_{i2}s_2(t) + \ldots + a_{ih}s_h(t), \quad i = 1, \ldots, m, \tag{3.2}$$

for $i = 1, \ldots, m$ and $t = 1, \ldots, n$. If we define the arrays

$$A = \begin{pmatrix} a_{11} & a_{12} & \cdots & a_{1h} \\ a_{21} & a_{22} & \cdots & a_{2h} \\ \vdots & \vdots & \ddots & \vdots \\ a_{m1} & a_{m2} & \cdots & a_{mh} \end{pmatrix},$$

$$y(t) = (y_1(t), \ldots, y_m(t))',$$

and

$$s(t) = (s_1(t), \ldots, s_h(t))'$$

then (3.2) may be written in compact form

$$y(t) = As(t) + \varepsilon(t), \quad t = 1, \ldots, n, \tag{3.3}$$

where the noise term $\varepsilon(t) = (\varepsilon_1(t), \ldots, \varepsilon_m(t))'$ may be possibly added. The assumption $h = m$, i.e. A is a square matrix, though not strictly needed is often introduced as simpler methods for solving (3.3) are available in this case. The independent component analysis (ICA) is concerned with (3.3) under the following hypotheses.

- The unobservable variables $\{s_j(t)\}$ are statistically independent.
- The variables $y(t)$, $s(t)$ (and possibly $\varepsilon(t)$) have nongaussian distributions not necessarily known.

Given a set of observations $\{y(t)\}$ these assumptions allow effective methods for estimating the sources $\{s(t)\}$ and the mixing matrix A to be developed up to a permutation of the rows of (3.3), the sign and a multiplicative constant. Without loss of generality it is assumed further that $\mathbb{E}\{s_j(t)\} = 0$ and $\mathbb{E}\{y_i(t)\} = 0$. Moreover the assumption $\mathbb{E}\{y_i(t)^2\} = 1$ is often held true to fix the order of magnitude of the solutions.

The ICA methods and problems are accounted for by Hyvärinen et al. (2001). Useful common applications are for instance the optimal visualization of high dimensional data, dimensionality reduction, filtering, detection of interesting features, e.g. structural changes and outliers. The ICA has been applied successfully in several fields such as biomedicine, speech recognition, signals processing and time series. For instance the blind source separation (BSS) problem is often tackled by ICA methods. However, the BSS does not necessarily imply the validity of the assumptions of the ICA. The ICA may be regarded as a variant of the projection pursuit (Huber, 1985; Friedman, 1987). Convenient projections are investigated for optimal data visualization, density estimation, regression models estimation, to name but a few applications. Unlike the ICA, however, the projection pursuit methods are not necessarily based on special model assumptions or on the statistical independence hypothesis, while the objective functions of most ICA algorithms may be considered in a sense as indexes for projection pursuit. The differences between the two approaches may be outlined for instance by comparing the methods suggested by Galeano et al. (2006) and by Baragona and Battaglia (2007) as far as the outlier identification problem in time series is concerned.

3.4.1 ICA algorithms

Statistical independence and nongaussianity are the basic principles that support the development of most ICA algorithms. Let f denote a probability density function. The independence between the sources s_i and s_j may be defined by the equality $f(s_i, s_j) = f(s_i)f(s_j)$. This latter equality implies in turn that

$$\mathbb{E}\{h_i(s_i)h_j(s_j)\} = \mathbb{E}\{h_i(s_i)\}\mathbb{E}\{h_j(s_j)\} \tag{3.4}$$

where h_i and h_j are some suitable nonlinear functions. As a special case, if h_i and h_j are the identity functions, (3.4) defines s_i and s_j as uncorrelated variables. In general (3.4) defines nonlinear decorrelation. Though it is only a necessary condition for independence, often the nonlinear decorrelation is assumed as the objective function for ICA algorithms and produces satisfactory solutions to the ICA problem.

The maximum nongaussianity is the other basic principle that allows effective algorithms to be developed. In practice independent components cannot be computed exactly and we may seek for approximated independence only. As sums of nongaussian variables are closer to gaussian than the original ones, according to the central limit theorem, the ICA problem may be formulated as the problem of finding the local maxima of nongaussianity of a linear combination $z_j(t) = \sum_i w_{ij} y_i(t)$ provided that the variance of $z_j(t)$ is constant. Clearly $z_j(t)$ will be maximally nongaussian if it equals a source s_{j_i} possibly with opposite sign. The coefficients w_{ij}'s will estimate some entries of some de-mixing matrix B which is supposed to approximate the inverse of the mixing matrix A up to a permutation matrix. Two examples of nongaussianity measures are the negentropy (Hyvarinen and Oja, 2000) and the mutual information (Bell and Sejnowski, 1995).

3.4.1.1 Negentropy

The nongaussianity measure negentropy is defined

$$J(z) = H_\varphi - H(z), \tag{3.5}$$

where the function $H(\cdot)$ is the entropy

$$H(z) = -\int f(z)\log f(z)\mathrm{d}z. \tag{3.6}$$

f denotes the probability density function of z and H_φ is the entropy of a gaussian variable. As the entropy of a gaussian variable is larger than the entropy of any variable with the same variance, the index defined by (3.5) is always greater than or equal to zero. Moreover, z is as more different from a gaussian variable as smaller its entropy, so that the index $J(z)$ may be thought of as an objective function to be maximized.

3.4.1.2 Mutual Information

This nongaussianity measure is defined as

$$I(z_1, \ldots, z_h) = \sum_{i=1}^{h} H(z_i) - H(z), \tag{3.7}$$

where the function $H(\cdot)$ is the entropy (3.6). The index I as defined in (3.7) is always greater than zero and it equals zero if and only if the variables z_i's are statistically independent. An algorithm that uses (3.7) as objective function has to minimize it.

Relationships between negentropy and mutual information are discussed in Hyvärinen et al. (2001, chapter 10).

The stochastic gradient descent algorithm (Bell and Sejnowski, 1995) minimizes an objective function which includes the general nonlinear relationship

$$J(w) = \mathbb{E}(g(w, y)), \tag{3.8}$$

where the dependence of the source estimate z from the unknown coefficients w is made explicit and g is some suitable nonlinear function. Given an initial value $w(0)$ the basic step of the algorithm is the move from iteration $t-1$ to iteration t which may be summarized by the following updating formula

$$w(t) = w(t-1) - \alpha(t)\frac{\partial}{\partial w}\mathbb{E}\left\{g(w, y(t))\right\}_{w=w(t-1)},$$

where $\alpha(t)$ controls the step size. Usually a pre-processing step is performed before the application of the optimization algorithm. This amounts in most cases to operate the following transforms on the data.

- Centering the variables, i.e. the $\{y(t)\}$ are replaced by $\tilde{y}(t) = y(t) - \mathbb{E}\{y(t)\}$ so that $\mathbb{E}\{\tilde{y}(t)\} = 0$.
- Whitening, that is the $\{y(t)\}$ are replaced by $\tilde{y}(t) = D^{-\frac{1}{2}}E'y(t)$, where $\mathbb{E}\{y(t)y(t)'\} = EDE'$, so that $\mathbb{E}\{\tilde{y}(t)\tilde{y}(t)'\} = I$, the identity matrix.
- Band-pass filtering, i.e. a linear filter is applied to $\{y(t)\}$ to yield $\tilde{y}(t)$ which has spectral density concentrated in the frequency band of interest.

3.4.2 Simple GAs for ICA

Numerical algorithms such as the stochastic gradient learning rule are widely used for estimation of the independent sources. However these algorithms may produce sub-optimal solutions. This circumstance motivates the introduction of genetic algorithms to seek for improved solutions.

A GAs-based procedure could be outlined as follows. Let us find the sources $\{z(t)\}$ and the de-mixing matrix B such that

$$z(t) = By(t) \tag{3.9}$$

where $\{y(t)\}$ is defined as in (3.2) and let $(w_1, w_2, \ldots, w_h)$ denotes the generic row of B such that $\sum_{i=1}^{h} w_i^2 = 1$. As a first step an appropriate encoding and a suitable fitness function have to be defined. As for encoding, it is well known that $h - 1$ angles suffice to completely and uniquely determine a point on the unit h-dimensional sphere. Let $0 \leq \phi \leq 2\pi$ and $0 \leq \theta_j \leq \pi$, $j = 1, \ldots, h-2$. Then

$$\begin{aligned} w_1 &= \sin(\theta_1)\sin(\theta_2)\ldots\sin(\theta_{h-2})\sin(\phi) \\ w_2 &= \sin(\theta_1)\sin(\theta_2)\ldots\sin(\theta_{h-2})\cos(\phi) \\ w_3 &= \sin(\theta_1)\sin(\theta_2)\ldots\cos(\theta_{h-2}) \\ w_4 &= \sin(\theta_1)\sin(\theta_2)\ldots\cos(\theta_{h-3}) \\ &\ldots \\ w_h &= \cos(\theta_1) \end{aligned} \tag{3.10}$$

are the unit norm coefficients needed to transform the observed data $\{y(t)\}$ into the independent component $z(t) = w'y(t)$, where $w = (w_1, \ldots, w_h)'$. Every feasible solutions that the GA may take into account may be coded as a sequence $\{\theta_1, \theta_2, \ldots, \theta_{h-2}, \phi\}$. A set of sequences of this type forms the population to be evolved through the pre-specified number of generations to reach the optimal solution. For instance we may consider optimality according to the simple nongaussianity criterion of kurtosis maximization. The fitness function in this case may be assumed

$$J(\theta_1, \theta_2, \ldots, \theta_{h-2}, \phi) = \frac{\mu_4}{\text{var}(z_t)^2} - 3,$$

where $\mu_4 = \mathbb{E}\{z_t - \mathbb{E}(z(t))\}^4$. The actual chromosomes are binary vectors of length ℓ obtained by standard binary coding of $\{\theta_1, \theta_2, \ldots, \theta_{h-2}, \phi\}$.

As an alternative we may seek for a linear transform that produces a data set with diagonal cross-cumulant matrices. Cardoso and Souloumiac (1993) suggested the joint diagonalization of the cumulant matrices and Ziehe and Müller (1998) proposed the simultaneous diagonalization of several time-delayed correlation matrices. For illustration purpose we may define as objective function the sum of the absolute value of the off-diagonal entries of the matrix of some cross cumulants of order higher than 2 of the transformed data (3.9). A GAs-based algorithm may be used to minimize an objective function of this type defined on the set of feasible de-mixing matrices B.

A matrix B may be encoded as a chromosome

$$\theta_1^{(1)}, \ldots, \theta_{h-2}^{(1)}, \phi^{(1)} | \theta_1^{(2)}, \ldots, \theta_{h-2}^{(2)}, \phi^{(2)} | \ldots | \theta_1^{(m)}, \ldots, \theta_{h-2}^{(m)}, \phi^{(m)}, \tag{3.11}$$

and decoding may be performed according to (3.10). The first $h-1$ genes give the first row $(w_1^{(1)}, \ldots, w_h^{(1)})$ of the matrix B, the second sequence of $h-1$ genes gives the second row $(w_1^{(2)}, \ldots, w_h^{(2)})$ of B, then each sub-sequence of the chromosome between a pair of vertical bars is scanned and decoded until the last row of B is decoded as $(w_1^{(m)}, \ldots, w_h^{(m)})$. Let s denote the population size. Then we may generate at random s chromosomes with structure (3.11) to initialize the GA algorithm and the initial population evolves through a pre-specified number of generations N by using the genetic operators selection, crossover and mutation. The exact definition of the genetic operators depends on the choice between the representation of the genes of the chromosome (3.11) as binary sequences or floating-point numbers. The population at each iteration includes the set of s matrices $\{B^{(1)}, B^{(2)}, \ldots, B^{(s)}\}$ and for each one the fitness function may be computed as the sum of absolute values of some of the off-diagonal cross-moments matrices. The choice of number and orders of such matrices may be left to the user or may be performed by using an auxiliary GA as suggested by Sun et al. (2006).

As an example, let us consider a set of 5 time series of length 100 generated by the following autoregressive recursive equations

$$s_i(t) = \phi^{(i)} s_i(t-1) + a_i(t), \quad i = 1, \ldots, 5, \quad t = 1, \ldots, 100, \tag{3.12}$$

where $(\phi^{(1)}, \ldots, \phi^{(5)}) = (0.5, -0.7, 0.2, 0.7, -0.5)$, and $\{a_i(t)\}$ is a sequence of independent identically distributed random variables with nongaussian probability density function f. This latter has been chosen from the class of the exponential power function distributions as a special generalization of the gaussian distribution

$$f(a) = \left\{ \frac{\beta}{2\alpha\Gamma(1/\beta)} \right\} \exp\left\{ -\frac{|a-\mu|^\beta}{\alpha^\beta} \right\},$$

where $\Gamma(\cdot)$ denotes the gamma function, and μ, α ($\alpha > 0$) and β ($\beta > 0$) are the location, scale and shape parameters respectively. We assumed $\mu = 0$ and $\alpha = \sqrt{2}$, and we set $\beta = 4$ so as to obtain a platykurtic distribution as a result. Methods for generating random numbers from $f(a)$ may be found in Chiodi (1986). The time series data provided by (3.12) have been standardized and decorrelated to yield the sources that have been mixed by using the matrix

$$A = \begin{pmatrix} 1 & 0 & 0 & 0 & 1 \\ 0 & 1 & 0 & 0 & 1 \\ 0 & 0 & 1 & 0 & 1 \\ 0 & 0 & 0 & 1 & 1 \\ 1 & -1 & 0 & 0 & 1 \end{pmatrix}$$

to produce the transformed time series data

$$y(t) = As(t)$$

that are assumed as the observed signals. A GA has been used to find the de-mixing matrix B such that the transformed time series data

$$z(t) = By(t)$$

approximate the set of sources $\{s(t)\}$ as closer as possible. Let $\{\tilde{y}(t)\}$ denote the uncorrelated zero mean and unit variance time series set obtained as $\tilde{y}(t) = Qy(t)$, where the matrix Q is computed as described at the end of Sect. 3.4.1. Let $\tilde{z}(t) = B\tilde{y}(t)$ and $z(t) = (z_1(t), \ldots, z_5(t))'$. Then the objective function has been chosen

$$J(B) = \sum_{i=1}^{4} \sum_{j=i+1}^{5} \left| \sum_{t=1}^{100} \tilde{z}_i(t)^2 \tilde{z}_j(t)^2/100 - 1 \right|.$$

As a matter of fact, if $z_i(t)$ and $z_j(t)$ have to be independent then the necessary condition (3.4) holds in particular if the h_i's are chosen the square functions. Note that the matrix B does not need to be orthonormal but the sum of the squared entries in each of its rows is equal to 1, and $y_i(t)$ has unit variance, so that $\sum_{t=1}^{100} \tilde{z}_i(t)^2/100 = 1$ for all i. In spite of its simplicity the objective function $J(B)$ has been found effective for driving the search towards a valuable approximation of the true de-mixing matrix $B = A^{-1}$. In the GAs context the fitness function has to be maximized so that its exact definition has been taken as $f = 1/J$. For encoding the entries of each proposal solution matrix B we assumed 20 bits to represent each real parameter so that the length of each chromosome is $\ell = 20 \times h(h-1)$. Then the usual selection, crossover and mutation have been employed as in the simple GA.

As a final step the sources $z(t)$ estimated by using the matrix B provided by the GA have been further transformed by whitening. The estimated sources have been assumed $\hat{s}(t) = Rz(t)$ where the matrix R has been computed as described at the end of Sect. 3.4.1. The estimated de-mixing matrix has been calculated by taking into account all transforms that have been applied to the data, i.e. $\hat{B} = RBQ$. However, the sources could be recovered exactly only if the permutation matrix and signs would be known. For our simulated data we selected the rows permutation and signs by comparing $\hat{s}(t)$ to $s(t)$ and $\hat{B}$ to A^{-1}. This is not possible when dealing with real data.

We obtained $\hat{B}$ and $\hat{s}(t)$ from the simulated data $y(t)$ by using the GA and by using the stochastic gradient descent algorithm. For comparison the original sources and the sources estimated by the GA are reported in Fig. 3.3. Likewise, the original sources and the sources estimated by the stochastic gradient descent algorithm are reported in Fig. 3.4. In both cases the original sources are recovered rather accurately, the de-mixing procedures seem to yield poor results only for the second and third time series as far as the GA is concerned and for the third and fourth for the stochastic gradient descent algorithm. The inverse of the mixing matrix A and the estimated de-mixing matrices are reported below.

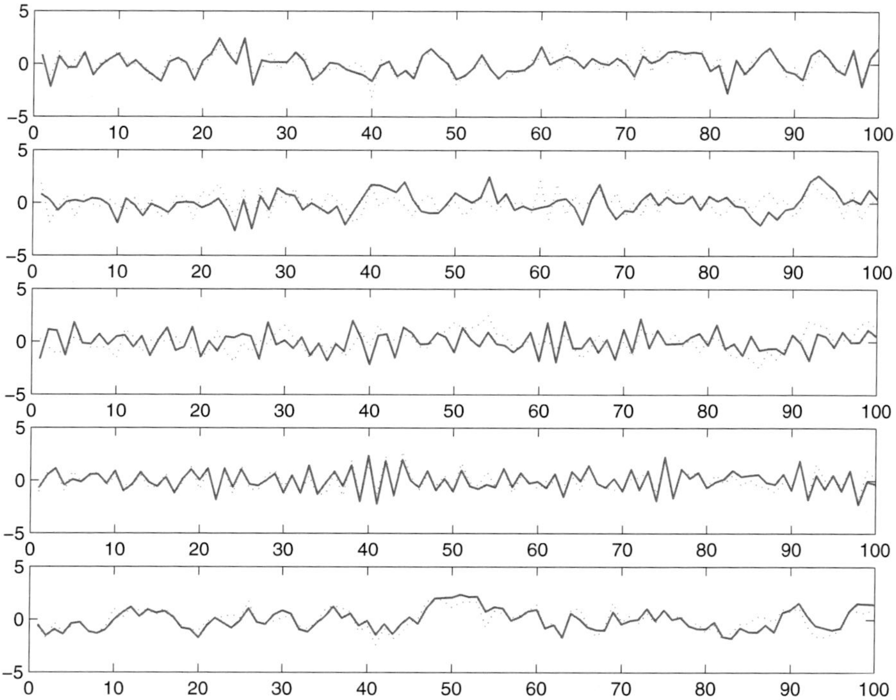

Fig. 3.3 Simulated nongaussian independent sources, original (*solid line*) and GA estimates (*dotted line*)

$$A^{-1} = \begin{pmatrix} 2 & -1 & 0 & 0 & -1 \\ 1 & 0 & 0 & 0 & -1 \\ 1 & -1 & 1 & 0 & -1 \\ 1 & -1 & 0 & 1 & -1 \\ -1 & 1 & 0 & 0 & 1 \end{pmatrix}$$

$$B_{\text{GA}} = \begin{pmatrix} 1.9 & -1.3 & 0.5 & -0.2 & -1.0 \\ 0.1 & 0.6 & 0.3 & -0.4 & -0.1 \\ 0.9 & 0.0 & 0.7 & -0.2 & 0.4 \\ 1.6 & -1.2 & 0.4 & 0.8 & -1.5 \\ -1.1 & 0.7 & -0.1 & 0.1 & 1.2 \end{pmatrix}$$

$$B_{\text{gradient}} = \begin{pmatrix} 1.6 & -0.8 & 0.3 & -0.3 & -0.7 \\ 2.0 & -1.0 & 0.1 & 0.5 & -1.8 \\ -0.3 & 0.2 & 0.7 & -0.5 & -0.1 \\ -0.2 & -0.1 & 0.4 & 0.5 & 0.1 \\ -1.1 & 1.5 & -0.5 & -0.4 & 1.1 \end{pmatrix}$$

The three matrices are similar with the exception of few entries that are considerably different from the corresponding entries of the matrix A^{-1}.

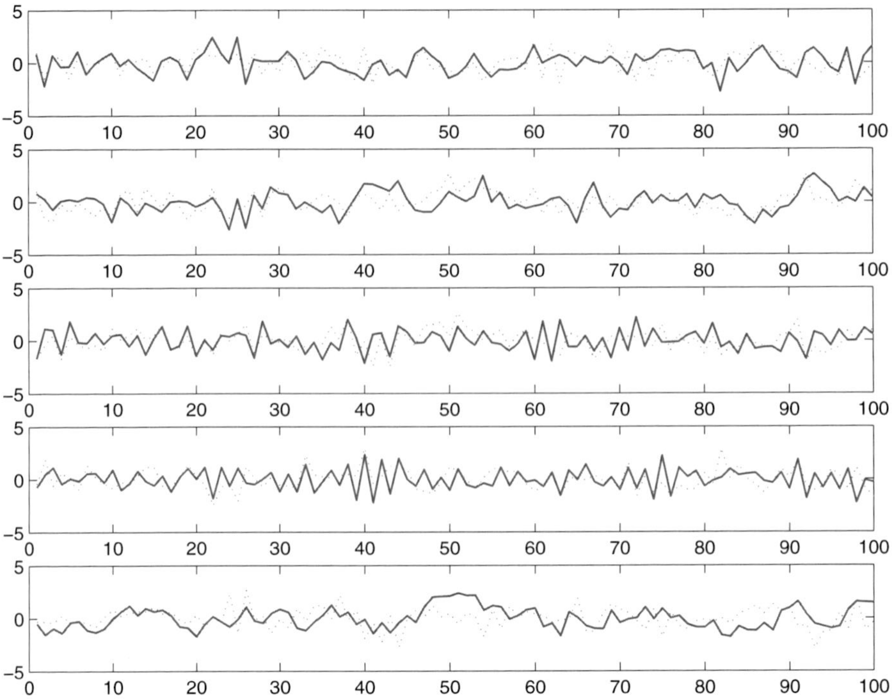

Fig. 3.4 Simulated nongaussian independent sources, original (*solid line*) and stochastic gradient descent algorithm estimates (*dotted line*)

The fitness function recorded in each of 1000 iterations of the GA is displayed in Fig. 3.5. The reciprocal of the final fitness function values is equal to 0.8329, i.e. the average entry of the lower half matrix of the fourth order cumulants that we considered in the definition of the fitness function is equal to 0.0833 which is a figure rather small (the fourth moment has been computed about 2.5 for each of the five estimated sources). The fitness function increases rather gradually unlike in most application cases. The steady improvement of the fitness function does not seem likely to be ascribed to mutation, as the rate of mutation $p_m = 0.0025$ is rather small. So we have to suggest that crossover is the most useful operator in this case though the rate of crossover $p_c = 0.7$ is not specially large. The crossover exchanges between a pair of proposal de-mixing matrices some of the weights that control the contribution of each observed time series data to the estimated sources and this device seems effective to improve the solution.

Table 3.2 displays the correlations between each of the five original sources and the corresponding ones estimated by the GA and by the stochastic gradient descent algorithm. The accuracy of the estimates may be appreciated for each single time series. For a synthetic comparison the average correlations may be computed equal to 0.7904 for the latter and 0.7298 for the second algorithm with a slightly better

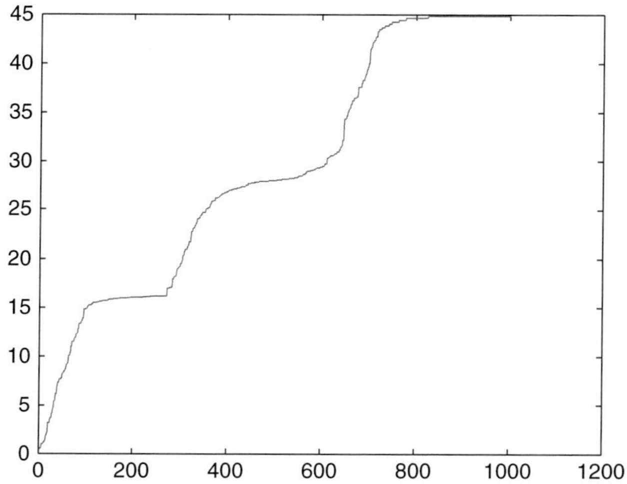

Fig. 3.5 Fitness function behavior against the number of iterations for the problem of finding the optimal de-mixing matrix in the ICA problem

performance of the GA. In this case the two approaches seem to produce comparable results, an extensive simulation study would be needed to address the issue properly.

Table 3.2 Correlations between original and estimated sources using a genetic algorithm and the stochastic gradient descent algorithm

	series 1	series 2	series 3	series 4	series 5
GA	0.8173	0.7087	0.7261	0.8487	0.8513
gradient	0.8980	0.8149	0.7347	0.5138	0.6874

3.4.3 GAs for Nonlinear ICA

In Sect. 3.4.1 the general case has been considered of a set of observed data $\{y(t)\}$ produced by the unknown nonlinear mixture of independent sources $\{s(t)\}$. Tan and Wang (2001) proposed a method that utilizes a GA to minimize an objective function as specified by (3.8) where it is assumed that g is a highly nonlinear and nonconvex cost function. Two special cost functions based on higher order statistics are introduced to evaluate the degree of the statistical independence of the outputs of the de-mixing system, i.e. the estimates of the unknown independent sources. The appropriate objective function should rely on the probability criterion of independence of random variables. Difficulties in estimating the probability density functions of unknown random variables may be overcome by resorting to higher order statistical moments. Then a first cost function may be built by considering all joint cross-moments of the outputs constrained to zero. This corresponds to fulfill a necessary condition for the independence of the outputs. A second cost function takes into account the mixed moments of any order weighted by a suitable window function. Parameter estimates, i.e. the estimates of the coefficients of the de-mixing matrix, are computed by a GA. Binary encoding, roulette wheel selection, multi-point crossover and binary mutation are found effective for achieving the proper recovery of the unknown sources and mixing nonlinear operators. These genetic operators characterize the simple GA excepted that the multi-point crossover (Spears and De Jong, 1991) is used instead of the one point crossover. The multi-point crossover generalizes the one point crossover allowing several cutting points to be chosen so that several fragments of the chromosomes in a pair may exchange instead of limiting the exchange only to the last genes of the chromosomes. The elitist strategy is recommended to improve the rate of convergence.

The two cost functions are used to implement two different GAs. A simulation experiment demonstrates that both GAs-based algorithms are able to provide accurate and robust results regardless of the initial values and with a rate of convergence superior to gradient-based approaches.

To improve further the performance of the GAs-based algorithms Gorriz et al. (2005) suggested a guided GA which includes statistical information inherent to the problem in the evolution process. In practice the GA is hybridized with gradient-based techniques to refine the solutions and improve the rate of convergence at the same time. Further improvements may be obtained by using an ICA algorithm in conjunction with the GAs, where the GAs aim at finding the optimal nonlinear function g in (3.8) and the ICA algorithm accomplishes the task of finding the optimal de-mixing matrix to be applied to the data transformed by the nonlinear function g. The usual GA operators, selection, crossover and mutation are modified accordingly. An example is discussed of an application to real data where the suggested GAs-based methods display encouraging results.

Chapter 4
Time Series Linear and Nonlinear Models

Abstract Modeling time series includes the three steps of identification, parameter estimation and diagnostic checking. As far as linear models are concerned model building has been extensively studied and well established both theory and practice allow the user to proceed along reliable guidelines. Ergodicity, stationarity and Gaussianity properties are generally assumed to ensure that the structure of a stochastic process may be estimated safely enough from an observed time series. We will limit in this chapter to discrete parameter stochastic processes, that is a collection of random variables indexed by integers that are given the meaning of time. Such stochastic process may be called time series though we shall denote a finite single realization of it as a time series as well. Real time series data are often found that do not conform to our hypotheses. Then we have to model non stationary and non Gaussian time series that require special assumptions and procedures to ensure that identification and estimation may be performed, and special statistics for diagnostic checking. Several devices are available that allow such time series to be handled and remain within the domain of linear models. However there are features that prevent us from building linear models able to explain and predict the behavior of a time series correctly. Examples are asymmetric limit cycles, jump phenomena and dependence between amplitude and frequency that cannot be modeled accurately by linear models. Nonlinear models may account for time series irregular behavior by allowing the parameters of the model to vary with time. This characteristic feature means by itself that the stochastic process is not stationary and cannot be reduced to stationarity by any appropriate transform. As a consequence, the observed time series data have to be used to fit a model with varying parameters. These latter may influence either the mean or the variance of the time series and according to their specification different classes of nonlinear models may be characterized. Linear models are defined by a single structure while nonlinear models may be specified by a multiplicity of different structures. So classes of nonlinear models have been introduced each of which may be applied successfully to real time series data sets that are commonly observed in well delimited application fields. Contributions of evolutionary computing techniques will be reviewed in this chapter for linear models, as regards identification stage and subset models, and to a rather larger extent for some classes of nonlinear models, concerned with identification and

R. Baragona et al., *Evolutionary Statistical Procedures*, Statistics and Computing,
DOI 10.1007/978-3-642-16218-3_4,

parameter estimation. Beginning with the popular autoregressive moving-average linear models, we shall outline the relevant applications of evolutionary computing to the domains of threshold models, including piecewise linear, exponential and autoregressive conditional heteroscedastic structures, bilinear models and artificial neural networks.

4.1 Models of Time Series

Let $\{y_t, \text{integer}\, t\}$ denote a time series, that is a stochastic process indexed by a discrete parameter which assumes the meaning of time. If no confusion is likely to arise, according to the context, a finite realization will be denoted without further specification by the array $y = (y_1, \ldots, y_n)'$, where n is the number of observations. Let $\{e_t, \text{integer}\, t\}$ denote a strictly white noise process, that is a sequence of independent random variables. Under stationarity assumption the white noise process has mean zero and variance σ^2 equal for all the e_t's. Following Priestley (1988), a model of the time series is a relationship between its elements, which produces a zero mean strictly white noise process:

$$h\,(\ldots, y_{t-2}, y_{t-1}, y_t, y_{t+1}, y_{t+2}, \ldots) = e_t\,.$$

If $\{e_t\}$ is a strictly white noise then all the dependence between values at different time points of y is explained by the function h. However, for physical reasons we shall assume that the series depends only on *past* values, and write the model in non-anticipative form:

$$h\,(y_t, y_{t-1}, y_{t-2}, \ldots) = e_t\,. \tag{4.1}$$

We shall assume the parametric approach, that is we want $h(\cdot)$ to depend on a finite set of parameters so that knowledge of parameter values yields a full account of $h(\cdot)$. In general the function $h(\cdot)$ is unknown and so are the parameter values. Moreover, the time series full joint distribution is not available and we may rest only upon the finite observed realization y. Then the model building procedure consists essentially in iteratively performing the three steps of identifying a model, estimating the parameters, checking the validity of (4.1). The procedure ends if (4.1) is fulfilled at least with adequate approximation, else the procedure starts anew with another iteration. Model identification is performed in general by choosing a mathematical specification of the function $h(\cdot|\theta)$, where θ is the parameter vector, according to some appropriate statistics. In an evolutionary computing framework we start with a set of tentative functions $\{h_1(\cdot|\theta), \ldots, h_s(\cdot|\theta)\}$ and evolve such a population towards closest approximation of (4.1). The parameter vector θ may either be included in the evolutionary searching procedure or be estimated whenever possible by special optimization algorithms. In this latter case we denote the evolutionary algorithm as a hybrid algorithm which combines the evolutionary computing devices with gradient-based optimization techniques, combinatorial optimization procedures and heuristic or meta-heuristic algorithms. The Gaussianity assumption on the white noise process allows us to use the maximum likelihood approach for parameter estimation. At this step we have to assume that the function $h(\cdot|\theta)$ is fully specified but for the vector parameter θ. The joint probability distribution of $e = (e_1, \ldots, e_n)'$ allows us to write the likelihood function that we have to maximize depending on the vector parameter value θ. Let $f(e)$ denote the density of e. We may use (4.1) and write the likelihood function L as follows

$$L(\theta|h, y) = f\{h(y|\theta)\}, \tag{4.2}$$

where the form of the function h is assumed known and y is the observed time series. This way the likelihood is a function of θ. The vector parameter θ may include either parameters that take values in a continuous space or parameters that are defined in some discrete set. Only in the former case gradient-based methods may be possibly used while such methods do not apply in the latter case as we cannot even define partial derivatives. Let $\theta = ({\theta_1}', {\theta_2}')'$ where θ_1 are continuous variables and θ_2 are discrete variable. According to (4.2) given $h(\cdot)$ and the observed data y the likelihood function may be written as a function of the parameter θ and the optimization problem consists in finding the estimate $\hat{\theta}$ defined as

$$\hat{\theta} = \arg\max_{\theta} \{L(\theta|h, y)\}. \tag{4.3}$$

If θ may be distinguished in the two arrays θ_1 and θ_2 then an iterative procedure is convenient that alternates the two step of maximizing (4.2) with respect to θ_1 given θ_2 and with respect to θ_2 given θ_1. For instance an evolutionary computing algorithm may be given the task of finding θ_2 and a steepest ascent algorithm the task of finding θ_1. Such a procedure defines a hybrid algorithm as well. Further more than two algorithms may be employed each of which may be devoted to solve the problem (4.3) with respect on a subset of the parameter set and conditional on the remaining parameters. For example (4.3) may be linear as far as some of the parameters are concerned so that maximization conditional on the other parameters is straightforward.

Such a procedure is very general but it may be very complicated too and hardly feasible in practice. Priestley (1988, chapter 5) suggests a specification for the function h which is both flexible enough to cover a wide range of functional forms and tractable in the context of the statistical analysis. Indeed model (4.1) is fairly intractable as an infinite dimensional model whilst the function h may be given a finite dimensional form by letting h to depend on the finite set $\{y_{t-1}, \ldots y_{t-p}, e_{t-1}, \ldots e_{t-q}\}$ for integers $p \geq 0$ and $q \geq 0$, so that we may write:

$$y_t = h\left(y_{t-1}, y_{t-2}, \ldots y_{t-p}, e_{t-1}, e_{t-2} \ldots e_{t-q}\right) + e_t.$$

By assuming further that a first order Taylor expansion for h exists, then the state dependent model (SDM) for the time series $\{y_t\}$ takes the form

$$y_t = \mu(z_{t-1}) + \sum_{j=1}^{p} \phi_j(z_{t-1}) y_{t-j} + e_t - \sum_{j=1}^{q} \psi_j(z_{t-1}) e_{t-j}, \tag{4.4}$$

where the array

$$z_{t-1} = (e_{t-q}, \ldots, e_{t-1}, y_{t-p}, \ldots, y_{t-1})$$

is called the state vector at the time $t-1$. Formally $h(z_{t-1})$ may be interpreted as the projection of y_t on the σ-algebra generated by $e_{t-1}, e_{t-2}, \ldots$ and is therefore the conditional expectation of y_t given the whole past, while e_t plays the role of innovations of the process. A large lot of models may be defined from (4.4) including the linear autoregressive moving-average models and many popular nonlinear models.

- *ARIMA models.* If μ, the ϕ_j's and the ψ_j's are independent of z_{t-1} then they are constant parameters and we obtain an ARIMA model. This is equivalent to assume that the model function $h(\cdot)$ is linear. Some additional assumptions have to hold, see, e.g., Box et al. (1994).
- *AR threshold models.* Assume that $\psi_j = 0$ for all j and that the state vector z_{t-1} reduces to the single variable y_{t-1}. Let $\mu(z_{t-1}) = a_0^{(i)}$ and $\phi_j(z_{t-1}) = a_j^{(i)}$ if $y_{t-1} \in R_i$ for $j = 1, \ldots, p$ and $i = 1, \ldots, k$. The R_i's defined as $R_i = (r_{i-1}, r_i]$ are k interval that partition the interval $(r_0, r_k]$ on the real axis This is the (self-exciting) autoregressive threshold (SETAR) model.
- *Piecewise linear models.* If we allow the parameters $a_j^{(i)}$ to vary linearly with y_{t-1} then we have the piecewise linear autoregressive threshold (PLTAR) model.
- *Exponential autoregressive models.* Assume that $\mu = 0$ and $\psi_j = 0$ for all j. If $\phi_j(z_{t-1}) = a_j + b_j \exp\left(-\gamma y_{t-1}^2\right)$, $j = 1, \ldots, p$, then we obtain the exponential autoregressive (EXPAR) model.
- *Bilinear models.* If μ and the ϕ_j's are constants independent of z_{t-1} and we let $\psi_j(z_{t-1}) = c_j + \sum_{i=1}^{\ell} b_{ij} y_{t-i}$, $j = 1, \ldots, q$, then model (4.4) is a bilinear (BIL) model. The parameters $\psi_j(z_{t-1})$ are linear functions of $\{y_{t-1}, \ldots, y_{t-\ell}\}$.

4.2 Autoregressive Moving Average Models

Models of the ARMA and ARIMA class are most popular in time series analysis essentially for two reasons: first, they are a natural generalization of regression models, and may be easily interpreted using similar concepts as in regression analysis; and, second, they may be seen as universal approximation for a wide class of well behaved stationary stochastic processes.

Let $\{x_t\}$ denote a second-order stationary purely non-deterministic process, i.e., with spectral measure $F(\lambda)$ everywhere differentiable with derivative $f(\lambda)$ strictly greater than zero for any λ. Assume also that the first and the second moments are finite and let $E(x_t) = \mu$. Then, the Wold's decomposition theorem states that the following equality holds in quadratic mean:

$$x_t = \mu + \sum_{j=0}^{\infty} h_j u_{t-j} \, . \tag{4.5}$$

That is, there exists a strictly white noise process $\{u_t\}$, with $E(u_t) = 0$ and $E(u_t^2) = \sigma^2$, and a sequence of constants $\{h_j\}$ with $h_0 = 1, \sum h_j^2 < \infty$, such that the squared difference between the left hand side and the right hand side of (4.5) has mean zero.

The Wold decomposition (4.5) is a very interesting and convenient result for theoretical analysis of stochastic processes, but as a model for representation it has the main drawback that it depends on an infinite number of parameters. By employing the so called "backward operator" B, such that $Bx_t = x_{t-1}$ and $B^k x_t = x_{t-k}$, (4.5) may be rewritten

$$x_t = H(B)u_t \quad ; \quad H(B) = \sum_{j=0}^{\infty} h_j B^j \, .$$

An operational model may be obtained by deriving an approximation to (4.5) based on a finite parameterization. The most obvious choice is truncating the infinite sum to a finite number of terms (which produces the moving average model): it amounts to substituting the power series $H(B)$ by its partial sums. A more efficient approximation, in terms of number of required parameters, consists in replacing the power series $H(B)$ by a ratio of two finite degree polynomials:

$$H(B) \simeq \Theta(B)/\Phi(B)$$

where

$$\Theta(B) = 1 - \theta_1 B - \cdots - \theta_q B^q \; ; \Phi(B) = 1 - \phi_1 B - \cdots - \phi_p B^p \, .$$

The resulting approximation of the Wold decomposition (4.5) gives the ARMA model:

$$x_t - \phi_1 x_{t-1} - \phi_2 x_{t-2} - \cdots - \phi_p x_{t-p} = c + u_t - \theta_1 u_{t-1} - \theta_2 u_{t-2} - \cdots - \theta_q u_{t-q} \tag{4.6}$$

where $c = \mu(1 - \phi_1 - \cdots - \phi_p)$. Equation (4.6) is called an ARMA(p, q) model and p and q are known as the autoregressive and the moving average *orders* of the model.

As it is probably already apparent, there is a general agreement in the literature concerning the crucial requirement of *parsimony*, the ability of obtaining a good approximation by employing the smallest possible number of parameters. The reason is that each parameter is an unknown to be estimated from the data, therefore any additional parameter may be the source of additional bias and sample variability. Moreover, all parameters are estimated basing on the same data, therefore their estimates might be correlated, and the bias could spread through the parameters.

Parsimony is universally accepted as precept among time series analysts, so that the ARMA model building problem may be seen as choosing the model with the smallest number of parameters given an approximation level. An additional way of reducing the number of parameters is considering incomplete models, where some of the parameters $\phi_1, \ldots, \phi_p, \theta_1, \ldots, \theta_q$ are constrained to zero. Such models are usually referred to as *subset ARMA* models.

The canonical model building procedure runs iteratively through the following three steps:

1. *Identification.* Selection of the orders p and q, and, if a subset model is considered, choice of which parameters are allowed to be non-zero. Such step is based on a function, called identification *criterion*, which assigns a loss to each possible choice of the orders and the parameters subset. Several different criteria have been proposed, some of them will be considered in what follows.
2. *Parameter estimation.* Conditional on identification, the estimation of parameters may be performed through classical statistical inference. In particular, a gaussianity assumption allows to derive maximum likelihood estimates. Essentially, it may be shown that, given the parameters (and some initial values), the data vector $\{x_t\}$ and the innovations vector $\{u_t\}$ given by

$$u_t = x_t - \phi_1 x_{t-1} - \cdots - \phi_p x_{t-p} + \theta_1 u_{t-1} + \cdots + \theta_q u_{t-q} = u_t(\phi, \theta)$$

are in a one to one correspondence; furthermore, the Jacobian of the transformation is equal to one. Therefore the likelihood of the data equals the likelihood of the innovations which, owing to normality and independence, depends essentially on the sum of squares of the innovations:

$$S(\phi, \theta) = \sum_t u_t^2(\phi, \theta) .$$

Thus, the maximum likelihood estimates of the parameters $(\hat{\phi}, \hat{\theta})$ are defined by:

$$(\hat{\phi}, \hat{\theta}) = \arg \min_{(\phi, \theta)} S(\phi, \theta)$$

a least squares problem. If the moving average order is $q = 0$, the least squares problem may be solved by equating derivatives to zero and solving the related linear system, while if there is a non zero moving average part the minimization problem is non linear, but efficient numerical optimization methods are available.
3. *Diagnostic checking.* Once the model is completely specified and estimated, it is customary to check whether it fits the data sufficiently well. This is generally accomplished by computing the residuals, which may be interpreted as estimators of the innovations: if the model fits good, the residuals should inherit the most relevant properties of the innovation process: zero mean, constant variance and, more important, whiteness. For this reason, the most widely used diagnostic

checking tools take into account the residuals and test the null hypothesis of whiteness on them. This may be performed both in the time domain (with test statistics based on the sum of squared autocorrelations for some initial lags) and in the frequency domain (checking the constancy of the estimated spectral density over frequency). If the model is not accepted as a satisfying representation of the data, the identification stage should be repeated, taking into account which kind of non whiteness has been found in the residuals.

4.2.1 Identification of ARMA Models by Genetic Algorithms

The most difficult step of the model building procedure is identification. The space of possible solutions is discrete and usually very large, and there is not, in general, any better way of comparing two of them than computing the identification criterion values. For such reasons, the ARMA model identification has been considered as a particularly suitable problem for meta-heuristic methods, and a few proposals employing genetic algorithms are found in literature. All papers are concerned with subset models, some of them also consider more complicated models such as multiplicative seasonal or multivariate models, and are addressed in the next Section. These papers always introduce hybrid algorithms, where the estimation is obtained through the least squares approach (maximum likelihood in the gaussian case). Though in principle the choice of the parameter values could be obtained by a purely genetic search, there is an unanimous agreement that the numerical optimization techniques developed for the classical model building procedure (as sketched previously) are more time-saving and computationally efficient. Some authors (see Gaetan 2000; Ong et al. 2005) use a simplified procedure rather than minimizing $S(\phi, \theta)$ numerically on the entire space of admissible (ϕ, θ) values. Such procedure is due to Hannan and Rissanen (Hannan and Rissanen, 1982) and consists in obtaining a first estimate of the residuals by fitting a high-order autoregression to the data. Then, conditional on the residual of that autoregression, the ARMA model (4.6) becomes linear in the parameters $\phi_1, \ldots, \phi_p, \theta_1, \ldots, \theta_q$, which may be directly estimated with least squares by simply solving the (linear) normal equations.

We turn now to consider the encoding methods proposed in the literature for ARMA identification. Each solution must represent a particular model structure, specifying the autoregressive order p, the moving average order q, and a set of lags (integer between 1 and p or q) that identify the non zero parameters of the autoregressive and the moving average part. Two different codings have been proposed, in either case a maximum search order has to be selected, both for the autoregressive part (P say) and for the moving average part (Q). The simplest coding amounts to reserving one gene to each possible lag, filling it with 1 if the parameter is free, and with 0 if the parameter is constrained to zero. For example, if we take $P = Q = 6$, the following subset model:

$$x_t = \phi_1 x_{t-1} + \phi_4 x_{t-4} + \phi_5 x_{t-5} + u_t - \theta_2 u_{t-2} - \theta_4 u_{t-4} - \theta_6 u_{t-6}$$

is coded by means of the following chromosome

$$\begin{array}{cc} 1\,0\,0\,1\,1\,0 & 0\,1\,0\,1\,0\,1 \\ \text{(AR lags)} & \text{(MA lags)} \end{array}$$

This coding system was adopted by most authors, and has the advantage of simplicity and fixed-length chromosomes, but it is not particularly efficient.

An alternative coding based on variable-length chromosomes, was proposed by Minerva and Poli (2001a). The chromosomes consist of two different gene subsets: the first one is devoted to encode the autoregressive and moving average orders, by specifying the number of relevant predictors, i.e., the number of non-zero parameters, respectively for the autoregressive part, p^*, and for the moving average part, q^*. This part consists of eight binary digits and encodes two integer numbers between 0 and 15 (therefore this coding allows for models that have up to 15 non-zero autoregressive parameters and 15 non-zero moving average parameters). The other genes subset is devoted to specifying the lags which the non zero parameters correspond to: it comprises $5(p^*+q^*)$ binary digits, and encodes, consecutively, p^*+q^* integer numbers between 1 and 32. Therefore, in the Minerva and Poli's implementation, $P = Q = 32$ and all models containing a maximum of 15 non zero parameters, both for the AR and the MA structures, may be coded. For example. the chromosome corresponding to the previous model is:

$$0011\ \ 0011\ \ \ 00001\,00100\,00101\,00010\,00100\,00110\ .$$

The first part of the chromosome contains 8 digits, while the second part has a variable length from zero (white noise) to 150 binary digits. Encoding with the same order limitations would require, in the fixed-length scheme introduced before, 64-digit chromosomes. It appears that the advantage of using the variable length scheme might be sensible if we are searching for relatively sparse models, because the average length depends directly on the number of non zero parameters (for example, a coding admitting no more that 4 non zero parameters in each AR or MA structure, with a maximum lag of 64, would require a fixed chromosome 128 long, and a variable length chromosome with 6–54 binary digits).

In any case, the structure of the genetic algorithm depends on the choice of a maximum possible order: it may be based on a-priori considerations, or even on the number of available observations. A more data-dependent choice of the maximum admissible lag could also be based on an order selection criterion computed only on complete models (with all parameters free) as proposed in Bozdogan Bearse (2003): in this case a relatively "generous" criterion like AIC seems advisable to avoid a too hard limitation of the solution space.

Since all proposed codings are binary, each proposal corresponds to usually slight modifications of the canonical genetic algorithm. The selection procedure is obtained by means of the roulette wheel methods, except for Bozdogan Bearse (2003) who adopt rank selection. The mutation operator is employed in its standard form, while for the cross-over operator some authors propose a random one cut point (Gaetan, 2000), others a random two point cross-over (Ong et al., 2005) or a uniform cross-over (Bozdogan Bearse , 2003). All authors use generation gaps equal to one, and slightly different elitist strategies: saving the best chromosome, or the two best chromosomes, or even the 10 % best chromosomes in the population. When dealing with the alternative coding based on subsets of genes that encode the AR and MA order, Minerva and Poli (2001a) suggest that the cross-over operator should be modified in order to apply on entire fields (representing the integer numbers denoting order or lag) rather to the single binary digits. Mutation and cross-over probabilities are generally in accordance with the literature on canonical genetic algorithms, proposed values are between 0.01 and 0.1 for mutation, and from 0.6 to 0.9 for cross-over. Not many suggestions are offered concerning the population size, and the chromosomes composing the initial generation (they are generally selected at random in the solution space). It may be reasonably assumed that a good starting point, with satisfying mixing properties, would require initial individuals which may exploit the fitting ability of each single possible parameter. Therefore, advantageous chromosomes in the initial population are those encoding models with just one non zero parameter (i.e., in the first coding scheme, chromosomes with only one gene equal to one). The minimum population size that allows to fully develop this idea is obviously equal to the total number of possible parameters, or $P + Q$.

Much more relevant differences are found in the literature on ARMA models building by means of genetic algorithms, as far as the fitness function is concerned. Essentially, the fitness function is linked to some version of identification criterion or penalized likelihood. A favorite choice is adopting one of the most popular identification criteria in time series, such as the AIC or the BIC (also called Schwarz) criteria:

$$\mathrm{AIC}(M) = N \log\{\hat{\sigma}^2_{(M)}\} + 2p(M)$$
$$\mathrm{BIC}(M) = N \log\{\hat{\sigma}^2_{(M)}\} + p(M) \log N$$

where N is the series length, $\hat{\sigma}^2_{(M)}$ is the residual variance estimate for model M, and $p(M)$ is the number of free parameters of model M. Alternatively, Bozdogan (1988) suggests the identification criterion called ICOMP. Rather than simply considering the number of non zero parameters, ICOMP measures the model complexity through a generalization of the entropic covariance complexity index of Van Emden (1971). The criterion ICOMP is computed by estimating the Fisher's information matrix for the parameters and by adding to the likelihood- proportional term, $N \log \hat{\sigma}^2$, the quantity $C(\hat{F}^{-1})$:

$$\mathrm{ICOMP}(M) = N \log \hat{\sigma}^2_{(M)} + C(\hat{F}^{-1})$$

where

$$C(X) = \dim(X) \log\{\mathrm{trace}(X)/\dim(X)\} - \log|X|\,.$$

A further different approach is linked to the theory of stochastic complexity (Rissanen, 1987, 2007) and is called *minimum description length* criterion. A model is seen as a possible explanation of the data behavior, so that, given the model, the complete description of the observed values requires less information than enumerating them individually. Therefore, given an alphabet and a data set, each possible model is associated to a code length MDL(M), which may be seen as the sum of two parts: the first one is the code required for describing the model (and is roughly a function of the free parameters of model M), and the second one is the length required for describing the residuals, which is shown to be equivalent to $N \log\{\hat{\sigma}^2_{(M)}\}$. Therefore the minimum description length criterion, though derived in a different framework, has a similar form to the preceding ones:

$$\text{MDL}(M) = N \log\{\hat{\sigma}^2_{(M)}\} + q(M)$$

with the correction term $q(M)$ computed as the code length of the model.

Finally, Minerva and Poli (2001a) use an AIC-like criterion where the residual variance is replaced by a prediction error variance:

$$s^2(\ell) \propto \sum_t [x_{t+\ell} - \hat{x}_t(\ell)]^2$$

where $\hat{x}_t(\ell)$ is the predictor based on the model. Obviously, for the forecast horizon $\ell = 1$ there is no difference with AIC, Minerva and Poli (2001a) try their criterion also for $\ell = 2$ and 3.

A common problem to all these implementations is that the proposed criteria are to be minimized, thus they cannot be employed directly as fitness function (which has, on the contrary, to be maximized). Two kinds solution have been proposed: Bozdogan Bearse (2003) avoid the problem of defining a fitness proportionate selection by adopting an ordered fitness selection rule: chromosomes are ordered according to the decreasing values of the ICOMP criterion, and each chromosome is selected with a probability proportional to its rank. An alternative is defining the fitness function by a monotonically decreasing transformation of the identification criterion. Most natural candidates are a simple linear transformation:

$$\text{fitness}(M) = W - \text{criterion}(M)$$

which is possible if an estimate of the worst possible value of the criterion, W, is available (Gaetan (2000) suggests to compute W on the current population), or a negative exponential transformation:

$$\text{fitness}(M) = \exp\{-\text{criterion}(M)/d\}$$

where d is a scaling constant. A Boltzman selection procedure is proposed by Gaetan (2000) using the last expression for the fitness, but with a progressively decreasing "temperature" $d_k = (0.95)^k$, where k is the generation number.

The simulation studies presented in literature suggest satisfying results of each implementation, with slight substantial differences, indicating that for univariate time series with most encountered series lengths, the genetic algorithm yields good models after just a few generations, and converges nearly always, though after many more generations, to the true simulated model.

4.2.2 More General Models

Generalizations of ARMA models in several directions have been proposed, and they are widely applied in several fields. Most of them may be identified by means of genetic algorithms with minor modifications to the procedures outlined in the previous Section.

Integrated (ARIMA) models are suitable for series with trends in mean, and are very popular in econometrics. The essential difference to an ARMA model is that the autoregressive polynomial $\Phi(B)$ is factorized in two terms:

$$\Phi(B) = (1 - B)^d \, \Pi(B) \tag{4.7}$$

where $\Pi(B)$ has all its zeroes outside the complex unit circle, and d is a non negative integer, usually not larger than two. Identification may be obtained following the same guidelines as ARMA models, but adding a pair of binary genes to encode the integer d.

Similarly, long-memory fractionally integrated ARMA models (usually ARFIMA) are also defined by an autoregressive polynomial factorized as in (4.7), but with d a real number greater than zero and not larger than 0.5. In that case also, the chromosome should be augmented by some binary genes in order to encode the fractional order d with sufficient precision.

Generalized models which are useful for seasonal data are the multiplicative seasonal ARMA models, where each of the two polynomials $\Phi(B)$ and $\Theta(B)$ are obtained as the product of two factor polynomials, in order to distinguish and combine the seasonal dependence (linking each observations to those which are in the same seasonal position at the previous years) and the usual dependence at smaller lags. A genetic algorithm for identifying seasonal ARMA models has been proposed by Ong et al. (2005). They consider subset models in all the components (AR, seasonal AR, MA and seasonal MA); suppose that maximum values for each of the four orders (maximum lag), p, P, q, Q, say, are selected, then the chromosome is made up of $p + P + q + Q$ binary genes, that sequentially indicate which parameters are allowed to be non zero. They use classical mutation, two random cut-point crossover, fitness-proportionate selection by means of roulette wheel, and elitist strategy saving the best chromosome. Parameters are estimated via the Hannan and Rissanen procedure, and the fitness function is based on the BIC criterion (what reversing transformation is used, is not explained in the paper). The experience reported by Ong et al. (2005) on simulated and real data sets shows that the genetic algorithm leads to satisfying models in a very small number of generations.

Finally, an important generalization of ARMA models is to multivariate time series (the so-called vector VAR or VARMA models). Such multivariate models may also be identified by means of genetic algorithms, and in this case the advantage over traditional identification strategies may be even larger, because of the strongly increasing number of involved parameters, and therefore much wider solution space.

Bozdogan Bearse (2003) consider the identification of subset vector autoregressive models by means of genetic algorithms, using a fitness function based on the ICOMP criterion. If $x(t) = [x_1(t), \ldots, x_m(t)]', t = 1, \ldots, , N$ denotes a multivariate time series with m components, a VAR model of order p is defined by:

$$x(t) = c + A_1 x(t-1) + A_2 x(t-2) + \ldots + A_p x(t-p) + u_t \tag{4.8}$$

where $\{u_t\}$ is a multivariate m-component white noise, and $A_1, A_2, \ldots, A_p$ are $m \times m$ matrices of parameters, and c is a m-vector of constant intercepts. Subset models are obviously specified by fixing what entries of each matrix are allowed to be non zero. Thus, a careful attention has to be reserved to encoding. Once a maximum autoregressive order P is selected, the number of possible parameters is $Pm^2 + m$ and several alternative codings are plausible. Bozdogan Bearse (2003) propose to consider sequentially the m separate equations of the model (4.8), each equation corresponding to a sub-string of $1 + Pm$ binary genes. In each sub-string the first position specifies if the intercept is present (gene = 1) or absent (gene = 0) in the equation: the following m portions, of P binary genes each, specify what parameters linking the variable to any fixed regressor are free (gene = 1) or constrained to zero (gene = 0). In other words, the inner loop scans the lags $1, 2, \ldots, P$, while the outer loop scans the position (row, column) of the parameters in the matrices A_i.

In their genetic algorithm implementation, Bozdogan Bearse (2003) adopted a rank selection based on the ICOMP criterion, with elitist strategy, standard mutation and uniform cross-over. They also employed the resulting models for detecting influential observations.

More recently, Chiogna et al. (2008) have addressed the identification of transfer function models by genetic algorithm. A transfer function model relates an output series to several input series through linear delayed dependence, where the output series follows an ARMA model:

$$\Phi(B)y(t) = \sum_{i=1}^{k} \omega_i(B)x_i(t) + \Theta(B)e_t$$

where $\{e_t\}$ is a white noise process, $\{x_i(t)\}$ are given inputs and $\omega_i(B)$ are polynomial in the backwards operator B, with different degrees. Chiogna et al. (2008) propose a genetic algorithm for simultaneously identifying the orders of the autoregressive and moving average parts $\Phi(B)$ and $\Theta(B)$ and those of the transfer function parts $\omega_i(B)$, also in the case when multiplicative seasonal behavior is allowed.

In the framework of meta-heuristics, the identification of subset vector autoregressive models was addressed by means of different optimization methods:

Baragona (2003b) used a hybrid simulated annealing, and Winker (2001) used the threshold accepting (see also Winker and Gilli, 2004).

4.3 Nonlinear Models

In this section parameter estimation of non linear time series models will be considered. There have been proposed many time series models that aim at dealing with some specific kind of non linearity. It is virtually impossible to take each and every model into account, so we shall limit ourselves to the most popular non linear time series models in statistical methods and applications and concentrate on models for which heuristic algorithms for computing parameter estimates have been used.

4.3.1 Threshold AR and Double Threshold GARCH Models

Threshold models are suitable for series whose behavior alternates among different types (the regimes) according to a condition originated by the series itself. The most popular of these models, the self-exciting threshold autoregressive (SETAR, see. e.g. Tong, 1990) is based on the assumption that the series is generated by several alternative AR models according to the values assumed by a past observation. The sample space is split into disjoint regions delimited by assigned borders, or thresholds, and each region is associated to an AR model. Then, if the past observation is included in the ith region, the ith AR model generates the next time series value.

In this section we consider GAs-based algorithms for building threshold models. The GAs are designed to determine the appropriate number of regimes and select the threshold parameters. These tasks are recognized to be the most important and most difficult steps in threshold models building procedures. If, for instance, a SETAR model is known to have only two regimes, then there is only one threshold to select among n candidate thresholds (we assume here, as usual in the literature, that thresholds may be searched among the observed time series values). In this case a grid search allows all possible thresholds be tried and the objective function may be computed for each of the n choices. If the number of regimes is unknown, and the only available information that may be supplied is concerned with the maximum number of regimes K, the thresholds are to be searched among a large number of alternatives (approximately, this number is $O[n^{(K-1)}]$). If the double threshold autoregressive heteroscedastic (DTARCH) model is considered (Li and Li, 1996), K and H regimes may be postulated for the average returns and variance respectively. The space of solutions may include $O[n^{(K+H-2)}]$ candidate thresholds. The size is so large, even for short time series, that using GA for threshold models building seems a well motivated choice. Pittman and Murthy (2000) and Wu and Chang (2002) proposed a GA to identify and estimate two – regimes SETAR models. Recently Davis et al. (2006, 2008) employed threshold autoregressive processes for modeling structural breaks, and used a GA for identifying the model. More general approaches based on GA have been developed by Baragona et al. (2004a) for SETARMA and subset SETARMA models and Baragona and Cucina (2008) for DTARCH models. The GA has been found quite effective through both simulation experiments and applications to real time series.

Let, for k and p given, the SETAR(p) model be assumed with the state vector $z_{t-1} = y_{t-d}$ for some integer $d \in [1, p]$ which is called the delay parameter

$$y_t = \sum_{j=1}^{p} c_j^{(i)} y_{t-j} + e_t \text{ if } r_{i-1} < y_{t-d} \leq r_i, \qquad i = 1, \ldots, k. \tag{4.9}$$

We have observed already that comparing the equations (4.9) and (4.4) the functions $\phi_j(\cdot)$ are assumed constant and equal to $c_j^{(i)}$ in each of the intervals $(r_{i-1}, r_i]$. Each coefficient $\phi_j(\cdot)$ exhibits a jump in each of the extremal points of the intervals. If we allow the variance of the SETAR model (4.9) to vary, then a convenient way for modeling the innovation variance is to define the conditional variance h_t given the past observations of the time series by the autoregressive heteroscedastic (ARCH) model

$$h_t = \sum_{j=1}^{q} \alpha_j e_{t-j}^2. \tag{4.10}$$

The parameters $\alpha_1, \ldots, \alpha_q$ have to be non negative and their sum has to be less than 1. Other assumptions have to be imposed on the α_j's to ensure higher moments to exist. A threshold structure may be postulated for the ARCH model (4.10) as well. A time series generated by a DTARCH model may be written

$$\begin{aligned} y_t &= c^{(i)} + \sum_{j=1}^{p} \phi_j^{(i)} y_{t-j} + e_t \text{ if } r_{i-1} < y_{t-d} \leq r_i, \qquad i = 1, \ldots, k \\ h_t &= \sum_{j=1}^{q} \alpha_j^{(i)} e_{t-j}^2 \qquad\qquad \text{if } u_{i-1} < e_{t-c} \leq u_i, \qquad i = 1, \ldots, h \end{aligned} \tag{4.11}$$

where $\{u_0, u_1, \ldots, u_{h-1}, u_h\}$ are the ARCH threshold parameters, $u_0 = -\infty$ and $u_h = \infty$, h is the number of regimes and c is the delay parameter. More restrictive assumptions are sometimes formulated for the threshold ARCH model, namely that the regimes depend on the time series $\{y_t\}$. In this case, a change in the regime of y_t implies a contemporaneous change in the regime of h_t.

The GA that is proposed here addresses the search for the regimes and threshold parameters. In general two vectors of threshold parameters have to be determined for the DTARCH model excepted if the change in the regime in the ARCH model is assumed to depend on the change in the regime of the SETAR model (4.9). Basically the algorithm structure remains the same, but searching for thresholds in the first line of (4.11) has to proceed in parallel with the searching for thresholds in the second line. Let n observations $\{y_1, \ldots, y_n\}$ be available and let n innovations be estimated by fitting a high order AR model to the data. Choose a minimum number m of observations in each regime. Then, arrange the observed data $\{y_1, y_2, \ldots, y_n\}$ in ascending order to obtain the sequence $\{y_{(1)}, y_{(2)}, \ldots, y_{(n)}\}$. Let us consider only the subsequence $\{y_{(m+1)}, y_{(m+2)}, \ldots, y_{(n-m-1)}, y_{(n-m)}\}$. As a matter of fact, the first and last m observations in the ascending sequence may be dropped because at least m observations in each regime are required. Let $\ell = n - 2m$ and w be a binary vector of length ℓ

$$w = (w_1, w_2, \ldots, w_\ell)'$$

and define the mapping $w_i \rightarrow y_{(i+m)}$, $i = 1, \ldots, \ell$. If $w_i = 1$, then $y_{(i+m)}$ is a threshold parameter, and $w_i = 0$ otherwise. The number of regimes in the SETAR model is given by $w_1 + w_2 + \cdots + w_\ell + 1$. Another binary vector v has to be defined which is mapped into the subsequence $\{e_{(m+1)}, e_{(m+2)}, \ldots, e_{(n-m-1)}, e_{(n-m)}\}$ of the innovations arranged in ascending order. The requirement that at least m observations have to belong to each regime obviously imposes a constraint on the number of regimes. It is more convenient, however, to define explicitly a maximum number K of regimes, so that $1 \leq k \leq K$. This simplifies somewhat the GA implementation. In the GA framework, given an integer s greater than 1, a set of vectors $\{w^{(1)}, w^{(2)}, \ldots, w^{(s)}\}$ and a set of vectors $\{v^{(1)}, v^{(2)}, \ldots, v^{(s)}\}$ form the population, in general a small subset of the set of all feasible threshold parameters sequences. The GA starts with an initial population, then proceeds through a pre-specified number of iterations, I, say. In each iteration the vectors in the current population are evaluated, namely the fitness function is computed for the vectors $w^{(i)}$, $v^{(i)}$ and its value is associated to $w^{(i)}$, $v^{(i)}$. The fitness function computation involves the estimation of the DTARCH model by assuming the number of regimes and threshold parameters as encoded in $w^{(i)}$, $v^{(i)}$. We are using a hybrid GA because all parameters other than the regimes and thresholds may be estimated using another optimization algorithm. In addition, the AR order is found by trying several values p in a pre-specified range $[1, P]$ and choosing the one which minimizes the AIC criterion. Moreover, the estimation is performed for each values of the delay parameter d in the range $[1, p]$. Computations are quite demanding, so it is important that the space of solutions be explored efficiently. The GA design aims at optimize the searching procedure. Basically the simple GA is used, but some special features are introduced to exploit the peculiarity of the present problem. The population in each iteration is processed by means of the usual genetic operators selection, crossover and mutation. A description of each of the three operators follows.

Selection. The well known roulette wheel rule is used. Each vector in the current population is assigned probability of survival proportional to its fitness function. Any vector in the population may be selected, even more than once, and placed in the population that will be processed in the next iteration. It may happen, however, that a vector is not selected, that is it does not survive and it is discarded. To avoid discarding best fitted solutions, the elitist strategy is adopted to amend the pure stochastic selection. A vector that has been discarded is reinserted in the new population if its fitness function is greater than the fitness function of each of the selected vectors. In this case, this best vector replaces the vector that in the new population has the worst fitness. This way the size s of the population remains unchanged through the iterations.

Crossover. Unlike selection, that implements the roulette wheel rule and the elitist strategy as commonly defined in canonical GA, the crossover is designed oriented to the present framework. A probability of crossover p_c has to be pre – specified. Then, in the current population, $[p_c s/2]$ vector pairs are selected at random. A vector may be selected more than once to enter a pair. The selected pairs are processed one at the time, and both vectors are updated soon after each crossover. Let $w^{(1)}$ and $w^{(2)}$ denote the two vectors in the pair. All bits of the two vectors are examined, and the indexes where the first one, or the second one, or both, have bit value equal to 1 are recorded. If there are no bits equal to 1 the crossover does not take place. Otherwise, let $\{i_1, \ldots, i_\mu\}$ denote the indexes of the bits equal to 1. An index is selected at random in this set, and let us denote the selected bit index i_α. Then, two cases are to be considered: (1) Either $w_{i_\alpha}^{(1)} = 1$ or $w_{i_\alpha}^{(2)} = 1$, but not both. If, for instance, $w_{i_\alpha}^{(1)} = 0$ and $w_{i_\alpha}^{(2)} = 1$, then we set $w_{i_\alpha}^{(1)} = 1$ and $w_{i_\alpha}^{(2)} = 0$. The number of regimes encoded in the second vector decreases by one, whilst a new regime adds to the number of regimes encoded in the first vector. (2) Both $w_{i_\alpha}^{(1)} = 1$ and $w_{i_\alpha}^{(2)} = 1$. In this case, the crossover does not take place. Note that the crossover may yield only one change of regime at most in each of the two vectors, either adding one, or deleting one. The proposed implementation seems convenient to avoid excessive change in the vectors that undergo the crossover. As a matter of fact, it obeys to a general rule that the vectors yielded by the crossover do not have to differ completely from the original vectors. The usual one – point crossover, for instance, has been found often to upset the vectors' structure and yield a vector with a number of regimes that exceeded the maximum K and the other one with only one regime. As a consequence, the first vector had to be discarded, while the other was likely to yield poor fitting. This circumstance is very unlikely to appear in the present crossover setting.

Mutation. As for crossover, for mutation too a peculiar implementation is designed that fits the problem better than the usual mutation operator. A probability of mutation p_m, usually quite small, less than 0.1, has to be pre – specified. A vector in the current population undergoes mutation with probability p_m. Let mutation have to occur for the vector $w^{(i)}$. A bit of this vector is chosen at random, $w_j^{(i)}$, say, and flips, that is $w_j^{(i)}$ is replaced by $1 - w_j^{(i)}$. If $w_j^{(i)} = 0$ then, after mutation, $w_j^{(i)} = 1$ and a new regime is added. If otherwise $w_j^{(i)} = 1$ then, after mutation, $w_j^{(i)} = 0$ and an existing regime is deleted. If we adopted the usual mutation operator, any bit of any vector would be allowed to flip with probability p_m. Due to the constraint on the number of regimes, this mutation operator is likely to yield new regimes while it is unlikely to delete some regimes. As a vector with more than $K - 1$ bits equal to 1 has to be discarded, the usual mutation in most cases would be an useless operator.

4.3.2 Exponential Models

The EXPAR(p) model may explicitly be written

$$y_t = \{\phi_1 + \pi_1 \exp(-\gamma y_{t-1}^2)\} y_{t-1} + \cdots + \{\phi_p + \pi_p \exp(-\gamma y_{t-1}^2)\} y_{t-p} + e_t. \quad (4.12)$$

The series generated according to this model alternates smoothly between two regimes, since for large values of y_{t-1}^2 it behaves essentially like an AR(p) model with parameters ϕ_j, and for small y_{t-1}^2 like an AR(p) model with parameters $(\phi_j + \pi_j)$ (see Haggan and Ozaki, 1981). Unlike linear models, a change of the error variance σ_e^2 by multiplying the $\{e_t\}$ by a constant k, say, does not imply that the $\{y_t\}$ turn into $\{ky_t\}$. The order of magnitude of $\{y_t\}$ in (4.12) depends on γ too, in the sense that we may obtain the time series $\{ky_t\}$ by both multiplying σ_e^2 by k^2 and dividing γ by k^2.

The ability of the EXPAR to account for limit cycles depends whether some conditions on the parameters in (4.12) be fulfilled. If the time series is believed to exhibit limit cycles behavior, then the estimation procedure needs to be constrained in some way.

A brief description of the basic parameter estimation procedure proposed by Haggan and Ozaki (1981) for the estimation of (4.12) follows. It may be considered as a natural benchmark for competitive alternatives because it is quite straightforward and unlike to fail to yield a solution. It does not ensure, however, that the limit cycles conditions be fulfilled.

The algorithm requires that an interval (a, b), $a \geq 0$, be pre-specified for the γ values in (4.12). This interval is split in N sub-interval, so that a grid of candidate γ values is built. Let $s = (b - a)/N$ and $\gamma = a$. Then, for N times, the following steps are performed.

1. Set $\gamma = \gamma + s$
2. Estimate ϕ_j e π_j by ordinary least squares regression of y_t on y_{t-1}, $y_{t-1}\exp(-\gamma y_{t-1}^2)\}$, y_{t-2}, $y_{t-2}\exp(-\gamma y_{t-1}^2)\}, \ldots$.
3. Compute the AIC criterion and repeat step 2 for $p = 1, \ldots, P$, where P is a pre-specified integer greater than 1.

Final estimated parameters are taken that minimize the AIC.

For the existence of limit cycles, the following conditions (see Priestley 1988, p. 88) are required to hold

(1) all the roots of

$$z^p - \phi_1 z^{p-1} \ldots - \phi_p = 0$$

lie inside the unit circle

(2) some of the roots of

$$z^p - (\phi_1 + \pi_1) z^{p-1} \ldots - (\phi_p + \pi_p) = 0$$

lie outside the unit circle

(3)

$$\frac{1 - \sum_{j=1}^{p} \phi_j}{\sum_{j=1}^{p} \pi_j} > 1 \text{ or } < 0.$$

The GAs may be used as well to cope with this estimation problem. A brief account of the genetic algorithm for model (4.12) parameters estimation will be given along the guidelines provided by Chatterjee and Laudato (1997). Note that any real parameter x is represented by a binary string c according to the formula

$$x = a + c(b - a)/(2^{\ell} - 1),$$

where x is assumed to belong to the interval (a, b) and ℓ is the pre-specified length of the binary string c. So, v parameters are represented by a sequence of v binary strings of length ℓ each. The steps of the genetic algorithm may be summarized as follows.

1. A positive integer s is chosen that represents the size of the population. The initial population is randomly generated to include s candidate solutions.
2. (tournament selection) The chromosomes are paired, and, in each couple, the one which possess the larger fitness function is copied into the other with a pre-specified probability p_s.
3. (cross-over) The chromosomes which survived the previous step may exchange some of their bits by means of the crossover operator. A probability p_c is pre-specified, so that $sp_c/2$ pairs are randomly chosen. For each pair, a cutting point k, say, is randomly chosen in the interval $(1, \ell - 1)$. The bits from $k + 1$ to ℓ of the first chromosome in the couple replace the corresponding ones in the second chromosome, and vice versa.
4. (inversion) For each chromosome in the population inversion may take place with pre-specified probability p_i as follows. Two cutting points are randomly chosen in $(1, \ell)$, k_1 and k_2, say, where $k_1 \leq k_2$. The bits between the two cutting points are taken in reverse order.
5. (mutation) The last operator is mutation, and may occur with pre-specified probability p_m per bit. The bit changes from 1 to 0 or vice versa.
6. The steps from 2 to 6 are repeated, independently for each model parameter, until some pre-specified criterion is met or the maximum number of generations N is attained.

The generalized exponential model (Chen and Tsay, 1993) is a further extension of model (4.12) where the γ coefficient is allowed to take different values in each term. The order p model may be written

$$y_t = \{\phi_1 + \pi_1 \exp(-\gamma_1 y_{t-d}^2)\} y_{t-1} + \cdots + \{\phi_p + \pi_p \exp(-\gamma_p y_{t-d}^2)\} y_{t-p} + e_t. \quad (4.13)$$

In Baragona et al. (2002) it is argued that, using model (4.13), some parsimony may be gained as far as the number of parameters is concerned, and the GA procedure is extended to identify such models.

4.3.3 Piecewise Linear Models

We consider that the functions $\theta_j(\cdot)$ are all zero while the functions $\phi_j(\cdot)$ may be written

$$\phi_j(z_{t-1}) = \phi_j(y_{t-d}) = \alpha_j^{(i)} + \beta_j^{(i)} y_{t-d} \text{ if } r_{i-1} \leq y_{t-d} < r_i, \qquad i = 1, \ldots, k. \tag{4.14}$$

The disjoint intervals (r_{i-1}, r_i) partition the real axis, as we assume that $r_0 = -\infty$ and $r_k = +\infty$. The resulting non linear model is called piecewise linear autoregressive (PLTAR). This model (see Baragona et al., 2004b) is an extension of the self-exciting threshold model, where we allow each parameter in each regime to be linearly varying with y_{t-d} rather than constant; it is also assumed that each parameter, as a function of y_{t-d}, is continuous everywhere.

If the parameters $\alpha_j^{(i)}$ and $\beta_j^{(i)}$ were not constrained in the proper way, the functions $\phi_j(y_{t-d})$, in general, would not be continuous. In order that the functions $\phi_j(\cdot)$ be continuous, the $k-1$ following conditions

$$\begin{aligned}
\alpha_j^{(1)} + \beta_j^{(1)} r_1 &= \alpha_j^{(2)} + \beta_j^{(2)} r_1 \\
\alpha_j^{(2)} + \beta_j^{(2)} r_2 &= \alpha_j^{(3)} + \beta_j^{(3)} r_2 \\
&\cdots \\
\alpha_j^{(k-2)} + \beta_j^{(k-2)} r_{k-2} &= \alpha_j^{(k-1)} + \beta_j^{(k-1)} r_{k-2} \\
\alpha_j^{(k-1)} + \beta_j^{(k-1)} r_{k-1} &= \alpha_j^{(k)} + \beta_j^{(k)} r_{k-1}
\end{aligned} \tag{4.15}$$

must hold.

In the equation system (4.15), by assuming $r_1, \ldots, r_{k-1}$ known real constants, there are $2k$ unknowns and only $k-1$ equations. So, computing the solutions would require that $k+1$ unknowns be given arbitrary values. Unfortunately, such a procedure would not ensure that the equation system (4.15) admit a unique solution. This latter, also, would seem rather meaningless, even if it exists.

In order to allow the parameter $\phi_j(\cdot)$ to increase or decrease linearly to join its next value, we introduced the following specification based on spline functions

$$\phi_j(y_{t-d}) = \lambda_j + \sum_{i=1}^{k} \nu_j^{(i)} S_i(y_{t-d}) \tag{4.16}$$

where

$$S_1(u) \qquad\qquad = u$$
$$S_i(u) = \begin{cases} 0 & u \le r_{i-1} \\ u - r_{i-1} & u > r_{i-1} \end{cases}, \qquad i = 2, \ldots, k.$$

The original PLTAR model parameters are easily recovered by using the formulas

$$\alpha_j^{(i)} = \lambda_j - \sum_{s=1}^{i} \nu_j^{(s)} r_{s-1} \qquad \beta_j^{(i)} = \sum_{s=1}^{i} \nu_j^{(s)}$$

that may be easily shown to fulfill conditions (4.15). Equation (4.14) outlines the functional coefficients specification

$$y_t = \sum_{j=1}^{p} \left\{ \sum_{i=1}^{k} (\alpha_j^{(i)} + \beta_j^{(i)} y_{t-d}) \mathrm{I}_{y_{t-d} \in (r_{i-1}, r_i]} \right\} y_{t-j} + \varepsilon_t,$$

while formula (4.16) shows that the model includes a linear AR and a nonlinear scheme

$$y_t = \sum_{j=1}^{p} \lambda_j y_{t-j} + \sum_{j=1}^{p} \sum_{i=1}^{k} \nu_j^{(i)} S_i(y_{t-d}) y_{t-j} + \varepsilon_t.$$

In Baragona et al. (2004b) the following procedure is presented that implement a hybrid version of the GA. A set of positive integers has to be chosen as potential delay parameters. Let the set $\mathcal{D} = \{d_1, d_2, \ldots, d_D\}$ be available where the elements of $\mathcal{D}$ are arranged in ascending order and, in general, d_D does not exceed the maximum order of the AR coefficients. Then for each and every $d \in \mathcal{D}$ the following steps are performed.

1. Generate at random s sequences of threshold parameters (initial population).
2. Run an N-generations genetic algorithm.
3. Each and every chromosome evaluation includes automatic AR orders identification and maximum likelihood estimation of the autoregressive coefficients (hybrid algorithm).
4. Choose as final solution the parameter set that minimizes the overall AIC criterion.

Step 2 involves a GA where the chromosomes are threshold sequences. The usual operators selection (roulette wheel rule), crossover (single cutting point) and mutation are adopted.

As far as chromosome encoding and fitness function computation are concerned some details have to be added.

Chromosome encoding

In this context a chromosome encodes a set of threshold parameters, that is a sequence of real numbers arranged in ascending order for convenience. We could encode the threshold parameters $r_1, \ldots, r_{k-1}$ directly either as real numbers, using a floating-point code (that is, each gene would be represented by a real number) or as binary strings, using the usual mapping from binary strings to real numbers. However, problems may arise because the solutions space becomes unnecessary large and the number of regimes is required to be pre-specified. The encoding used by Baragona et al. (2004b) consists in ordering the time series observations and defining the map

$$(y_{(1)}, y_{(2)}, \ldots, y_{(n)}) \Leftrightarrow (b_1, b_2, \ldots, b_n),$$

where b is a binary string and $b_i = 1$ if $y_{(i)}$ is a threshold parameter and $b_i = 0$ otherwise. The number of regimes may be computed $k = b_1 + b_2 + \ldots + b_n + 1$. This encoding has the advantage that the solutions space is much smaller without loss of generality. As a matter of fact, if we consider only the in-sample observations then a threshold between $y_{(t)}$ and $y_{(t+1)}$ could be any value less than or equal to $y_{(t+1)}$.

Fitness function computation

In every fitness function evaluation the structural parameters d, k, $r_1, \ldots, r_{k-1}$ are assumed known though actually they are tentative thresholds provided by the GA and a delay parameter from the set $\mathcal{D}$. Let $p_{\max}$ be the maximum AR order. The AIC is computed for $p = 1, \ldots, p_{\max}$ and the order p that minimizes the AIC is assumed

$$\text{AIC}(p, d, k, r_1, \ldots, r_{k-1}) = \{n - p(k+1)\}\log\sigma_\varepsilon^2 + 2p(k+1).$$

Once the appropriate order p is found the fitness function is set to

$$f(r_1, \ldots, r_{k-1}|d) = \exp(-\text{AIC}(p)/c)$$

Note that the parameters λ_j and $\nu_j^{(i)}$ are estimated by minimizing the residual sum of squares since the model is linear in those coefficients:

$$\text{SSQ} = \left\{ y_t - \sum_{j=1}^{p} \lambda_j y_{t-j} - \sum_{j=1}^{p} \sum_{i=1}^{k} \nu_j^{(i)} S_i(y_{t-d}) y_{t-j} \right\}^2 .$$

Results from a simulation experiment reported by Baragona et al. (2004b) demonstrate that the GAs-based PLTAR building procedure is able to identify and estimate the parameters of a time series generated according to a PLTAR model. Standard errors of the estimates are computed as well.

4.3.3.1 Piecewise Linear Approximation to Multiregime Models

Threshold models reported in Sect. 4.3.1 and the EXPAR model reported in Sect. 4.3.2 both are autoregressive models of the time series y whose parameters are allowed to vary depending on y_{t-d}. This latter is assumed as the state variable

$z = z_{t-1}$. In the former case the functions $\phi(z)$ are not continuous as they have a jump in each and every threshold while in the latter case they are continuous functions of the state variable. The EXPAR models belong to the wide class of the smooth transition autoregressive (STAR) models. The AR parameters $\phi(z)$ of a STAR model are requested to be smooth functions of z, that is continuous with continuous derivative. Halfway between TAR and STAR models the PLTAR models require less demanding assumptions about the parameter function $\phi(z)$ that retains continuity but not necessarily differentiability and notwithstanding it may offer a useful approximation to both classes.

Model parameters estimation will be performed by minimizing the root mean square error (RMSE) of the residuals. These latter are computed as usual as the difference between y_t and the value predicted by the model for any given choice of model parameters. In the sequel for estimating PLTAR and TAR models we shall use GAs because the residual RMSE will be a non differentiable function of some of the parameters. In case of TAR models not only derivatives cannot be computed but the RMSE will not be a continuous function of some of the parameters. On the contrary, for STAR models, and EXPAR models in particular, we shall use a quasi-Newton method with numerical evaluation of the derivatives of the objective function. In fact, in general the RMSE computed from models in this class will be differentiable though derivatives for some parameters are difficult to compute. For the GAs parameters we shall assume population size $s = 10$, number of iteration $N = 30$. For threshold time points identification we shall use a binary array of length $\ell = n$, where n is the number of observations of the time series y. For real parameters the precision will be assumed $\ell = 20$, that is a binary string of length 20 will be used to represent real numbers. For a given interval (a, b) this choice will allow numbers far apart more than $(b - a)/(2^\ell - 1)$ to be distinguishable. For instance, in $(0, 1)$ a precision 20 implies that numbers in the interval will be from zero to one with step $1/(2^{10} - 1)$, i.e. 6 significant (decimal) digits. The generational gap is assumed $G = 0.9$, the probability of crossover $p_c = 0.7$ and mutation probability $p_m = 0.7/n$. In spite of the small genetic pool and short generations evolution, we shall see that the GAs are able to yield more than satisfactory results.

Our starting point is the consideration that a continuous piecewise linear function may in practice approximate analytic functions to any degree of accuracy. As a first example, consider the logistic STAR (LSTAR) model (see Teräsvirta, 1994)

$$y_t = \sum_{j=1}^{p} \phi_j^{(1)} y_{t-j} + G(y_{t-d}) \sum_{j=1}^{p} \phi_j^{(2)} y_{t-j} + e_t \tag{4.17}$$

where

$$G(y_{t-d}) = (1 + \exp(-\gamma(y_{t-d} - c)))^{-1}$$

and $\{e_t\}$ is a sequence of independent identically distributed random variables with mean zero and variance σ^2. Let us compare models (4.14) and (4.17) by simulating an artificial time series generated by the LSTAR model (4.17), see Fig. 4.1. We assumed the number of observations $n = 100$, $\sigma^2 = 1$, $d = 1$, $p = 1$, the AR parameters $\phi_1^{(1)} = 0.7$ and $\phi_1^{(2)} = -1.2$, $\gamma = 2$ and $c = 0$. Variance and standard deviation of the simulated time series may be computed equal to 1.6652 and 1.2904 respectively. Assuming d and p known, the LSTAR model parameters $\phi_1^{(1)}$, $\phi_1^{(2)}$, γ and c have been estimated by using the quasi-Newton BFGS method. Then, assuming $d = 1$ and $p = 1$, a PLTAR has been estimated by using the GAs-based procedure. Results are displayed in Table 4.1. The LSTAR estimates are rather accurate as far as the autoregressive parameters are concerned, but are biased as regards the coefficients of the logistic function. In fact, the LSTAR model is linear in the former parameters while is non linear in the latter ones, so that the derivative numerical computation is relatively easy in the former and difficult in the latter case. The estimated PLTAR model includes $k = 3$ regimes in each of which a first order polynomial represents the behavior of the AR parameter as a function of the state variable y_{t-1}. In Fig. 4.2 the variable AR parameter of the LSTAR model (4.17) is plotted along with the piecewise linear AR parameter of the PLTAR model (4.14). The approximation provided by the PLTAR parameter seems adequate to match the logistic curve of the LSTAR parameter or at least comparable with the estimated LSTAR parameter curve. Moreover, the one-step-ahead forecasts have been computed from the LSTAR and the PLTAR models and plotted in Fig. 4.1 along with the original time series. There is evidence that there is a close agreement between the two predicted time series, and both seem able to reproduce fairly well the observations generated from model (4.17). The root mean square errors (RMSE) are 0.9464 and 0.9254 for LSTAR and PLTAR models respectively (Table 4.1). The performance of the two models may be considered similar. Note that the RMSE computed from the estimated PLTAR model is less than that computed from the LSTAR model at the expense of a slight increase of the number of parameters. As a matter of fact, the LSTAR model has 4 estimated parameters while the estimated parameters of the PLTAR model are actually 6, not 8, because 2 model parameters are constrained by (4.15). Estimated parameters, according to (4.16) are the two thresholds $\hat{r}_1$, $\hat{r}_2$, and the coefficients λ_1 and $\nu_1^{(1)}$, $\nu_1^{(2)}$ and $\nu_1^{(3)}$. The further and remarkable advantage in using the PLTAR model resides in that there is non need to specify in advance any special functional form for the AR parameters.

An example of modeling a time series generated from an EXPAR model by fitting a PLTAR model may be considered as well. An artificial time series y of 100 observations has been simulated from model (4.12) by assuming an EXPAR(2), i.e. $p = 2$, with delay parameter $d = 1$, $\gamma = 2$, the variance of the white noise $\sigma^2 = 1$ and autoregressive coefficients $\phi_1 = -1.1$, $\phi_2 = 2$, and $\pi_1 = -0.9$, $\pi_2 = -0.1$. These latter have been chosen so as to meet conditions 1–3 in Sect. 4.3.2. The simulated time series y has variance equal to 4.6504 and standard deviation 2.1565 (see Fig. 4.3). An EXPAR(2) model has been fitted to y by using the BFGS algorithm. Estimates are reported in Table 4.2. Two estimated parameters are severely biased,

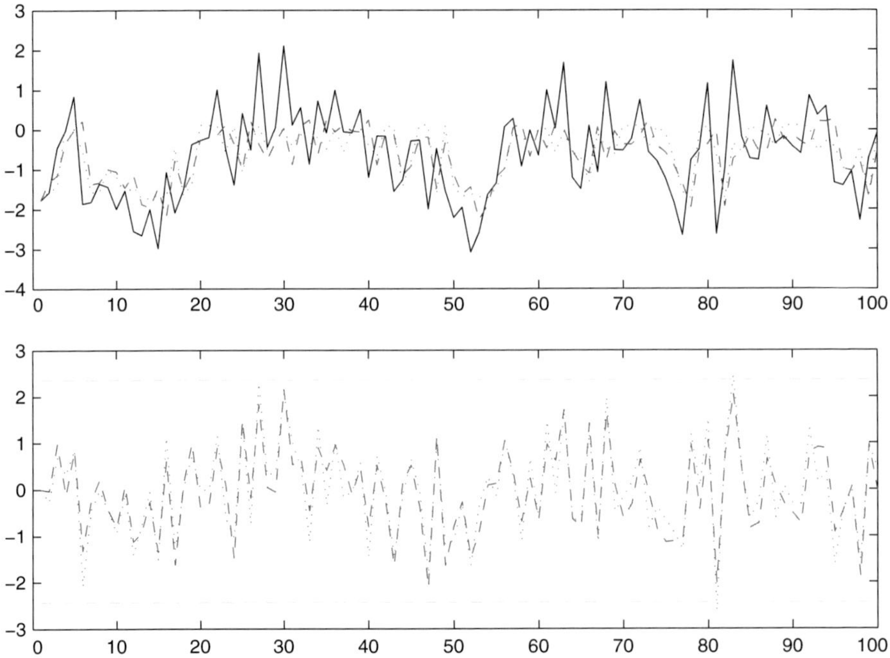

Fig. 4.1 *Top panel*: artificial time series generated by a LSTAR model (*solid line*) and one-step-ahead forecasts yielded by an LSTAR model (*dashed line*) and a PLTAR model (*dotted line*) – *Bottom panel*: residuals computed from the LSTAR model (*dashed line*) and from the PLTAR model (*dotted line*)

Table 4.1 Model estimates comparison from a order 1 LSTAR and a PLTAR fitted to 100 artificial time series data generated from a LSTAR model

Model	Parameters				RMSE
LSTAR(1), true values	$\phi_1^{(1)} = 0.7000$	$\phi_1^{(2)} = -1.2000$	$\gamma = 2.0000$	$c = 0.0000$	1.0000
LSTAR(1), estimates	$\hat{\phi}_1^{(1)} = 0.7361$	$\hat{\phi}_1^{(2)} = -1.2087$	$\hat{\gamma} = 2.7567$	$\hat{c} = 1.0$	0.9464
PLTAR(1), estimates	$\hat{\alpha}_1^{(1)} = 1.3047$	$\hat{\beta}_1^{(1)} = 0.2463$	$\hat{r}_1 = -1.5308$		0.9254
	$\hat{\alpha}_1^{(2)} = -0.7423$	$\hat{\beta}_1^{(2)} = -1.0909$	$\hat{r}_2 = 0.1260$		
	$\hat{\alpha}_1^{(3)} = -0.9235$	$\hat{\beta}_1^{(3)} = 0.3471$			

namely $\hat{\pi}_1$ and $\hat{\gamma}$ while the remaining estimates are rather accurate. The one-step-ahead forecasts closely reproduce the behavior of the time series y and we obtained the residual RMSE equal to 1.0450. Then a PLTAR of order 2 and delay parameter 1 has been fitted to the same data by using the GAs. Results are reported in Table 4.2 as well. The estimated PLTAR model has 4 regimes and the RMSE equals 1.0179. The RMSE from the PLTAR model is smaller than that from the EXPAR model. The artificial time series is displayed in the top panel of Fig. 4.3 along with the

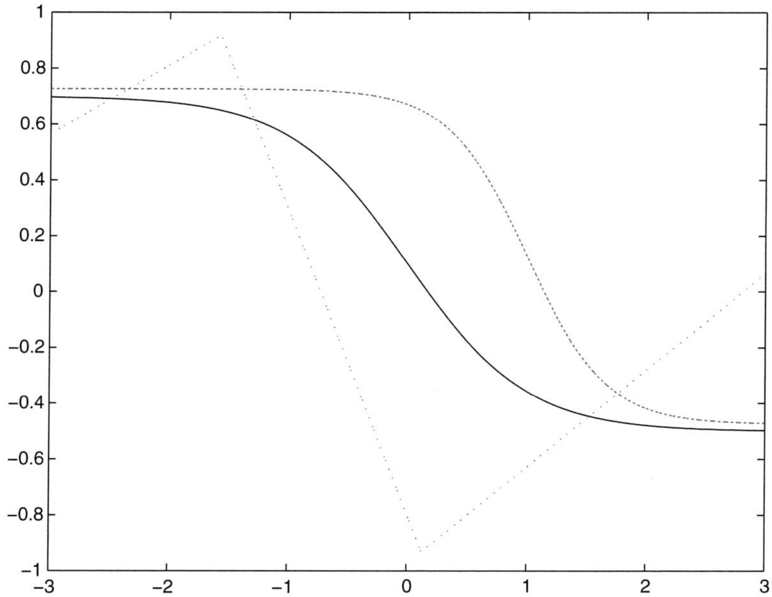

Fig. 4.2 First order AR parameter for a LSTAR model (true value, *solid line*, and estimate, *dashed line*) and a PLTAR model estimate (*dotted line*) plotted against the state variable

Table 4.2 Model estimates comparison from an order 2 EXPAR and an order 2 PLTAR fitted to 100 artificial time series data generated from a EXPAR(2) model

Model	Parameters			RMSE
EXPAR(2),	$\phi_1 = -1.1000$	$\pi_1 = 2.0000$	$\gamma = 2.0$	1.0000
true values	$\phi_2 = -0.9000$	$\pi_2 = -0.1000$		
EXPAR(2),	$\hat{\phi}_1 = -1.0009$	$\hat{\pi}_1 = 1.0000$	$\hat{\gamma} = 1.6768$	1.0450
estimates	$\hat{\phi}_2 = -0.7637$	$\hat{\pi}_2 = -0.0879$		
PLTAR(2),	$\hat{\alpha}_1^{(1)} = -0.8081$	$\hat{\beta}_1^{(1)} = 0.0712$	$\hat{r}_1 = -0.9609$	1.0179
estimates	$\hat{\alpha}_2^{(1)} = -0.5823$	$\hat{\beta}_2^{(1)} = 0.0997$		
	$\hat{\alpha}_1^{(2)} = -0.0887$	$\hat{\beta}_1^{(2)} = 0.8199$	$\hat{r}_2 = 0.4135$	
	$\hat{\alpha}_2^{(2)} = -0.8352$	$\hat{\beta}_2^{(2)} = -0.1634$		
	$\hat{\alpha}_1^{(3)} = 0.7927$	$\hat{\beta}_1^{(3)} = -1.3117$	$\hat{r}_3 = 1.4055$	
	$\hat{\alpha}_2^{(3)} = -1.0248$	$\hat{\beta}_2^{(3)} = 0.2953$		
	$\hat{\alpha}_1^{(4)} = -1.0276$	$\hat{\beta}_1^{(4)} = -0.0165$		
	$\hat{\alpha}_2^{(4)} = -0.4576$	$\hat{\beta}_2^{(4)} = -0.1083$		

one-step-ahead forecasts computed from the EXPAR and PLTAR models. The time series values predicted by the PLTAR model are in good agreement with both the predicted values from the EXPAR model and the original time series. The residuals from the two models shown in the bottom panel of Fig. 4.3 are rather close each other. Figures 4.4 and 4.5 display the behavior of the autoregressive parameters of order 1 and 2 respectively computed by using the true values and estimates for

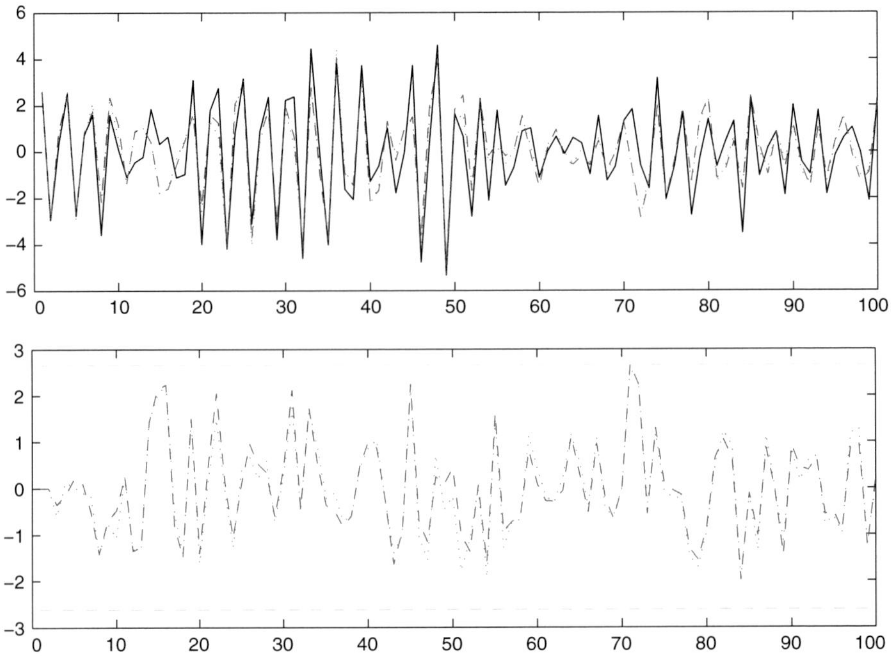

Fig. 4.3 *Top panel*: artificial time series generated by an EXPAR model (*solid line*) and one-step-ahead forecasts yielded by estimated EXPAR (*dashed line*) and PLTAR (*dotted line*) models – *Bottom panel*: residuals computed from the EXPAR model (*dashed line*) and from the PLTAR model (*dotted line*)

models PLTAR and EXPAR. Both the PLTAR and the EXPAR estimated coefficients are closer to each other than to the true coefficient but the overall shape is very similar. The first order parameter estimates seem to constitute a better approximation than the second order ones. Though the bias is rather large for $\hat{\pi}_1$ the curve is in close agreement with the true parameter behavior. However, the bias is not negligible if the state variable is near zero.

Note that the estimated EXPAR(2) model has 5 parameters while the estimated PLTAR(2) model totalizes 13 parameters to be estimated, i.e. 3 thresholds, 2 coefficients $\hat{\lambda}_j$ $(j = 1, 2)$ and 2 coefficients $\hat{\upsilon}_j^{(i)}$ $(j = 1, 2$ and $i = 1, \ldots, 4)$. The large number of parameters makes the PLTAR model to have a residual RMSE smaller than the residual RMSE computed for the EXPAR(2) model. So a PLTAR model should be preferred possibly by reason that a special functional form has to be pre-specified before a LSTAR or EXPAR model could be estimated while this identification step is avoided if we want to fit a PLTAR model. As a matter of fact, prior knowledge needed to choose between a LSTAR or EXPAR model properly may not be available while a PLTAR model may fit time series generated by several

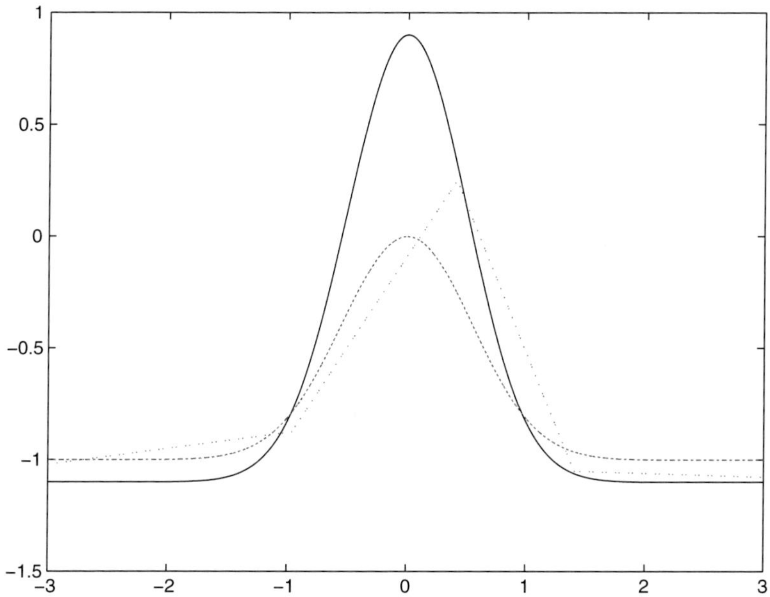

Fig. 4.4 First order AR parameter of an EXPAR model (true value, *solid line*, and estimate, *dashed line*) and its PLTAR estimate (*dotted line*) plotted against the state variable

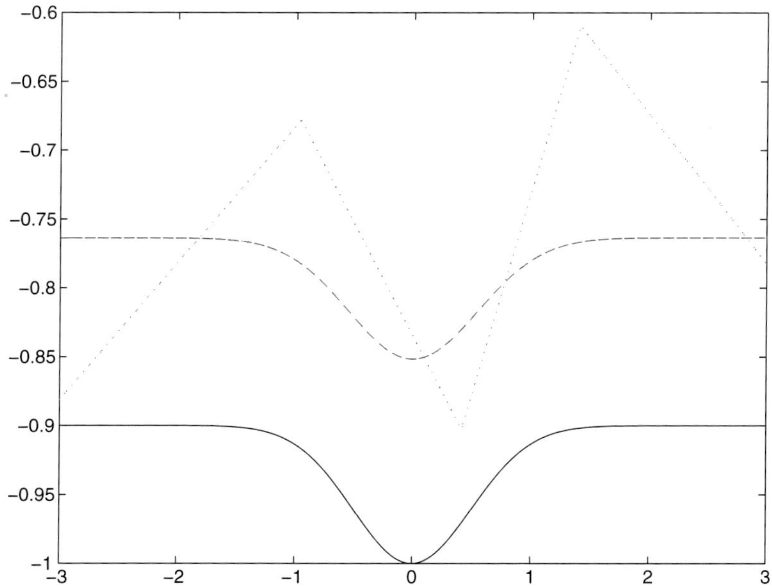

Fig. 4.5 Second order AR parameter of an EXPAR model (true value, *solid line*, and estimate, *dashed line*) and its PLTAR estimate (*dotted line*) plotted against the state variable

different random processes. Using PLTAR modeling could prevent us from using the wrong model and this advantage has to be taken into account.

A comparison between a TAR and a PLTAR model may support the use of the latter to fit time series that are actually generated by the former model. In this case it may seem unlikely that a PLTAR model could be able to provide a good approximation to a step model, but the following example shows that such an approximation may be both accurate and useful. Let $n = 100$ observations be generated by a two-regimes TAR model that follows an AR(1) for both regimes with autoregressive coefficients $c_1^{(1)} = 0.8$ if $y_{t-1} \leq 0$ and $c_1^{(2)} = -0.8$ if $y_{t-1} > 0$. A zero mean unit variance white noise drives such random process. The artificial time series y has variance and standard deviation equal to 2.1978 and 1.4825 respectively (see Fig. 4.6). We fit a TAR model to the data by assuming that $d = 1$, $p = 1$ and $k = 2$ are known and by estimating the autoregressive coefficients and the threshold parameter. We do not use a gradient-based optimization algorithm as the objective function is not continuous. Instead we use a GA to estimate all three unknown parameters. Then we estimate by another GA the parameters of a PLTAR where we assume that $d = 1$ and $p = 1$ are known but all remaining parameters, including the number of regimes k, have to be estimated. Results are reported in Table 4.3. The

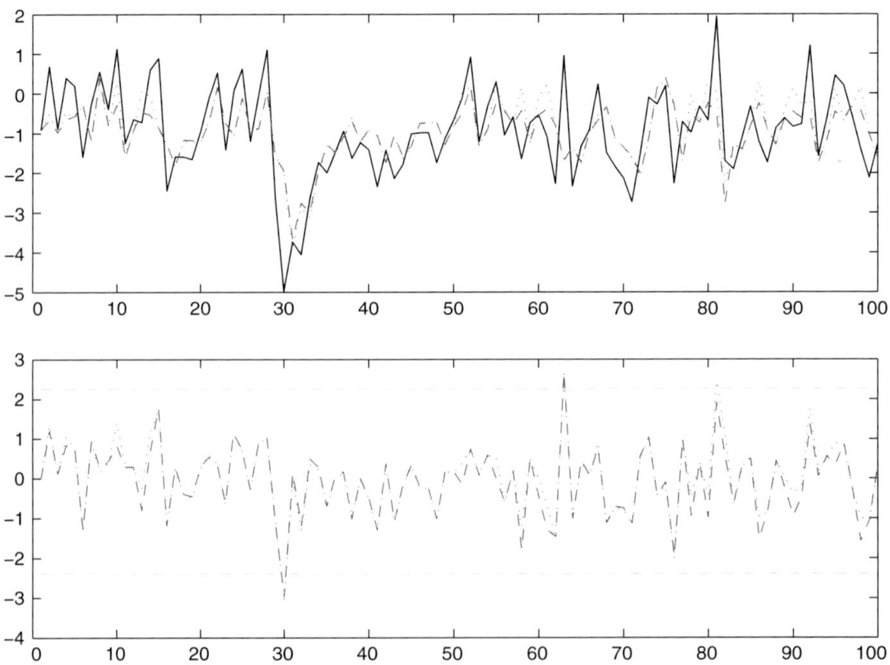

Fig. 4.6 *Top panel*: artificial time series generated by a TAR model (*solid line*) and one-step-ahead forecasts yielded by a TAR model (*dashed line*) and a PLTAR model (*dotted line*) – *Bottom panel*: residuals computed from the TAR model (*dashed line*) and from the PLTAR model (*dotted line*)

Table 4.3 Model estimates comparison from a order 1 TAR and a PLTAR fitted to 100 artificial time series data generated from a TAR model

Model	Parameters			RMSE
LSTAR(1),	$c_1^{(1)} = 0.8000$		$r_1 = 0.0000$	1.0000
true values	$c_1^{(2)} = -0.8000$			
LSTAR(1),	$\hat{c}_1^{(1)} = 0.7388$		$\hat{r}_1 = -0.3206$	0.8965
estimates	$\hat{c}_1^{(2)} = -1.4400$			
PLTAR(1),	$\hat{\alpha}_1^{(1)} = 0.7442$	$\hat{\beta}_1^{(1)} = -0.0071$	$\hat{r}_1 = -0.9860$	0.8978
estimates	$\hat{\alpha}_1^{(2)} = -1.7406$	$\hat{\beta}_1^{(2)} = -2.5273$	$\hat{r}_2 = -0.0312$	
	$\hat{\alpha}_1^{(3)} = -1.6538$	$\hat{\beta}_1^{(3)} = 0.2550$		

PLTAR approximate the TAR structure with a continuous piecewise linear function that changes its slope in three intervals of the state variable. The RMSE computed from the estimated PLTAR model compares favorably with the RMSE computed from the estimated TAR model. In this latter case we have 3 parameters while in the former one there are 6 estimated parameters. The increase in the number of parameters is compensated in this case by a decrease of the RMSE. In addition, we do not need to know that the functional form of the model is a step function because the PLTAR model allows us to obtain an adequate fit of time series generated from a wide class of models. In Fig. 4.7 the agreement between the true and estimated TAR autoregressive coefficient and the estimated PLTAR coefficient is displayed. It is apparent that for a piecewise linear coefficient to approximate a step coefficient 3

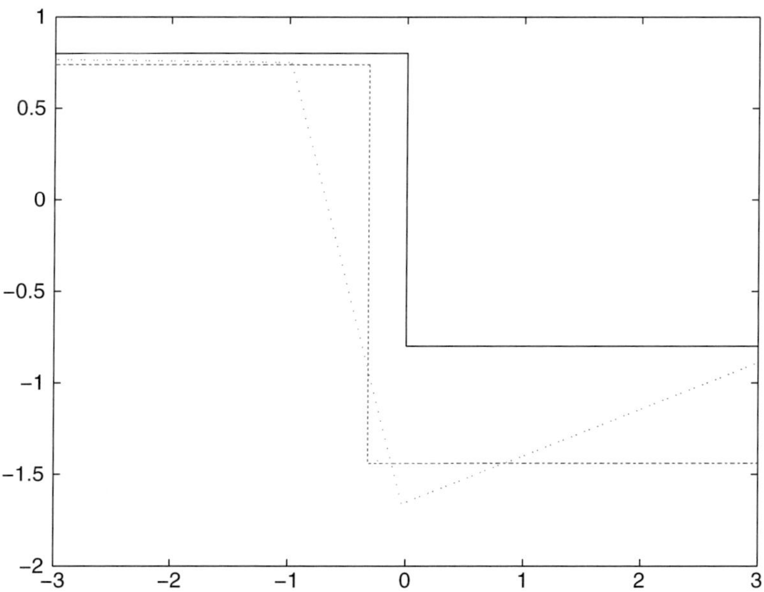

Fig. 4.7 First order AR parameter for a TAR model (true value, *solid line*, and estimate, *dashed line*) and a PLTAR model estimate (*dotted line*) plotted against the state variable

regimes at least are necessarily needed. Both estimated models are able to provide close one-step-ahead predictions of the original time series values. In Fig. 4.6 the predicted and original time series are displayed in the top panel. In the bottom panel the residuals from TAR and PLTAR models are displayed.

Many other complicated non linear models may be approximated by a PLTAR model satisfactorily. We may mention only one further example, the polynomial exponential. The polynomial exponential model of order 2 may be written

$$y_t = a_1(y_{t-d})y_{t-1} + a_2(y_{t-d})y_{t-2} + e_t, \tag{4.18}$$

where

$$a_1(y_{t-d}) = \alpha_0^{(1)} + (\alpha_1^{(1)} + \alpha_2^{(1)} y_{t-d}) \exp(-\gamma y_{t-d}^2),$$
$$a_2(y_{t-d}) = \alpha_0^{(2)} + (\alpha_1^{(2)} + \alpha_2^{(2)} y_{t-d}) \exp(-\gamma y_{t-d}^2),$$

and $\{e_t\}$ is a sequence of independent identically distributed random variables with mean zero and variance σ_e^2. Model (4.18) has been originally suggested by Ozaki (1982) to fit the well known Canadian lynx data and has been used for simulation purpose in Cai et al. (2000). Results from a simulation experiment reported in Baragona et al. (2004b) support the use of PLTAR models to fit time series generated by a polynomial exponential model.

4.3.4 Bilinear Models

The bilinear model obtained from the SDM model form (4.4) by assuming that the parameters $\psi_j(z_{t-1})$ are linear in $\{y_{t-1}, y_{t-2}, \ldots, y_{t-\ell}\}$ is as follows:

$$y_t = \mu + \sum_{j=1}^{p} \phi_j y_{t-j} - \sum_{j=0}^{q} c_j e_{t-j} - \sum_{i=1}^{\ell} \sum_{j=0}^{q} b_{ij} y_{t-i} e_{t-j} \tag{4.19}$$

(with $c_0 = 1$). It is apparent that (4.19) is a generalization of the usual ARMA model obtained by adding the last term in the right hand side of the equation, which is bilinear in (y, e). This simple additional term allows the model to reproduce some typical non linear behavior such as sudden changes and "bursts".

Bilinear models for time series were introduced by Granger and Andresen (1978), and the analysis was extended by Subba Rao (1981) who derived also stationarity and invertibility conditions, and expression for the covariances. The estimation of the parameters in (4.19) may be obtained, assuming normality, by numerical maximization of the likelihood; a simpler method (similar to the Hannan-Rissanen procedure) consists in estimating first the innovations $\{e_t\}$ by fitting a high order autoregression to the data, and then substituting the estimated innovations into (4.19), which becomes linear in the unknown parameters so that they may be simply estimated by least squares. On the other hand, the identification of a bilinear model involves similar difficulties as ARMA models, and may be addressed by genetic algorithms, especially when we allow subset models.

Chen et al. (2001) proposed a GA approach for building subset bilinear time series models. Their model is slightly more general than (4.19) since the bilinear term and the term linear in e_{t-j} are allowed to have a different order:

$$y_t = \mu + \sum_{j=1}^{p} \phi_j y_{t-j} - \sum_{j=0}^{q} c_i e_{t-j} - \sum_{i=1}^{\ell} \sum_{j=0}^{r} b_{ij} y_{t-i} e_{t-j} \tag{4.20}$$

and some parameters may be constrained to zero. A maximum value for each order p, q, ℓ, r is assumed, and the model is identified by choosing which lag corresponds to non zero parameters in the first, second, third and fourth summation in (4.20).

If the maximum orders are chosen equal to P, Q, L, R respectively, any such structure may be described by $P + Q + L + R$ bits denoting whether at each lag the associated parameters are zero or not. For example, if $P = Q = 5$ and $L = R = 3$ (and with an additional first bit for the constant μ), we have a vector with 17 bits, logically split into five segments: the first bit relates to the mean, the next five bits to the AR part, the next five to the MA part, and the last two 3-bit segments relate respectively to the lagged observations and the lagged innovations appearing in the bilinear term. For instance, the vector

$$1:1\,0\,0\,0\,0:0\,1\,0\,0\,0:0\,1\,0:1\,0\,0$$

identifies a model with μ, a linear term in y_{t-1}, a linear term in e_{t-2} and only a bilinear term with lag 2 in the data and lag 1 in the innovations, or:

$$y_t = \mu + \phi_1 y_{t-1} + e_t - c_2 e_{t-2} - b_{21} y_{t-2} e_{t-1}$$

and the vector

$$0:0\,1\,1\,0\,0:1\,0\,0\,1\,0:1\,1\,0:0\,1\,0$$

identifies the model

$$y_t = \phi_2 y_{t-2} + \phi_3 y_{t-3} + e_t - c_1 e_{t-1} - c_4 e_{t-4} - b_{12} y_{t-1} e_{t-2} - b_{22} y_{t-2} e_{t-2}.$$

This coding system is assumed by Chen et al. (2001) for the chromosomes, whose length is therefore $1 + P + Q + L + R$. Note that, differently from the linear models, the number of bits equal to 1 in the chromosome is not equal to the number of parameters to be estimated, because the b_{ij} appear in a double summation: thus, the number of b_{ij} parameters is the product of the number of 1's in the fourth segment times the number of 1's in the fifth segment.

Chen et al. (2001) use the uniform crossover of Syswerda (1989), and regular mutation operator. For the fitness function, they adopt identification criteria such as AIC or BIC, and use rank selection. Therefore, the chromosomes are sorted in decreasing order of AIC, and their rank is used for computing the selection probabilities.

A simulation study suggested that the method performs well in specifying the bilinear parts, while the true order of the linear AR and MA parts are sometimes underestimated; Chen et al. (2001) conclude recommending genetic algorithms for bilinear subset model selection.

4.3.5 Real Data Applications

We present applications of some of the non linear models described in the preceding sections to two well known real time series data, i.e. the Canadian lynx data and the sunspot numbers. These data sets have been widely studied and many different models have been tried for fitting and forecasting purpose. We shall display several comparisons among results reported in the literature and results that have been obtained by using the GAs for estimating non linear time series models.

4.3.5.1 The Canadian Lynx Data

The Canadian lynx data consists of the annual records of the number of lynx trapped in the Mckenzie River district of North-west Canada from 1821 to 1934. The number of observations is $n = 114$. We downloaded the data from *Hyndman, R.J. (n.d.) Time Series Data Library, http://robjhyndman.com/TSDL. Accessed on 15 November 2010.* This time series has been extensively studied (see, for instance, Tong (1990), pp. 380–381, table 7.5). The data are transformed as $\log_{10}$(number recorded as trapped in year 1820+t), $t = 1, \ldots, 114$. We used the first 100 observations, from 1821 to 1920, for estimating the parameters and then we computed the multi-step forecasts from 1921 to 1934, that is the time origin was assumed the year 1920, and lead times were $1, 2, \ldots, 14$.

In Table 4.4 EXPAR, generalized EXPAR models of order 2, 6 and 11 and the best PLTAR obtained with delay 1 (3 regimes, order 2) are compared with respect to the in-sample residual variance, the AIC criterion and the MSE of multi-step forecasts. In Fig. 4.8 forecasts from EXPAR(6) models with a single γ and with

Table 4.4 Canadian lynx data: comparison between EXPAR, generalized EXPAR and PLTAR

Model	Residual variance	AIC criterion	Multi-step forecasts MSE
EXPAR(2) one γ	0.0498	−289.97	0.0437
EXPAR(2) 2 γ's	0.0479	−291.86	0.0419
EXPAR(6) one γ	0.0416	−286.36	0.0857
EXPAR(6) 6 γ's	0.0399	−284.89	0.0412
EXPAR(11) one γ	0.0296	−306.00	0.0597
EXPAR(11) 11 γ's	0.0267	−296.31	0.0719
PLTAR(3, 2)	0.0433	−260.63	0.0224

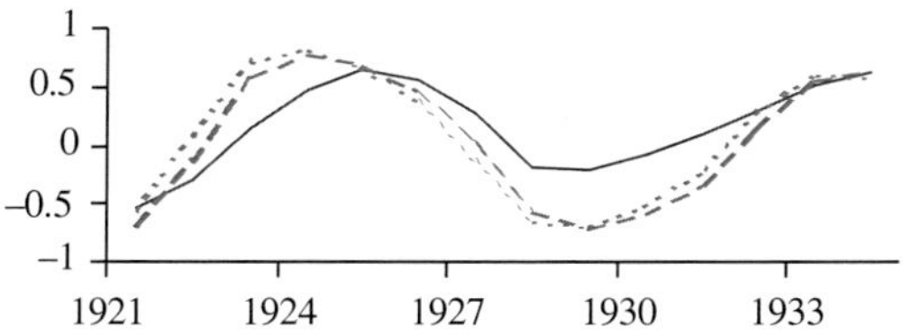

Fig. 4.8 Canadian lynx data forecasts. *Solid line*: original data. *Dotted line*: forecasts from the EXPAR(6) model with a single γ parameter. *Dashed line*: forecasts from the generalized EXPAR(6) model with 6 γ's

6 γ's are compared. Allowing for more γ's obviously makes the residual variance to decrease. The residual variance is decreasing as well if we consider the models in increasing orders. The forecast MSE, however, does not exhibit this behavior, and best forecasts are yielded by the EXPAR(6) model with 6 γ's, though the EXPAR(2) model with two γ's is only slightly worse. This circumstance seems to suggest that the adherence of the model to the sample data does not ensure more accurate multi-step forecasts. Note that we considered out-of-sample forecasts, so that the parameter estimates did not take into account the last 14 observations. These latter are better predicted by the EXPAR(6) model, in spite of the fact that the smallest residual variance is yielded by the EXPAR(11) model with 11 γ's. The former model forecasting ability is possibly due to the fact that it describes well the overall behavior of the time series. Finally, the PLTAR model has a larger residual variance, but the forecast MSE is considerably smaller.

4.3.5.2 The Sunspot Numbers

The sunspot numbers (see Tong, 1990, chapter 7, pp. 419–429) have been investigated as well by using several models and estimation methods. We made out computations on the mean-deleted transformed data $2\{(1 + y_t)^{1/2} - 1\}$ as suggested in Tong (1990), p. 420. We considered the AR(9) model reported by Tong (1990), p. 423, and the self-excited threshold autoregressive SETAR(2; 11, 3) model proposed by Ghaddar and Tong (1981), p. 247. Then, we took into account the EXPAR(2), the EXPAR(6) and the EXPAR(9) models with one γ and with 2, 6 and 9 γ's respectively. For estimating the parameters of each model we used the observations from 1700 to 1979, while the observations from 1980 to 1995 were reserved for the multi-step forecasts. The data were taken from the web site http://sidc.oma.be (RWC Belgium World Data Center for the Sunspot Index). The results are displayed in Table 4.5. Models are compared by means of the residual variance and the forecasts MSE. Time origins are 1979, 1984, 1987 and lead times $1, 2, \ldots, 8$. Some forecasts from 1980 to 1992 are plotted in Fig. 4.9.

The best forecasts not always are obtained by using models that have the least residual variance. The EXPAR(9) model with 9 γ's, for instance, yields the smallest residual variance, but the SETAR(2; 11, 3) model provides the best multi-step forecasts for the years 1980–1987. The results change, however, if different time

Table 4.5 Sunspot numbers: comparison among AR, SETAR, EXPAR and generalized EXPAR

Model	Residual variance	*mse* 1980–1987	*mse* 1985–1992	*mse* 1988–1995	*mse* 1980–1992
AR(9)	4.05	3.60	16.5	9.01	16.19
SETAR(2; 11, 3)	3.73	1.82	33.51	17.34	22.27
EXPAR(2) one γ	4.90	7.08	65.28	31.39	32.97
EXPAR(2) 2 γ's	4.83	3.77	85.33	29.32	38.46
EXPAR(6) one γ	4.47	7.64	54.74	19.46	21.11
EXPAR(6) 6 γ's	4.34	11.85	42.01	20.62	21.89
EXPAR(9) one γ	3.66	4.99	20.43	8.21	13.02
EXPAR(9) 9 γ's	3.57	2.62	16.34	10.65	10.27

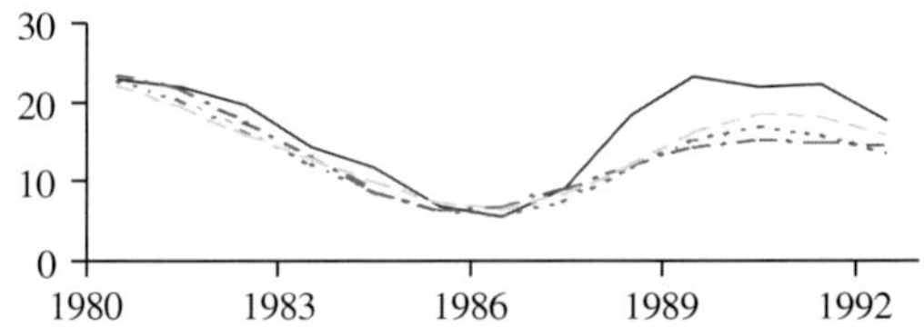

Fig. 4.9 Sunspot numbers forecasts 1980–1992. Original data: *solid line*. Forecasts: AR(9) *dotted line*; SETAR(2;11,3) *dash Ǘdotted line*; EXPAR(9), 9 γ's, *dashed line*

intervals are considered. Thus, the least mean square forecasts error is observed for the EXPAR(9) with 9 γ's in 1985–1992, for the EXPAR(9) with a single γ in 1988–1995. In the wider time span 1980–1992, the EXPAR(9) with 9 γ's is able to produce the best multi-step forecasts. The cyclical behavior of this time series is changing over time, and our models may describe it better in certain years than others. It seems that the EXPAR(9) model with 9 γ's almost always yields the most accurate forecasting performance.

4.3.6 Artificial Neural Networks

A different specialization of the general non linear autoregressive time series model

$$y_t = f\,(y_{t-1}, y_{t-2}, \ldots) + e_t \tag{4.21}$$

is offered by the artificial neural networks (ANN). These devices have been developed in fields different than statistics, such as artificial intelligence, machine vision, pattern recognition, classification of medical images, decision making and forecasting. Notwithstanding the special terminology which strictly refers to the chief applications and the analogy somewhat loose with models of the human brain or nervous system, in the recent past the ANNs have been added to the statistical methods available for discriminant analysis, non linear regression, time series modeling and forecasting (see, for instance, Hornik and Leisch (2001) and Sarle (1994)).

Let us define the residual sum of squares (SSQ) for model (4.21) as

$$\mathrm{SSQ} = \sum_{t=p+1}^{n} \left(y_t - f(y_{t-1}, \ldots, y_{t-p})\right)^2,$$

where the observed time series values $y = (y_1, \ldots, y_n)'$ are available and the positive integer p denotes the model order. A common measure of model performance is the mean square error (MSE)

$$\hat{\sigma}_e^2 = \frac{1}{n-p}\mathrm{SSQ}. \tag{4.22}$$

Note that SSQ is a decreasing function of the number of lagged variables used in model (4.21), so that it would be possible to obtain smaller values of the MSE (4.22) by increasing the model order p. So usually model comparison is done according to the parsimony principle, i.e. best optimal results have to be obtained by minimizing the number of lagged variables and restricting to those that are strictly needed for significant model improvement.

4.3.6.1 Multilayer Perceptron Backpropagation Model

The basic elements of an ANN are the processing units called neurons. A neuron is a device which transform a combination of inputs to an output by means of a non linear function. Early processing units have been introduced by McCulloch and Pitts (1943) and Rosenblatt (1958) as

$$x \mapsto g(\alpha' x + \delta), \tag{4.23}$$

where x denotes the input vector, the array α and the threshold δ are in general unknown parameters and g is the activation function. Function g does not need to be differentiable and it may yield a binary output, for instance. Equation (4.23) has been presented as a simple model for classification or for implementing Boolean functions. A comprehensive method for assembling neurons to build flexible models useful in many applications has been introduced by Rumelhart et al. (1986) who provided guidelines for combining units (4.23) to form a neural network and an algorithm to estimate the unknown parameters. The multilayer perceptron is the neural network basic system including an input x, a hidden layer of neurons and an output y. The activation functions in the hidden layer are non linear differentiable and the resulting model is genuinely non linear, i.e. non linear in the parameters. An ANN based on a single hidden layer may be written as the non linear model

$$y^* = f(x, w) = \sum_{j=1}^{h} \beta_j g(\alpha_j{}' x + \delta_j), \tag{4.24}$$

where h is the number of hidden units (neurons), the parameter vector w includes all unknown parameters

$$w = [\beta_1, \ldots, \beta_h, \alpha_1, \ldots, \alpha_h, \delta_1, \ldots, \delta_h], \tag{4.25}$$

and the function g may be chosen among several proposal functions of sigmoid type, for instance the logistic function. For example, the ANN displayed in Fig. 4.10 is the graphical display of model (4.24) with $p = 2$, i.e. two inputs here represented by the lagged observed time series data y_{t-1} and y_{t-2}, a hidden layer with $h = 3$ neurons and a single output. This latter is to be compared to the target y_t, that is the observed time series data at the current time t. The activation functions are of identical logistic shape in each neuron and non linearly transform a linear combination of the inputs plus a threshold constant. A linear combination of the values yielded by the hidden layer computing devices produces the single valued output.

The backpropagation algorithm is based on the gradient descent algorithm which aims at minimizing a function of the difference between the output y^* obtained by propagating the input throughout the neural network and the target (observed) output y. This difference is called the residual and as the residual depends on the parameters w we may denote $E = E(w)$ the objective function. Let $w^{(i)}$ denote a tentative value of the vector parameter w, then from the input x the output y^* may be computed throughout (4.24) and compared to the target value y. The parameters w are updated according to the rule

$$w^{(i+1)} = w^{(i)} - \eta \frac{\partial E}{\partial w},$$

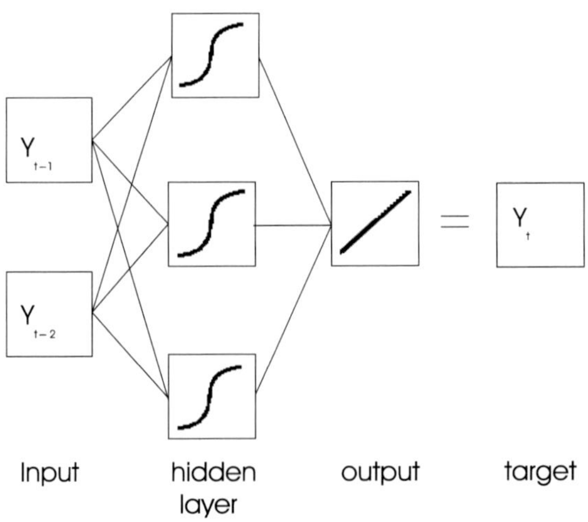

Fig. 4.10 Graphical display of an ANN for non linear modeling of time series data

where $\frac{\partial E}{\partial w}$ is the gradient of E and η is a proportionality constant called learning rate. The procedure is iterated until a maximum pre-specified number of iterations is attained or if some stopping rule is met. Usually the data are split into a training set, a test set and a validation set. Estimation is performed on the training set only, while the test set is used for model selection and the validation set is used for evaluating the out-of-sample performance of the estimated model.

An ANN for modeling the non linear time series (4.21) may include a sequence of vector $z_{t-1} = \{y_{t-1}, \ldots, y_{t-p}\}$ as input ($t = p+1, \ldots, n$) and the observed time series $y = (y_{p+1}, \ldots, y_n)'$ as target, where n is the number of observations and p is the model order. For a single hidden layer with h neurons, (4.24) becomes

$$y_t^* = \sum_{j=1}^{h} \beta_j g({\alpha_j}' z_{t-1} + \delta_j), \quad t = p+1, \ldots, n,$$

and the usual objective function is the MSE (4.22)

$$E(w) = \frac{1}{n-p} \sum_{t=p+1}^{n} \left(y_t - y_t^*\right)^2 .$$

The approximation property of the multilayer perceptron model has been shown to hold by Hornik (1993) provided that some mild assumptions on the activation functions g are fulfilled. This is always the case with the most common activation functions used in the applications. Usually the activation function g (as, for instance, the logistic one) is a sigmoidal shaped function that allows the input unit to impact the output unit significantly if the combination of the inputs exceeds the given threshold.

In Hornik and Leisch (2001) a comparison between some AR and ANN models to fit the sunspot numbers time series is reported. Sunspots in the years 1700–1988 have been used, so that the available observations are $n = 289$. For estimating the parameters 200 observations have been used, while 50 have been used as test set and the remaining 39 as validation set. According to the results displayed by Hornik and Leisch (2001) the ANNs compare favorably with respect to the AR models. The computed MSEs are smaller for the ANNs than the AR using several model orders and, for the ANNs, different numbers of hidden units. The best result is obtained for an ANN with 6 inputs, an hidden layer with 2 neurons and a single output. For this latter ANN the MSE computed on the validation set is equal to 387 while the MSE computed on the validation set for an AR(9) model is equal to 653. In evaluating these results, however, two circumstances have to be taken into account.

- The ANN models include a much larger parameter set that an AR model so that estimation problems are likely to occur unless a large data set is available.
- Unlike statistical time series models such as the autoregressive ones, the interpretation of model structure and parameters of an ANN model yields information

of limited value excepted at most consideration about the number of lags of the inputs.

So a good motivation for using ANNs resides in that this class of models is able to yield accurate out-of-sample forecasts.

Many extensions and improvements of the basic multilayer perceptron model have been proposed in the literature (Mandic and Chambers, 2001). For computing the parameter vector w numerical optimization methods such as the quasi-Newton algorithms have been proposed in place of the gradient descent method. However, a great deal of research has been involved to introduce different neural network structures to allow for more flexibility and to cope with specific practical issues. Shortcuts and feedback connections seem the most innovative features of more complicated neural networks.

- Shortcuts connections between inputs and outputs allow linear relationships to be added to the non linear model structure. This is motivated in time series models, for instance, because most non linear models include a linear structure as well.
- Recurrent neural network models allow feedback connections among units. This is not permitted in the conventional feed-forward structure where input, hidden layers and output influence each other only along the direction from input to output. In robotics and language recognition, for instance, often recurrent neural networks are found useful.

For whatever extension of the multilayer perceptron the most common method for estimating the parameter vector is the backpropagation algorithm. However some drawbacks are known that have to be taken into account in deciding for adoption of the method and in evaluating the estimates. As a gradient descent algorithm the backpropagation algorithm typically has a slow rate of convergence so that a large number of iterations have to be performed to obtain an accurate estimate. Moreover, the estimates depend on the starting points and it is advisable to run the algorithm several times with different initial values. This device obviously further increases the computation time. Finally there are no definite rules on how many hidden layers and processing units in each layer have to be chosen for optimal results.

4.3.6.2 Neural Networks and Genetic Algorithms

Methods based on a mixture of ANN and GAs have been proposed and found effective in a wide range of applications, from hydrological systems to financial data (Delgado and Prat, 1997; Minerva and Poli, 2001b; Versace et al., 2004; Kim and Shin, 2007). The most attractive feature of GAs as processing tools for the ANN structure is the availability of automatic searching for optimal ANN structure. In general, the ANN structure requires the number of hidden layer to be pre-specified and, for each hidden layer, the number of neurons has to be decided. In particular, for a non linear time series model the order p is the most important parameter that has to be chosen to define the number of input units, i.e. how many lagged variables have to be used to minimize the SSQ and at the same time to fulfill the parsimony principle.

Though several other choices have to be performed for an ANN to be completely identified, e.g. the activation function, the connection type and the combination that yields the output, we shall confine the discussion to the model order p and to the number of neurons h in a single layer perceptron environment to illustrate the GAs-based ANNs modeling. In this framework the GAs-based methods for parameters estimation will be considered as well.

The GAs for searching for optimal ANNs structure include in general the following issues.

- The network structure and parameters have to be encoded in a chromosome that represents a potential solution to the modeling problem. Given the assumptions, a chromosome encodes a completely specified ANN and the population, that is the current set of chromosomes, is a set of proposal ANNs.
- The evolution process has to be designed as far as the genetic operators selection, crossover and mutation are concerned. At each step of such iterative process the ANNs that form the past generation may change to originate the set of ANNs that form the new generation.
- The evolutionary dynamics is driven by the fitness function which associates a numerical positive value to each ANN in the current population. The fitness function value has to be as greater as better the proposal ANN is able to fit the data.
- A convergence criterion has to be specified, for instance the iterations may stop if the diversity in the population is practically negligible or if the improvement of the maximum of the fitness function values is smaller than a given threshold. A common alternative device in the GAs framework consists in avoiding specification of any convergence criterion and choosing a number of iterations instead that have to be performed irrespective of the fitness distribution in the current population.

For instance, the multilayer perceptron displayed in Fig. 4.10 may be encoded by the following binary chromosome

010|011|0001 0100 0101|1010 1000 0111|1001 1110 1010|1010 1110 1100

We reserve 3 digits for both the number of inputs and the number of neurons in the hidden layer. In this way we assume implicitly 8 as the maximum number of inputs and neurons, decoding conventionally the all-zero string as 8 to avoid potential solutions with neither inputs nor neurons. The digits that follow the first 6 encode, with 4 binary digits precision, each tentative estimates of the coefficients included in vector w as specified in (4.25). So the first 3 digits encode a number of inputs equal to 2 and the digits 4–6 a number of neurons equal to 3. Then, assuming coefficients α's and β's in the interval $(-1, 1)$ and threshold constants δ's in $(0, 1)$ tentative estimates may be decoded as $\alpha_1 = (-0.87, -0.47)$ and $\delta_1 = 0.33$, $\alpha_2 = (0.33, 0.07)$ and $\delta_2 = 0.47$, $\alpha_3 = (0.2, 0.87)$ and $\delta_3 = 0.67$. Finally the output is given by the linear combination of the 3 values yielded by the hidden layer with coefficients $\beta_1 = 0.33$, $\beta_2 = 0.87$ and $\beta_3 = 0.6$.

The GAs-based approach implies that ANNs with different number of neurons in the hidden layer have to be compared. In this respect the MSE does not allow an equal comparison and the fitness function had better chosen as a model selection criterion, for example the Asymptotic Information Criterion (AIC), the Information Complexity criterion (ICOMP), the Minimum Description Length (MDL) or one of the several variants of these and other methods (Wong and Li, 1998; Bozdogan Bearse , 2003; Rissanen, 2007). If, for instance, the usual AIC is used, the fitness function may be assumed

$$f(w) = \exp\left\{-\left(n\log(\hat{\sigma}_e^2) + 2(p+2)h\right)\right\},$$

where $\hat{\sigma}_e^2$ is the MSE as defined by (4.22) and $(p+2)h$ is the number of unknown parameters in (4.24), i.e. h arrays α's of p entries each, h thresholds δ's and h coefficients β's. All parameters are included in the array w as defined in (4.25) which assumes the meaning of chromosome in a GAs context. Note that w is a variable length chromosome because the GA population includes ANNs that may differ as regards the model order p and the number of neurons h. GAs with variable length chromosomes have been often considered in the literature (Minerva and Poli, 2001a, among others) and specialized genetic operators are widely available.

An extensive simulation experiment is reported in Delgado and Prat (1997) that compares the performance of ARIMA and seasonal ARIMA models and GAs-based ANNs in fitting several artificial time series generated by ARIMA and seasonal ARIMA models. Comparable results are displayed according to the MLD criterion as performance evaluation index and fitness function. In the ANN implementation neurons specialized for autoregressive representation and neurons specialized for the moving-average part are included to support the interpretation task and to allow a close comparison between estimates obtained by the ARIMA and the GAs-based ANNs modeling. As an application to a real data set the sunspot numbers time series is considered from 1700 to 1935 ($n = 236$ observations). Two ARIMA models , that is a subset AR model with three parameters at lags 1, 2 and 9, and a subset ARIMA models with AR lags 1, 2, 3, 4 and 8, 9, difference of order 11 and an MA parameter at lag 11, are compared with an ANN with 12 inputs, an hidden layer of 4 neurons and a single output. The variances of the residuals are reported 206, 195 and 184 but such small variances are obtained at the expense of a large number of parameters specially as far as the two latter models are concerned.

Modifications and considerations of further detail, such as subset lag choice, that may improve the model structure and contribute to reduce the number of parameters may be included in the GAs along similar guidelines without requiring major revision of the code and of the genetic operators.

Chapter 5
Design of Experiments

Abstract In several research areas, such as biology, chemistry, or material science, experimentation is complex, very expensive and time consuming, so an efficient plan of experimentation is essential to achieve good results and avoid unnecessary waste of resources. An accurate statistical design of the experiments is important also to tackle the uncertainty in the experimental results derived from systematic and random errors that frequently obscure the effects under investigation. In this chapter we will first present the essentials of designing experiments and then describe the evolutionary approach to design in high dimensional settings.

5.1 Introduction

In developing a scientific theory, testing a research hypothesis or getting insights into the process underlying an observable phenomenon, several questions may be addressed by experimental research. In conducting experiments, most of the system elements are supposed to be under the control of the investigator, who can then strongly affect the accuracy of the experimental result. The investigator plans (designs) the experiments, and then takes decisions on what has to be experimentally evaluated and how the experiments should be conducted. These decisions frequently are not easy and are certainly not innocuous. The validity of the interpretation of the experimental results strongly depends on the elements selected for the analysis and on the laboratory protocols chosen to conduct the experimentation. In several research areas, experimentation is complex, expensive and time consuming, so an efficient plan of experimentation is necessary to reach reliable results and avoid unnecessary waste of resources. An statistical design of the experiments is essential also to tackle the uncertainty in the experimental results derived from systematic and random errors that may obscure the effects under investigation. In this chapter we will first present the essentials of designing experiments and then describe the evolutionary approach to design in high dimensional settings. High dimensionality occurs when a large number of variables may affect the result of the experiments, and the available knowledge about the system does not allow a clear a priori choice of a small number of critical variables. High dimensionality is becoming a common

R. Baragona et al., *Evolutionary Statistical Procedures*, Statistics and Computing,
DOI 10.1007/978-3-642-16218-3_5,

and crucial problem in scientific and technological research, and conventional statistical procedures to design and analyze experiments do not address adequately the problem. In this chapter, we will describe a way to design experiments based on the Darwinian paradigm of evolution: the design is not chosen a priori, but is evolved through a number of "generations", using genetic operators modeled on biological counterparts. In this approach, the design, consisting of a collection of experimental points with different structure compositions, is regarded as a population that can evolve: a population of experimental points that changes through generations according to the evolutionary paradigm and the target defined by the investigator. This population is very small with respect to the size of the space of possible designs, but it changes through generations, "learning" from one generation to the next and thus exploring in an intelligent way the search space. We will present the basic structure of the Evolutionary Design of Experiments (EDoE), and describe how to use EDoE in high dimensional problems. Statistical models will then be invoked to identify the information obtained at each generation and to determine its significance. Incorporating this additional information from models in the evolutionary procedure makes the search much more efficient and effective. We will consider three variants of the general EDoE procedure: the Evolutionary Neural Network design (ENN-design), the Model-based Genetic Algorithm design (MGA-design), and the Evolutionary Bayesian Network design (EBN-design). In describing these approaches, our main concern will be biochemical experimentation, where the space of the variables involved is generally large, where the initial knowledge is frequently poor, and where a complex network of interactions among components characterize the system under study.

5.2 Experiments and Design of Experiments

An experiment is an empirical investigation of a particular system, whereby the investigator has the control on most of the elements and conditions that may affect the result of the experimentation. Objectives for conducting an experiment may be the comparison of different treatments or compositions (in medical or agriculture experiments), the study of the emergence of new entities or functionalities (in biochemical or material science experiments), or the optimization with respect to a defined target of the experimental unit compositions and laboratory protocols. An experimental design represents a strategy adopted by the investigator to conduct experiments and infer from the observed results accurate and useful information to reach the defined objectives. If the design, or the logical structure of the experiments is complete (accounting in an appropriate way for all the relevant elements affecting the results) valid inferences could be drawn from the results but if the design is faulty the interpretations on the results are also faulty (Fisher, 1935). Design of experiments (DoE) is nowadays a rich area of statistical research, employed in a variety of fields including medicine, agriculture, pharmacology, biochemistry, and material science (Cox, 1953; Cox and Reid, 2000; Fan et al., 2000; Wu and Hamad, 2000;

Lazic, 2004; Montgomery, 2009; Atkinson et al., 2007; Bailey, 2008). A scientific approach to experimentation involves both the design of each single experiment, and the analysis and modeling of the observed results. More specifically, an experimental design can be described as a selected set of experimental points (also named tests, trials, or just experiments) where different compositions and different laboratory conditions are compared to understand the results and frequently to optimize these results with respect to a particular target. Formally, an experimental design can be written as an n-dimensional vector

$$\mathbf{X} = (\mathbf{x}_1, \ldots, \mathbf{x}_n)'$$

where n is the number of selected experimental points and each element $\mathbf{x}_i$ is a p-vector

$$\mathbf{x}_i = (x_{i1}, \ldots, x_{ip}) \text{ with } i = 1, \ldots, n$$

describing the particular combination of p factors that under defined conditions may yield the experimental results

$$\mathbf{y} = (y_i), \text{ with } i = 1, \ldots, n.$$

Further, each factor x_k, $k = 1, \ldots, p$ may assume different levels that can vary among factors both in number and domain.

In a common and schematic way the system under study may be represented as follows:

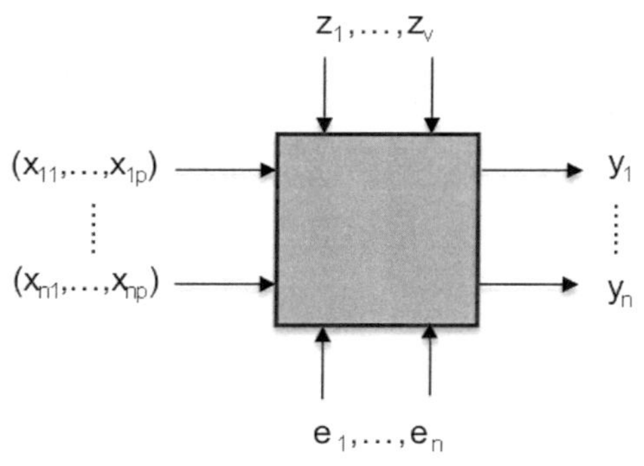

Fig. 5.1 General representation of a system

where the **x** vectors describe the set of variables selected as the relevant factors that independently or in relations among them (interactions) can affect the result of the experimentation. In this scheme the factors z_u, $u = 1, \ldots, v$, represent variables that can affect the results of the experimentation but are not under the control of the investigator, and the elements e_i, $i = 1, \ldots, n$, describe the experimental errors. Finally the results, or responses of the experimentation, are denoted by $y_1, \ldots, y_n$.

In designing the experiment the investigator is asked to determine the number of experimental points (n) to test for achieving reliable results; how many factors should be considered (p); which factors should be selected in a larger set of possible affecting factors; which and how many factors levels should be considered; and also which factor interactions should be investigated. In analyzing and modeling the resulting data the investigator is further asked to infer which factor and factor interactions are the most influential on the responses; which combination can optimize the response (uni or multi objectives optimization); which combination gives the smallest variability in the response; and finally, given the systematic and random errors in the experimentation, which level of uncertainty characterizes the estimation of relevant parameters and overall interpretation of the results.

Design and analysis are consequently strictly connected: statistical methods and models to analyze data and formulate interpretations on the underlying process depend on the design chosen, but the design depends on the questions of the investigator, on the structure of the problem, and on the possible settings of the process.

5.2.1 Randomization, Replication and Blocking

In designing experiments some basic and general principles have been introduced into the literature to increase the accuracy of the response; in particular the principles of randomization, replication, and blocking.

Randomization. In order to avoid bias or systematic errors the allocation of each factor level combinations to the experimental units and the order in which the individual experiment units are performed are randomly determined. Methods of allocation of factor combinations to units that involve arbitrary choice of the investigator are frequently subject to bias. A random allocation instead, prior to the start of the experiments, ensures that selections less plausible may be considered and the favored selections are not over-represented because of a systematic selection. Randomization can be achieved in different ways, but the most frequently adopted uses the random number generator, a computer program that produces strings of digits with no discernible tendency to produce systematic patterns.

In an increasing number of research fields randomization is now realized through a technology that using robot machines can allocate combinations to units in a random way. Typically in biochemistry research the high-throughput experimentation is conducted with microwell technology where a robotic device dispenses in a random way the different combinations to the different test tubes. Randomization is also required by most statistical methods of analysis that treat the observations as independently distributed random variables.

Replication. With the aim of determining an estimate of the experimental error and obtaining more precise estimates of the parameters of the chosen model, experimentation on each factor level combination is repeated a number of times (replications) in an independent and identical way.

It is worth noticing that replication is different from *repetition* of the measurement. In this last case different measurements are taken on the same experimental units, but these observations are not independent. Repeated measurements inform on the variability of the measurement systems, and replicated experiments inform on the variability between units and within units.

Blocking is a procedure to avoid haphazard errors that can occur during the development of the investigation. Haphazard errors may represent known intrinsic variations of the experimental units, variations in the elements (materials) of the compositions, variations in the development of the investigation, errors in measuring the response. For improving precision it may be possible to consider more uniform experimental conditions and materials, improving measuring procedures, or blocking the experiment. Blocking an experiment consists in dividing the experimental units into blocks, in such a way that the units in each block present similar experimental conditions. Frequently these divisions are already present in the structure of the problem: age and sex are natural blocks in experiments on people or animals; different batches of chemicals, possibly even from different providers, are blocks in chemical experimentation; plots of land different in fertility, composition, or sun exposition, are blocks in agricultural experiments. As a general rule blocks should all have the same size and be large enough to consider at least once each factors level combination.

These three basic principles should always be considered for whatever design the experimenter decide to construct.

5.2.2 Factorial Designs and Response Surface Methodology

We frequently encounter the problem of designing an experiment where several different factors can affect the response of the experiment, and we are interested in measuring their influence on the response and assessing the network of factors interactions relevant in determining this response. The design of these experiments, consisting of all possible combinations of the levels of the factors, with an equal number of replications, is generally named *factorial design* (Cox and Reid, 2000). In this structure each factor is characterized by a number of levels that may be qualitative, as for medical procedures, or quantitative, as for concentration, temperature, reaction time. If the number of factors and levels of each factor is high, the number of experimental units to investigate can be very high. For instance, selecting just 3 explanatory factors with 5 levels each, we should investigate 125 (5^3) experimental units in order to evaluate each combination, and 375 experimental units if we decide to replicate the evaluation three times.

Designing factorial experiments we may be interested in estimating the main factor effects, which are the averaged effects of each factor over all the units. Formally we can describe any experimental observation by an additive model. In a 3 factors problem, for instance, we can represent the observed response as

$$Y_{ijk,s} = \mu + \alpha_i + \beta_j + \gamma_k + \varepsilon_{ijk,s} \qquad i = 1, \ldots, a, \; j = 1, \ldots, b, \; k = 1, \ldots, c, \; s = 1, \ldots, m$$

where we assume that the factors, denoted A, B, C, at level i of A, j of B and k of C, affect the response $Y_{ijk,s}$ in the s replicate, with $s = 1, \ldots, m$, and in an additive way. The *main factor effects* on the response, represented by α_i, β_j, γ_k, describe the positive or negative deviation of the response from the constant μ when the factor is present. They are named main effects because they are regarded as the primary factors of interest in the experiment (Montgomery, 2009). In this representation the element $\varepsilon_{ijk,s}$ describes the random error component (unconsidered variables, experimental noise) and is generally assumed to have a Normal probability distribution with the form $\varepsilon_{ijk,s} \sim N(0, \sigma^2)$.

Factors may interact and these *interactions* can play a key role in affecting the behavior of the response of the experiment. We may in fact notice that the difference in response between the levels of one factor is not the same at all levels of other factors. This phenomenon is very common in pharmaceutical or biochemistry experiments, where compound reactions may produce abrupt changes in the response caused by variations in the factor level combination. The observed response $Y_{ijk,s}$, in a 3 factors problem, may be modeled as

$$Y_{ijk,s} = \mu + \alpha_i + \beta_j + \gamma_k + (\alpha\beta)_{ij} + (\alpha\gamma)_{ik} + (\beta\gamma)_{jk} + (\alpha\beta\gamma)_{ijk} + \varepsilon_{ijk,s}$$

where two and three level interactions are introduced in the dependence relation.

When the problem involves quantitative factors we can describe each experimental observation with a regression model

$$\begin{aligned} Y_{ijk,s} = {} & \beta_0 + \beta_1 x_{1i} + \beta_2 x_{2j} + \beta_3 x_{3k} + \beta_{12} x_{1i} x_{2j} + \beta_{13} x_{1i} x_{3k} + \beta_{23} x_{2j} x_{3k} \\ & + \beta_{123} x_{1i} x_{2j} x_{3k} + \varepsilon_{ijk,s}. \end{aligned}$$

The estimate of the parameters is generally derived with the least square method (Dean and Voss, 1999; Montgomery, 2009), and the analysis of variance (ANOVA) involving comparisons of measures of variations is also conducted to confront different levels and forms of variability. In the model above presented the sources of variations are the 3 factors chosen by the modeler to affect the response of the system. Tests of hypothesis to assess the relevance of factors or combinations of factors in influencing the response are also conducted (for a detailed analysis see, among others, Dean and Voss (1999) and Bailey (2008)).

When the main objective of experimentation is to optimize the response of the system, the *response surface methodology* is commonly adopted. This methodology explores the shape of the dependence relation of the response on a set of quantitative factors and uncovers the particular combination of factors levels that yields the maximum or minimum response. Suppose for instance, that two kind of molecules, x_1 and x_2, taken at different levels of concentration, x_{1i} with $i = 1, \ldots, a$, and x_{2j} with $j = 1, \ldots, b$, can give rise to a particular biological functionality. This functionality represents the response of the system (the target of the experimentation) and it is measured by an identified variable y. The dependence relation between the factors and the response can be described by

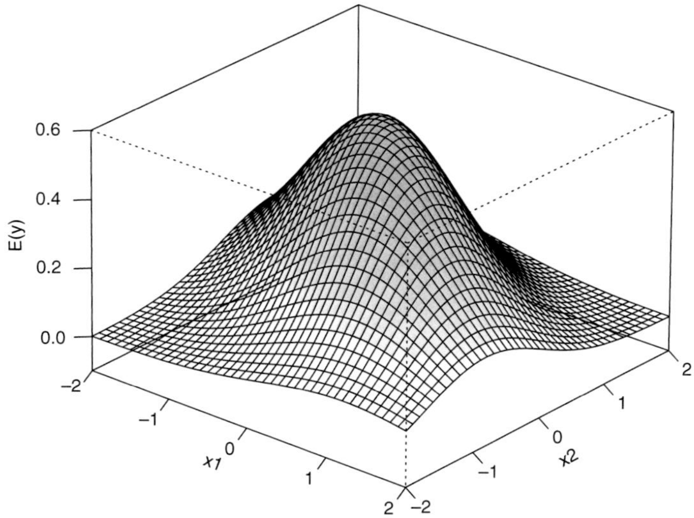

Fig. 5.2 A response surface for two factor design

$$y = f(x_1, x_2) + \varepsilon$$

where f may be a smooth function of x_1 and x_2 , and ε represents a random noise in the observable response. The expected response function $E(y) = f(x_1, x_2)$ is called *response surface*, and may have a graphical representation as in Fig. 5.2 where $E(y)$ is plotted on the two factors x_1 and x_2.

To determine the factor level combination that yields the maximum (or minimum, depending on the problem) one should adopt an experimental design that includes all possible factor level combinations and then achieve an experimental result for each location of the surface grid. This would involve a complete exploration of the chosen experimental space.

This design, involving all possible combinations, may be difficult to adopt when the number of experimental units to test is high. To estimate the response surface and determine the combination that give rise to the system optimum in such cases, a number of approaches have been proposed in the literature (Myers et al., 2004; Baldi Antognini et al., 2009). The most common way is to explore the space approximating the function with a first-order polynomial model,

$$y = \beta_0 + \beta_1 x_1 + \beta_2 x_2 + \ldots + \beta_p x_p + \varepsilon \tag{5.1}$$

where p factors are supposed to affect the response in a linear way without interactions; for each k, $k = 1, \ldots, p$, the parameter β_k measures the influence of factor k on y, and the error variable is assumed to be $N(0, \sigma^2)$.

When the surface shape is supposed to have curvature a second-order model may be more appropriate:

$$y = \beta_0 + \sum_{i=1,\dots,p} \beta_i x_i + \sum_{i=1,\dots,p} \beta_{ii} x_i^2 + \sum\sum_{i<j} \beta_{ij} x_i x_j + \varepsilon.$$

The approach of least squares estimates for the β parameters is then generally used and the adequacy of the fitted surface is evaluated with the ANOVA methodology.

However it is not generally the case that a polynomial model can approximate in an accurate way the response function on the entire experimental space. A common way to proceed is then to explore just a small area of the space, usually suggested by the experimenter, and approximate the dependence function with a first-order polynomial model (as in (5.1)). This model structure is usually appropriate for a small region of the factor space. In order to move from this region and reach the set of values where the optimum is located the *method of steepest ascent* is generally adopted when the optimum is the maximum value of the estimated response surface, or the *method of steepest descent* when the optimum is the minimum value of the surface.

The method of steepest ascent consists in selecting the direction in the space where the estimated response, namely $\hat{y} = \hat{\beta}_0 + \sum_{i=1,\dots,k} \hat{\beta}_i x_i$, increases more rapidly, with steps along the path towards the maximum that are proportional to the regression coefficients (Montgomery, 2009) . At any step the adequacy of the first order polynomial model is investigated with hypothesis tests both on the parameters and the variations through the analysis of variance. The procedure, which can be considered as “climbing a hill”, continues in the path of steepest ascent until a lack of fit of the first order model is encountered. This is considered as a hint that one is in the region of the maximum, so a second order polynomial model, incorporating curvatures, is chosen to approximate the response surface in this region. The identification of the set of factors levels $(x_{1i}, x_{2j}, \dots, x_{kr})$ that optimize the estimated response, is then achieved through calculus: the estimated response of the stationary point (the k-dimensional point for which the partial derivatives of the estimated response $\frac{\partial \hat{y}}{\partial \hat{x}_i}$ is zero) will provide the optimum value.

The selection of the designs to approximate the polynomial models can be chosen in a variety of ways. For a first order model a common procedure consists in selecting the class of designs that minimizes the variances of the regression coefficients; these are called the orthogonal first-order designs. For a second order model, the most popular choice is the class of central composite designs which consist of the first order design points augmented by a number of points selected at a specified distance from the design center in each factor direction.

5.3 The Evolutionary Design of Experiments

5.3.1 High-Dimensionality Search Space

Many areas of experimental research are characterized by large sets of parameters that can affect the result of the experimentation. Examples are expression profiles microarray studies, chemical microwell plate investigations, and biological organization analysis. In these fields the huge libraries of biological or chemical compounds now available, the different ways one can create compositions, and the great variety of laboratory protocols have produced a dramatic expansion of the number of parameters that scientists can control in developing their experiments; and the outcomes of their experiments, like discovering new drugs, new materials or new biological functionalities, may depend on not imposing a priori restrictions, to the dimensionality of the spaces through which their experiments must search (Minervini et al., 2009).

Conventional experimental approaches adapt with difficulties to this new setting of experimentation (Cawse, 2003): a classical factorial design for 10 factors and 5 levels for each factor prescribes a set of 9765625 (5^{10}) different experimental points to test, compare, and evaluate, and adding replications this number would at least triple. When experiments are costly and time consuming classical designs do not seem an appropriate way to plan experimentation. Fractional factorial experimental designs, denoted l^{p-j}, where the number of variables is reduced to $(p - j)$, have been proposed as a practical way to address this problem: the search space is reduced a priori, under the assumption that just a small group of variables and a small number of level interactions influence the response. However the selection of these variables and interactions before conducting any experiments may be difficult and misleading. Moreover in estimating main factors and interaction effects, alias effects may emerge generating ambiguities in interpretations that require difficult and quite complex analysis to resolve.

The high dimensionality problem is also encountered in the analysis of observed large data sets, and the conventional procedures for variable selection and feature extraction based on criteria such as Cp, AIC or BIC meet with difficulties because of the high computational time they required, which increases exponentially with the dimensionality. More recent approaches based on penalized likelihood methods (Greenshtein, 2006; Greenshtein and Ritov, 2004; Meinshausen and Bühlmann, 2006; Fan and Li, 2006), on wavelet decomposition (Donoho and Johnston, 1994) and on algebraic statistics (Pistone et al., 2000), have been recently proposed. These new approaches for variable selection and feature extraction have been so far applied to high dimensional data analysis, but they may find applications in the future in experimental design as well.

An alternative approach for experimental design in high dimensional spaces, already under active development is the subject of this chapter: the evolutionary approach (Forlin et al., 2008; De March et al., 2009a,b; Pepelyshev et al., 2009; Pizzi et al., 2009; Slanzi et al., 2009a,b; Slanzi and Poli, 2009; Borrotti et al., 2009) where the Darwinian evolutionary paradigm is used to formulate simple and efficient experimental design strategies.

5.3.2 The Evolutionary Approach to Design Experiments

Addressing the process of planning experiments in order to confirm a scientific hypothesis or compare different compositions the experimenter is asked to take a decision on a set of parameters that can affect the experimentation. As described in Section 5.2, the decision may concern a large set of parameters: *how many* and *which* factors should be considered in the investigation, given a known set of possible candidates; *how many* and *which* levels for each factor; *which* interactions among factors; and *which* experimental technology and laboratory protocols to employ. When the number of all these elements is high, the experimenter will not be able to proceed with the statistical designs involving all (or most of) the possible combinations of elements, and will make a selection of a small number of experimental units to test based generally on experience, previous knowledge or pilot experiments. This decision may or not lead to reliable and good results.

One way to address high dimensional search is to adopt the *evolutionary paradigm*. According to this approach the investigator can select an initial design consisting of a very small set of experimental points and test a selection of parameters (factors levels, laboratory protocols) chosen in a random way. Randomness (instead of just prior knowledge) allows the exploration of the space in areas not anticipated by prior knowledge but where interesting new effects may possibly reside. This initial design, or the first generation of experimentation, will then be conducted and their response observed. Following the principles of the evolution of living systems a second generation of tests is proposed with the factor and levels structure constructed according to a set of genetic operators that emulating natural systems behavior transform and evolve the design according to a defined target. The design is then achieved in a sequence of generations of experimentation where the information collected in one generation can feed the construction of the subsequent generation in order to achieve more and more valuable information with respect to a defined target.

The evolutionary approach represents an interactive process where the dialogue between design and laboratory experimentation at each generation creates a path in the combinatorial search space that may lead toward a region of optimality. This approach to experimental design has several nice features. Generation by generation, the evolving design requires a very small number of experimental points to test, and consequently a very small investment in resources. The small number of tests make very fast each phase of experimentation and it is always possible to monitor how much improvement there is from generation to generation. As this improvement slows, the entire procedure may be brought to a halt. Experience suggests that the procedure frequently reaches the optimality region in a surprisingly small number of generations. So it is an *easy, fast, low-cost and effective way* to design experiments.

In the following we will present different procedures in which the evolutionary approach has been developed. In particular, in this section, we consider the Genetic Algorithm design (GA-Design) and in the next section we will introduce the evolutionary model based design for which the evolutionary paradigm is combined with the statistical modeling, which can direct the search towards the most informative experimental points with respect to the specified target. On evolutionary design of experiments, we refer in particular to Poli (2006); Forlin (2009); Zemella and De March (2009).

5.3.3 The Genetic Algorithm Design (GA-Design)

For most optimization problems, experiments are designed to uncover the best factor level combinations that achieve a goal of interest. The design, as a set of combinations to be tested, can be regarded as a population of possible solutions to the problem. Each individual of this population is in fact an experimental point, or test, with a particular factor level combination that yields an experimental response.

A population-based design can be formulated in the following way.

Let $X = \{x_1, \ldots, x_p\}$ be the set of experimental factors, with $x_k \in L_k$, where L_k is the set of the factor levels for factor k, $k = 1, \ldots, p$. The experimental space, represented by Ω, is the product set $L_1 \times L_2, \ldots, \times L_p$. Each element of Ω, namely ω_r, $r = 1, \ldots, N$, is a candidate solution, and the experimenter is asked to find the best combination, ω_τ say, i.e. the combination with the maximum (minimum) response value.

Addressing the problem of finding ω_τ, the evolutionary approach can be adopted and a genetic algorithm can be constructed to design the experiments. Genetic Algorithms (GAs) (see Chap. 2, this volume; Blum and Roli, 2003; Heredia-Langner et al., 2003; De Jong, 2006; Schneider and Kirkpatrick, 2006) are iterative procedures inspired by nature capability to evolve living systems that learn and adapt to their environment. The GA in this case evolves populations of experiments through successive generations, adopting genetic operators that emulate nature in generating new solutions.

Building a GA an initial population at time 1, namely the design $\mathcal{D}^1$, is created generally in a random way: each element m of this population in the generation is described as a vector of symbols from a given alphabet (binary or decimal or other), and represents a candidate combination to be tested in this first population $\mathcal{P}^1$,

$$\mathcal{Y}^1 = \{\mathbf{x}_m^1\} = (x_{m1i}^1, \ldots, x_{mpr}^1) \qquad \text{with } m = 1, \ldots, n_1$$

and i, r as levels of the chosen factors.

In binary code this solution can be represented as a sequence of 0,1 digits, where 0, 1, expresses the absence or presence of a particular factor.

Using the terminology of biology, each experimental point is represented as a chromosome and each level of a particular factor is represented as a gene.

The size n of this population is generally taken to be very small with respect to the whole number of candidate solutions of the space Ω. Initially it is a randomly selected population because the algorithm should be able to explore the whole space and not be constrained in some areas of it (often the favorite areas of the experimenter).

Each element of this population ($m = 1, \ldots, n_1$), regarded as a candidate solution, is then evaluated in terms of its capacity to solve the problem: this evaluation is supposed to be measurable and represents the value of a fitness function f. Frequently the fitness function is the response of the test at the experimental point or a transformation of this measure. This first design $\mathcal{P}^1$ is expected to give some basic information to provide the construction of successive designs. The transition to the next generation (next population of experimental points) is in fact realized through a set of genetic operators that learn from the achieved information and process this information to obtain better solutions. Although a number of different operators have been suggested to realize the evolution the operators of selection, recombination and mutation are generally the most frequently employed. The *selection* operator chooses the experiments for next generation with respect to their fitness function: best experiments should have in fact high probability to be considered in the next generation (at the expense of the worst that do not seem to have a promising composition to reach the target). This operator corresponds to the principle of survival of the fittest living organisms in natural evolution. The proportional selection (or roulette wheel) is the most applied procedure and consists in selecting a member of the population with probability proportional to its fitness: the probability p_m^1, of the combination $\mathbf{x}_m^1$ is then assessed as

$$p_m^1 = \frac{f(\mathbf{x}_m^1)}{\sum_m f(\mathbf{x}_m^1)}$$

This procedure does not preclude low-fitness combinations to be part of the next generation, it just assigns them a very low probability to be selected. The reason for not simply selecting the combinations with highest values is that in each combination there may be some components which can become relevant in the future for their interaction with other components that arise in other generations.

Once selection has been completed, the *recombination* operator (or *cross−over* operator) can be applied. This operator recombines pieces of information present in different tests with the assumption that their interaction in a new test can give different (higher) fitness function values. The recombination operator randomly selects two members (parents) of the selected population and then breaks them at the same randomly chosen position. Afterwards it recombines the first part of one parent with the second part of the other, building in this way two offspring with different fitness values. The recombination can be realized also with two or more points of exchange according to the target of interest. In building a new population of test points, recombination can be very important to discover relevant interactions of components that at some specific unknown levels may produce great variation in the experimental response. This operator is generally applied with high probability and can deeply change the structure of the population and its associated fitness function values.

Selection and recombination operate on the existing compositions achieved and transformed from a previous population. In order to explore other areas of the experimental space the *mutation* operator can be applied. Mutation changes the factors and their levels in some members of the population: the operator randomly selects a few elements in the vector representation of each experimental composition (genes in the chromosome representation) and changes their values with different ones. This operator then assigns a positive probability to any candidate factor and respective level to be considered in a composition of the design. The main motivation of this operator is to introduce randomly some new components not yet selected or achieved in the previous process to become part of the design. As an example in a binary coding the mutation will transform the value 0 to a 1 or vice versa. Different coding will require a different transformation. If no other operator is applied then the new population of experimental points is ready to be conducted and evaluated, and the response of each element (the fitness function value) will be then used as the driving force for the evolutionary process.

The GA-design can be represented in the following way:

$\mathcal{D}^1 \leftarrow$ Randomly select an initial design from Ω
Conduct the experimentation testing each member of $\mathcal{D}^1$
    and derive its fitness function value
while termination conditions not met **do**
    $\mathcal{D}_1^1 \leftarrow$ Select($\mathcal{D}^1$)
    $\mathcal{D}_2^1 \leftarrow$ Recombine($\mathcal{D}_1^1$)
    $\mathcal{D}_3^1 \leftarrow$ Mutate($\mathcal{D}_2^1$)
$\mathcal{D}^2 \leftarrow$ Conduct the experimentation testing each member of $\mathcal{D}_3^1$
    endwhile

The convergence rate of the algorithm mainly depends on the code chosen for representing the factors level combinations and the probability of each genetic operator.

This iterative recursive procedure where the design identifies the experimental compositions to be tested and the evolution processes the test results to achieve the subsequent design, is the key concept to explore in a successful and easy way large experimental spaces.

It is worth noticing that the very positive feature of the GA-design is that the experimenter can avoid to reduce dimensionality by ad hoc procedures, which may mislead the search and hide fundamental components or interactions, and move in the entire search space along a path of improvement toward the optimality region. Randomness and evolution trace the path.

Example

As an example, we report an experimental study conducted in the biochemistry area (Bedau et al., 2005; Theis et al., 2008). This study aimed to find a molecular composition that can best generate vesicles: small and enclosed compartments that store or transport substances within a cell. Getting insight into this process is of scientific interest and can lead to important technological applications in several fields, including medicine and pharmacology.

From the literature it is known that certain amphiphilic molecules in particular environments may self-assemble and construct a variety of molecular aggregations such as vesicles, micelles or oil droplets. To study the emergence of vesicles the experimenter must select a set of candidate molecules from a large library of molecules, choose their level of concentration, and finally determine the laboratory protocol to conduct the experiments. These choices produce a very high dimensional search space.

A single experimental test consists in mixing a set of molecules taken at certain levels of concentration, under specified structural and process conditions. The response is recorded as a turbidity measure read by a fluorescent microscope, since turbidity is highly correlated to the vesicle volume.

From a library of amphiphilic molecules the experimenter selects 16 molecules, denoted and labeled as follows:

- Cholesterol, CHOL: X_1;
- 1,2-Dioleoyl-sn-Glycero-3-Phosphocholine, DOPC: X_2;
- 1,2-Dipalmitoyl-sn-Glycero-3-Phosphocholine, DPPC: X_3;
- 16:0PG or 1,2-Dipalmitoyl-sn-Glycero-3-[Phospho-rac-(1- glycerol)](Sodium Salt), DPPG: X_4;
- L-a-Phosphatidylcholine, Soy, PC: X_5;
- 1,2-Di-O-Octadecenyl-sn-Glycero-3-Phosphocholine, DIPC: X_6;
- Phytosphingosine (Saccharomyces cerevisiae) 4-Hydroxy- sphinganine, YPHY: X_7;
- 1,2-Dioleoyl-sn-Glycero-3-Phosphate (Monosodium Salt), PA: X_8;
- 1,2-Dioleoyl-sn-Glycero-3-Phosphopropanol (Sodium Salt), PPRO: X_9;
- 1-Oleoyl-2-Hydroxy-sn-Glycero-3-Phosphocholine, LPC: X_{10};
- 1,2-Diphytanoyl-sn-Glycero-3-Phosphocholine, MEPC: X_{11};
- 1,1',2,2'-Tetramyristoyl Cardiolipin(SodiumSalt), CARD: X_{12};
- 1,2,3-Trioleoylglycerol (Triolein), TRIO: X_{13};
- 1-Palmitoyl-2-Oleoyl-sn-Glycero-3-[Phospho-rac-(1-glycer- ol)](Sodium Salt), POPG: X_{14};
- L-all-rac-α-Tocopherol ($\geq$ 97%), VITE: X_{15};
- (2S,3R,4E)-2-acylaminooctadec-4-ene-3-hydroxy-1-Phos- phocholine(Egg, Chicken), SPM: X_{16}.

The experimentation have been conducted at Protolife Laboratory (Venice).

The vector $(X_1, X_2, \ldots, X_{16})$ represents the set of factors that the experimenter assumes will affect the response of the experiment. For their structure these experiments are known in the literature as *mixture experiments* (Cornell, 2002) since their factor levels $(x_{1i}, x_{2j}, \ldots, x_{pr})$ are chosen under the constraints $0 \leq x_{uv} \leq 1$ and $\sum_{uv} x_{uv} = 1$, with $u = 1, \ldots, p$ and v as an indicator of factor levels. According to the experimenter it is in fact the proportion of each factor in the mixture that affects the result, and not the total amount of the mixture. In this representation each element x_{uv} represents the number of the volume units of the molecule x_u. For technical reasons the experimenter introduced the constraint that each test can contain at most 5 different amphiphilic molecules. To design the experiment the natural questions are then:

- which amphiphilic molecules should be considered in the experiments?
- at which level will each be?
- which interactions among different amphophilic molecules will be relevant in generating vesicles?

To answer these questions, the experimenter could follow the classical Simplex Lattice Design (Cornell, 2002; Montgomery, 2009); but this design requires testing 15504 different combinations, which was not feasible for several reasons, including cost and time. Adopting instead the evolutionary approach a very small number of tests could be suggested and evaluated, and the results could be achieved in a quick and easy way.

In this research the evolutionary design was derived building a GA. This algorithm randomly selects a first population of 30 different mixture compositions. These mixtures have been tested in the laboratory, and three replicates per mixture have been conducted, in order to obtain information on the experimental noise. The size of the design, 30 tests replicated three times, derives from the structure of the technology used, a 96-microwells plate. As an example, the vector $(x_{5i} = 0.20; x_{7j} = 0.20; x_{11k} = 0.40; x_{15l} = 0.20)$ represented in the sequence

0.0	0.0	0.0	0.0	0.2	0.0	0.2	0.0	0.0	0.0	0.4	0.0	0.0	0.0	0.2	0.0

is a mixture of this initial design. Once the experimentation has been completed the response of each mixture is recorded. The response values, regarded as fitness values, drive the evolutionary process.

In this experiment selection, recombination and mutation operators have been applied.

The *selection* has been realized with the proportional probability criterion and mixtures with higher fitness result more represented in the new generation, at the expense of the ones with lower fitness. This operator raises the average fitness value of the new generation of mixtures, increasing the number of the good solutions but leaving their structure unchanged. The next operators work instead transforming the structure of some mixtures.

The *recombination* operator broke some selected mixtures in two or more parts to create new ones by recombining these in different ways. In this research, the constraint of being mixture experiments (the sum of the factors levels concentration is equal to one) leads to the following procedure: randomly select two mixtures and a number of volume units, say z in the interval [1–4] from one of them; then randomly select z volume units from the first mixture and v, with $v = 5 - z$, volume unit from the second mixture and recombine these elements to achieve a new mixture. The remaining elements from the two initial mixtures also recombine and form the second new mixture (in the terminology of the GA two children replace the two parents). The rate of the recombination used was 0.40.

The *mutation* operator moved one volume unit from a position of a mixture composition to another randomly chosen position of the same composition with the rate 0.40.

In addition to these standard operators, the experimenter also employed an *innovation* operator, which randomly generated new mixtures, with innovation rate 0.20.

This algorithm derived 5 generations of experimentation, testing 150 different mixtures (no mixture could occur more than once in all the generations). The total number of conducted tests represents then less than 1% of the whole space (0.96%). In spite of this extremely small number of tests, compared to the whole set of candidate combinations, the GA-design displays a good performance: the value of the average fitness increases from 0.161 of the first generation to 0.270 of the fifth generation and the highest fitness value in the generation (the response value of the best combination) increases from 0.477 to 0.748. The following Fig. 5.3 exhibits the responses of all the tests conducted.

With the GA-design it was possible to uncover populations of factor levels combinations with higher and higher performance, analyzing just a very small number of experimental points.

Modeling the relation between the response of the tests and the factors levels combinations the following polynomial interaction model have been derived (on the construction of the model see Forlin et al. (2008)),

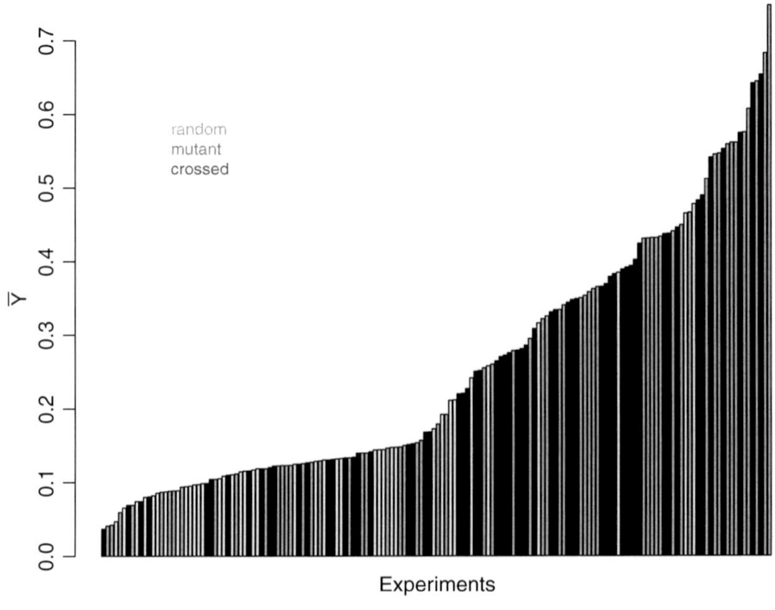

Fig. 5.3 Responses of the conducted tests

$$Y_m = \sum_{i=1}^{16} \beta_i x_{im} + \sum_{i=1}^{16} \sum_{k,i<k} \beta_{ik} x_{im} x_{km} + \sum_{i=1}^{15} \sum_{k,i<k} \beta_{ik4} x_{im} x_{km} x_{4m} + \sum_{i=1}^{15} \sum_{k,i<k} \beta_{ik8} x_{im} x_{km} x_{8m} + \sum_{i=1}^{15} \sum_{k,i<k} \beta_{ik13} x_{im} x_{km} x_{13m} + \varepsilon_m$$

where Y_m denotes the system response in the m mixture, x_{im} is the number of volume units of the ith amphiphilic molecule in the mth mixture, β_i describes the response to pure factor i, the remaining coefficients β describe the response to either the synergistic or antagonist blending and finally ε is a Gaussian noise component to represent the experimental error. The model is fit under the constraint $\sum x_i = 1$ on the component proportions, and the problem of identifiability of the parameters β_i and β_{ij}, introduced by the constraint on the sum of the x_i terms, has been addressed by omitting the intercept term, as suggested by Cornell (2002).

To infer the model parameters from the data a combined forward and backward stepwise regression has been used and evaluated with the ANOVA procedure. The main achievement from the estimated model has been to discover that some particular molecules, at some concentration levels and interacting with other molecules are present in mixtures with high response levels, as x_4, x_7, x_8, x_{13}. Deriving the contours plots it has been possible also observe in easy way the change of interaction effect through generations. Selecting the factors interaction x_4, x_8, x_{13}, the contour plots in Fig. 5.4 show the increase of the effect of the interaction from the second to the fifth generation.

To get more insights on the evolutionary process of the design and know if and how this procedure gets close to the optimal response, a simulation platform has been created adopting a data generating model with the same structure obtained in modeling the experimental results.

Conducting the simulation (Forlin et al., 2008) an initial random population of 30 mixtures was selected, and a fitness function value, derived from the estimated

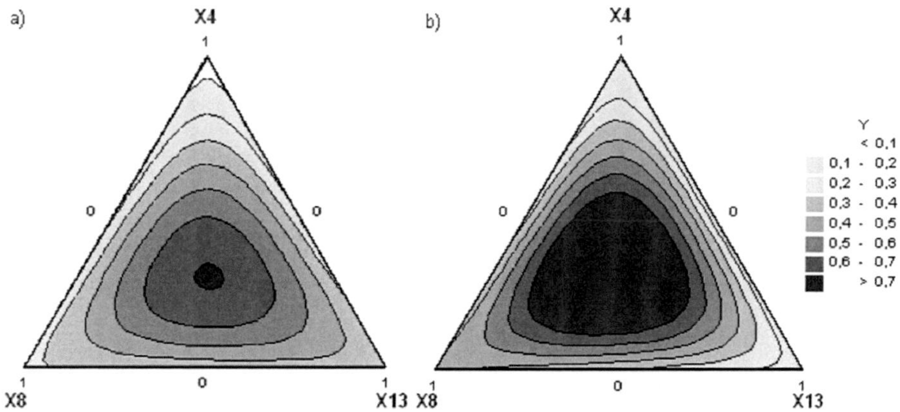

Fig. 5.4 Contour plots of the factors interaction x_4, x_8, x_{13} at the second generation (**a**) and at the fifth generation (**b**)

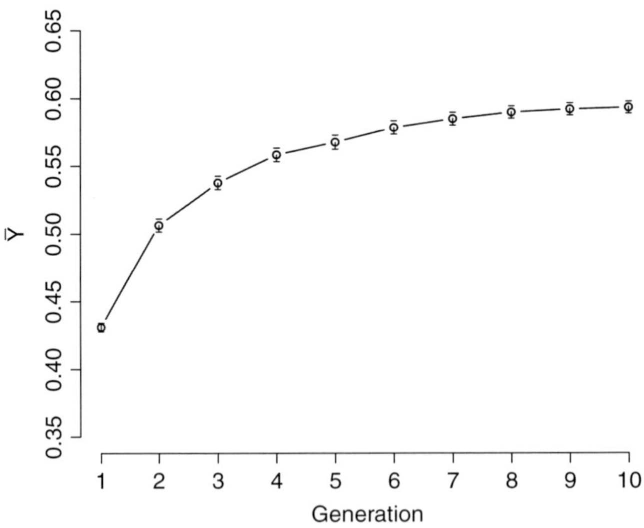

Fig. 5.5 The average response value at each generation achieved with the GA-Design

regression model, is assigned to each mixture. On this population the algorithm develops the iterative process, which involves selection, recombination, and mutation according to the same structure proposed for the real experimentation. The evolution is developed for 10 generations, and concerns 500 simulations.

The most interesting results from this simulation study are the behaviors of the average response and the best response through generations. As represented in Fig. 5.5, the average simulated response increases in a monotonic way from the first to the tenth generation, and the box-plots at each generation shows a very small variability of the average values.

The behavior of the average of the best response at each generation is also increasing, reaching the highest value in the 9th generation (no mixture is in fact allowed to be considered more than one time in the study) with very small variability, as described in Fig. 5.6.

Finally, to evaluate how the GA-design is able to uncover the best tests of the whole simulated space a frequency distributions of the responses is obtained and the 99th quantile is derived. This quantile is the left bound value of the 1% best experiments interval. The GA-design is able to enter in this interval in the second generation and then it continues to uncover an increasing number of the best experiments, reaching 12.4% in 10 generations. This search is illustrated in the Fig. 5.7.

Thus, as this example shows, the evolutionary design derived with a simple genetic algorithm can reach good results testing just a small number of experimental points. The procedure is fast, easy and reduces greatly the cost and time required to explore high dimensional experimental spaces, in comparison with classical designs.

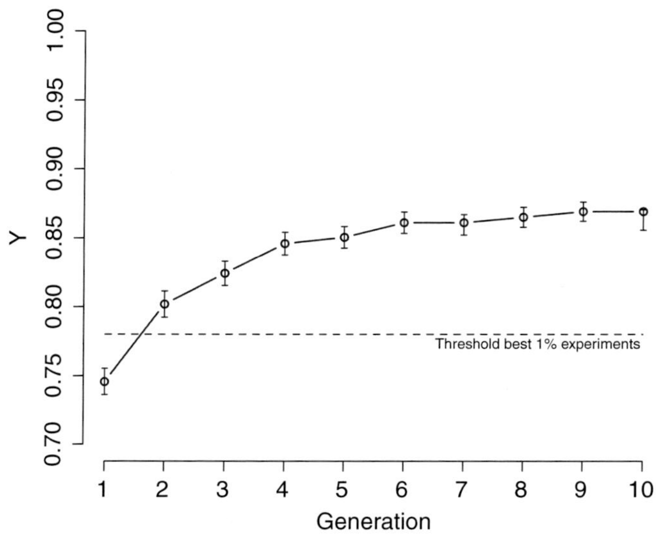

Fig. 5.6 The best response value at each generation achieved with the GA-Design

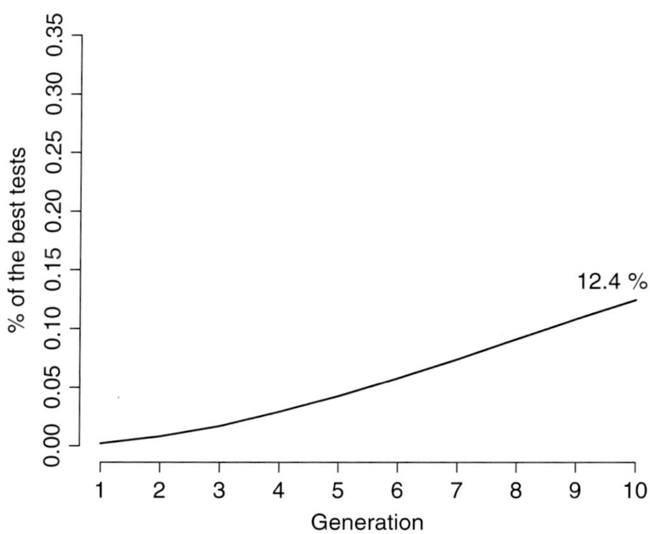

Fig. 5.7 The proportion of the best tests uncovered by the GA-Design in 0.01 right tail area of the response distribution

5.4 The Evolutionary Model-Based Experimental Design: The Statistical Models in the Evolution

At any generation the evolutionary design supplies the experimenter with a data set that consists of the structure and the laboratory response of each single test belonging to the population of that generation. This data set leads the evolution of the design, since at any generation test structures and responses are processed to build the next test generation. The information in one data generation can then affect deeply the composition of the next generation.

However, the relevant information that is contained in these data sets is much more than what is generally considered in an evolutionary procedure: the special role played by some factors and some particular levels, or the effect of different order factor interactions, should not be ignored, but identified and used to construct the next generation design. Modeling is the best way to extract this information from data. Models can in fact uncover and estimate the main relevant factors, detect and weigh the main interactions, measure the reliability of noisy results, and make predictions about unexplored regions of the search space. Therefore models can supplement the result data bases to make the evolutionary process more efficient and effective, discovering and communicating information between successive populations of experiments.

In the following sections we will describe and discuss some evolutionary model-based procedures. In particular we will present the Evolutionary Neural Nets design (ENN-design), the Model-based Genetic Algorithm design (MGA-design), and the Evolutionary Bayesian Networks design (EBN-design).

5.4.1 The Evolutionary Neural Network Design (ENN-Design)

The concept of evolution driven by neural network modeling inspires the Evolutionary Neural Network design (ENN-design), introduced by De March et al. (2009a). Neural networks models are known to be a powerful way to address complex and high dimensional systems. Neural network models have also been shown to be excellent tools for prediction (Apolloni et al., 2009; Poli and Jones, 1994) given their approximating properties and their capacity to deal with nonlinear relationships. The evolutionary design of experiments can be derived by exploiting the capacity of these models to predict the behavior of complex processes and by incorporating the achieved information in an iterative procedure.

Initially the predictive neural network design selects in a random way a population of experimental points and candidate sets of parameters (factors, levels, process conditions, ...) determining the structure of the first test population. These tests are carried out, and a response is measured for each of them. On the data set that includes both the experimental structures and the results, a neural network model is then constructed. A simple three layers architecture network with a feed-forward dynamics is used (De March et al., 2009a). The connection strengths of the network are evaluated on a subset of the population, identified as a training set, and the model is selected on a different set of data, the validation set. The predictive capacity of the model is finally tested and the accuracy of the predictions selects the best model. This model is then adopted to explore the whole unknown space of candidate tests, and for each of them derives a predicted response. A small set of those tests with the best predicted responses is then added to the initial population creating the second generation of tests to be conducted and from which to achieve the response (second design). A data set for this generation is now available: it includes the initial population of tests and the best predicted tests. On this second larger data set a predictive neural network model is then estimated and adopted to uncover the best predicted structures in the experimental space; the set of these best structures will then be added to the second generation. The procedure continues for a number of generations until a stopping rule criterion is reached. This is an evolutionary and adaptive design: a small set of experiments is evolved through a sequence of generations with a neural net model that, learning from data and predicting the unexplored experimental space, can achieve the relevant information to improve the design and intelligently adjust the way to reach the optimality region.

Example

The predictive neural network design has been applied in a simulation study to evaluate its performance and develop comparisons with other competitive approaches (De March et al., 2009b; Forlin et al., 2007). The problem that has been considered and examined in the previous Section involves experiments with a mixture structure, as described in Theis et al. (2008). Each experimental test is a composition of 16 candidate factors that can assume 6 different levels, $x_i = (x_{i1}, \ldots, x_{i16})$, $i = 1, \ldots, 6$, and involves an experimental search space that under a factorial (full or fractional) design consists of a huge number of combinations to be tested. The goal of the experiment is to find the combination that yields the highest response value. The ENN-design initiates the search selecting in a random way a first generation of 30 compositions to represent the first design in the evolution. Each composition receives a response from a stochastic generating process derived by Forlin et al. (2008), (the stochastic generator process play the role of the laboratory experimentation in providing the response). On this data set, that includes experimental test structures and responses, a three-layer neural network model is proposed and its connections estimated on a training set (80% of the data set). The network with the minimum predictive error computed in the validation set is then considered as the best predictive net and adopted to predict the response of all the possible tests of the experimental space. The best 30 predicted experiments are further selected and added to the first random population. The iterative procedure then restarts considering this new generation of experiments, that includes the initial set and the best predicted set achieved with the neural network model. Each generation of experiments is supposed to contain more information with respect to the previous one, and the model from these data is supposed to give more and more accurate predictions. This simulation study has been developed in 10 generations and 500 simulations. The main results are summarized in the following figures. The behavior of the average

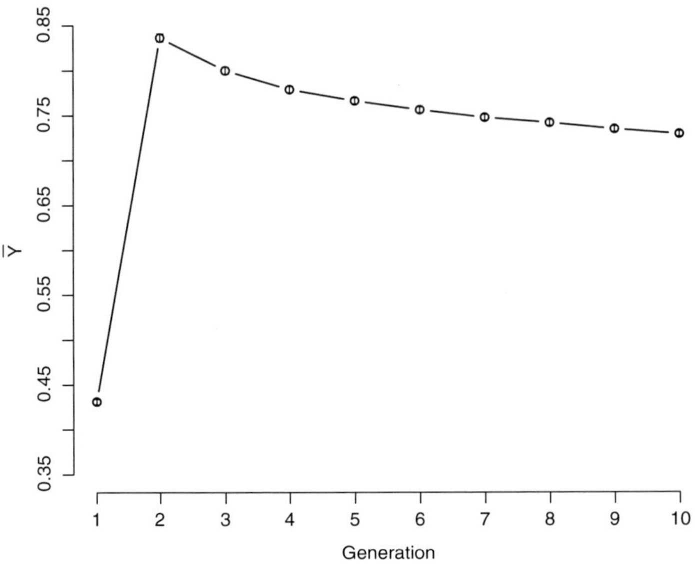

Fig. 5.8 The average response value at each generation achieved with the ENN-Design

response value, as described in Fig. 5.8, show a very strong increase at the second generation and after that a monotonic decrease: the ENN-design seems to uncover the best compositions in the second generation, and since no composition is allowed to be considered more than one time, the average values decrease.

The behavior of the best composition, as described in Fig. 5.9, confirms the previous comments: the neural net model selects the best solution at the second generation, afterwards the successive generation best solutions present lower values. No solution better than the one found in the second generation emerges in the following

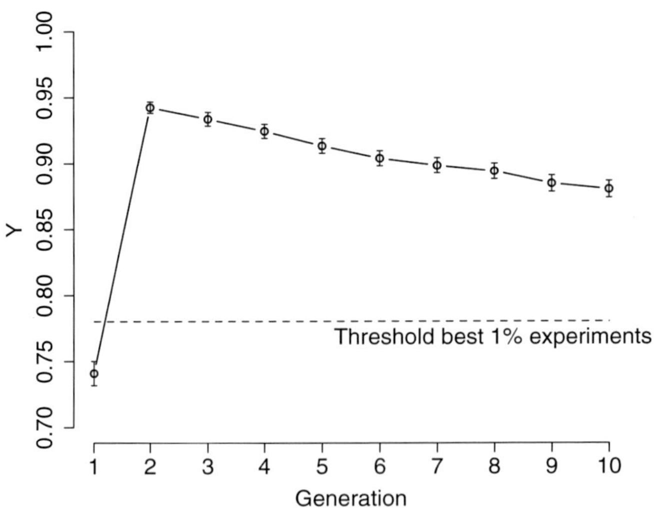

Fig. 5.9 The best response value at each generation achieved with the ENN-Design

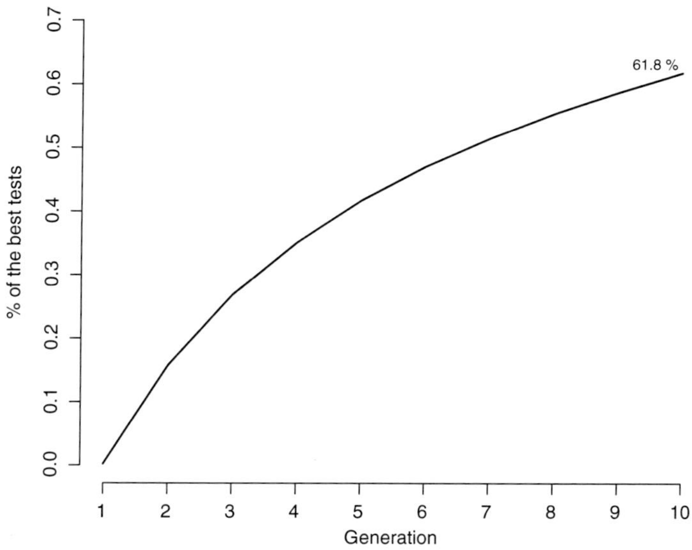

Fig. 5.10 The proportion of the best tests uncovered by the ENN-design in 0.01 right tail area of the distribution

ones. The dashed line gives the value of the 99th quantile of the distribution of the experiments, and shows that the best solution found by the evolutionary procedure is always grater than this value, which is by definition an extremely high value.

In evaluating the performance of the design it is also important to derive the proportion of the experiments passing the threshold of the 99th quantile of the distribution, that is the set of excellent experiments that have been discovered by the procedure. In Fig. 5.10, the behavior of this proportion shows that at the tenth generation the procedure discovers 61.8% of the best tests (the 1% best combinations of the whole experimental space). This is an excellent result, given the extremely small size of the design.

5.4.2 The Model Based Genetic Algorithm Design (MGA-Design)

The evolutionary design derived with genetic algorithms, as described in Sect. 5.3.3, can address the search problem in high dimensional spaces using few resources and achieving good results. In this design the evolution of test populations through generations is led by the responses of each tests and a set of genetic operators. However, more information could be obtained at each generation by modeling the data sets of experimental test compositions and responses, and then embedding this information in the genetic evolutionary process. The Model-based Genetic Algorithm design (MGA-Design) is constructed according to this principle (Forlin et al., 2007; De March et al., 2009a,b). Modeling the data set at any generation of the algorithm provides supplementary information that can guide the action of the genetic operators creating a more intelligent evolutionary dynamics.

The MGA-Design starts by selecting an initial population of tests. This population is chosen randomly and its size, n, is very small compared to the size of the whole experimental space. The tests of this first design, coded as a sequence of digits (as described in Sect. 5.3.3) are then conducted in the laboratory and the response of each experiment is recorded. On the obtained data set, that includes the composition and response of each test, a model is selected and estimated to make predictions. Polynomial models, nonlinear regression models, or other nonlinear models may be used to represent the relation and formulate predictions. The selection operator is then applied to the population according to the proportional probability criterion (other selection criteria might be chosen instead). From this selected population two compositions, regarded as parent compositions, are chosen and broken in two pieces at the same cut point and *for all possible cut points* of the sequence. For each cut point the first piece of the first composition is then recombined with the second piece of the second composition giving rise to a new composition (child) for the next generation; recombination is then applied to the remaining parts of the two parents giving rise to another composition (child). Thus, each cut point yields two different children, and so each pair of compositions can generate $2 \times (M - 1)$ new compositions (where M is the compositions length). We illustrate the operator in Fig. 5.11.

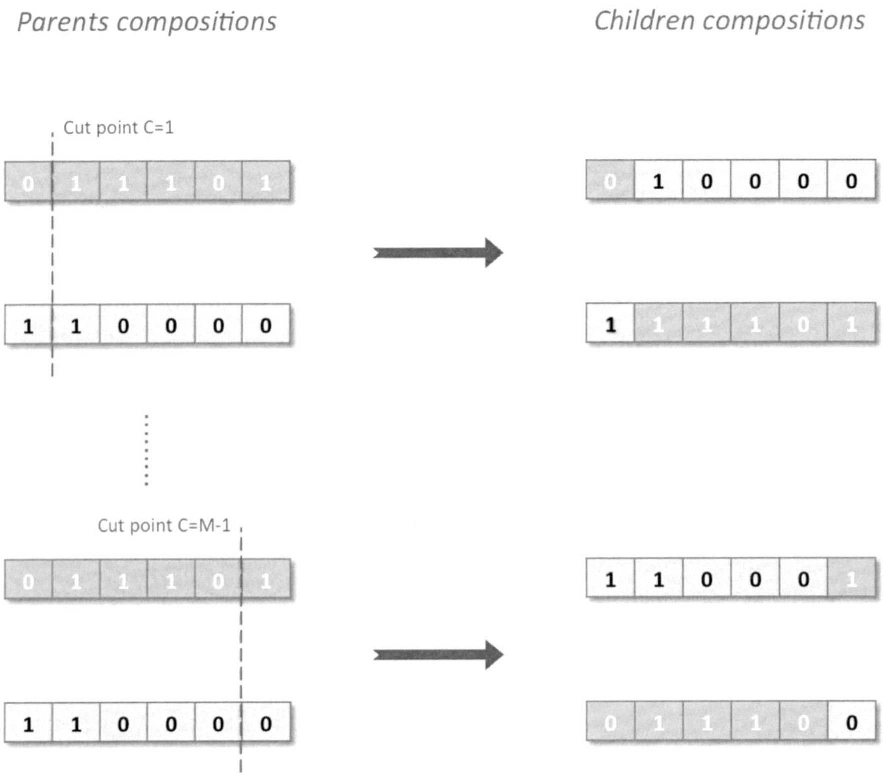

Fig. 5.11 The cross-over operator of the MGA-Design

Therefore, from the selected pair of compositions a population consisting of all the possible different combinations of sub-sequences is derived, namely all the possible different children that the couple can originate with these operators. In order to choose the best two new compositions for the next generation the estimated model is adopted to predict their responses (instead of conducting these populations of tests in the laboratory). For each parent pair, the two children with best responses are selected as candidates to replace their parents in the next generation. This procedure is repeated for *n* selected pairs, and the resulting "best children" comprise the next population (Forlin et al., 2007). Further genetic operators, such as mutation, could also be employed on this set of compositions before obtaining the "final" population to perform in laboratory. The foregoing procedure then iterates until a stopping rule criterion is satisfied.

The evolutionary procedure of the MGA-design is represented in Fig. 5.12. Making faster and more intelligent the evolution of the GA-Design, statistical models can be estimated on the resulting data to derive the next generation of experiments. Modeling these experiments we can in fact develop a sequential learning procedure which can lead the evolution process.

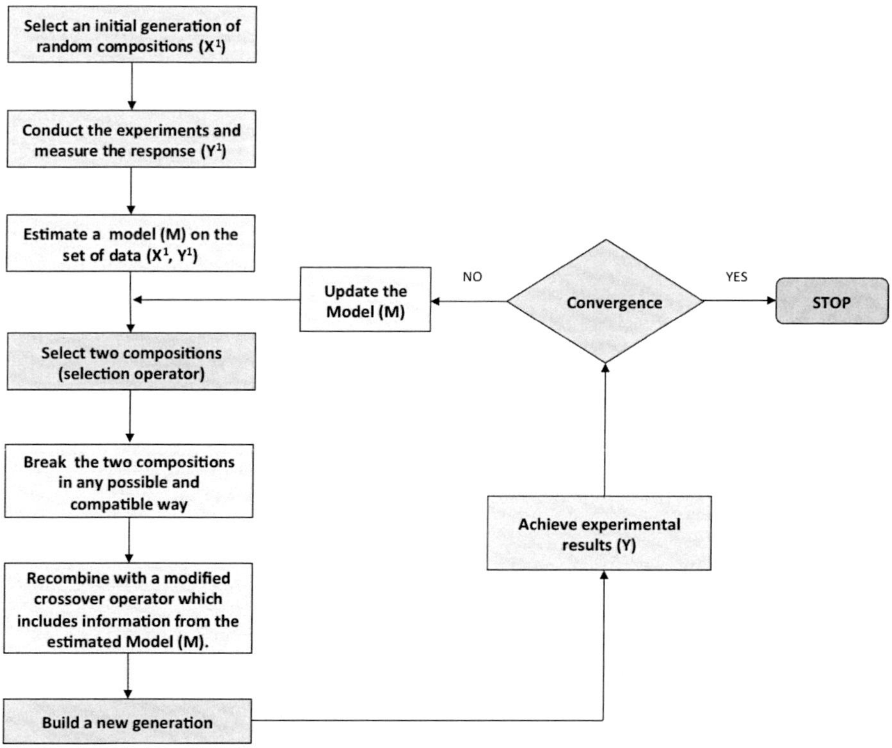

Fig. 5.12 The evolutionary procedure of the MGA-Design

Example

A simulation study has been conducted to evaluate the performance of the MGA-design for high dimensional experimental problems (Forlin et al., 2007). In order to develop a comparison with the simple GA-design the same structure of experimentation that has been considered in the example of Sect. 5.3.3 is proposed, namely 16 factors that can assume 6 different levels. The goal of the experimentation is to uncover the particular composition that obtains the highest response value. In the simulation analysis a first population of 30 random mixtures is selected, with representation ($\mathbf{X}^1$) matrix with size (30×16). A stochastic generator process is then used to assign a response (Y^1) to each row of X (the stochastic generator process plays again the role of the laboratory experimentation in providing the response). On this data set ($\mathbf{X}^1$, Y^1) a model in the form of a third order polynomial regression model is chosen and estimated in order to formulate accurate predictions. The selection operator is then applied with a proportional probability, and a generation of compositions is achieved for recombination. The recombination operator, acting with a probability $p_r = 0.90$, selects two compositions, breaks them in two parts a number of times as the number of any possible cut-points (as above described) and then recombines each first part of a composition with the second part of the other composition. The result is the "children-population" achieved by a couple of compositions acting as "parents". The procedure continues deriving the response of all these compositions by predicting them with the model selected on the previous population. The two best predicted children-compositions are then chosen to be part of the new generation. The recombination is repeated for all the couples of compositions (parent compositions) and the resulting generation (30 compositions) is tested recording the responses. This iteration is repeated for 10 generations, with 500 simulations. The main results of this design are represented in their evolution in the following Figs. 5.13, 5.14, and 5.15. The average behavior of the experimental

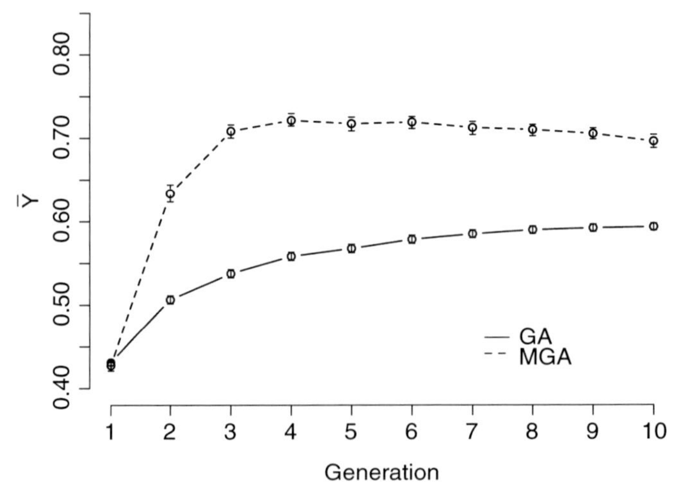

Fig. 5.13 The average response values at each generation achieved with the GA-Design and MGA-Design

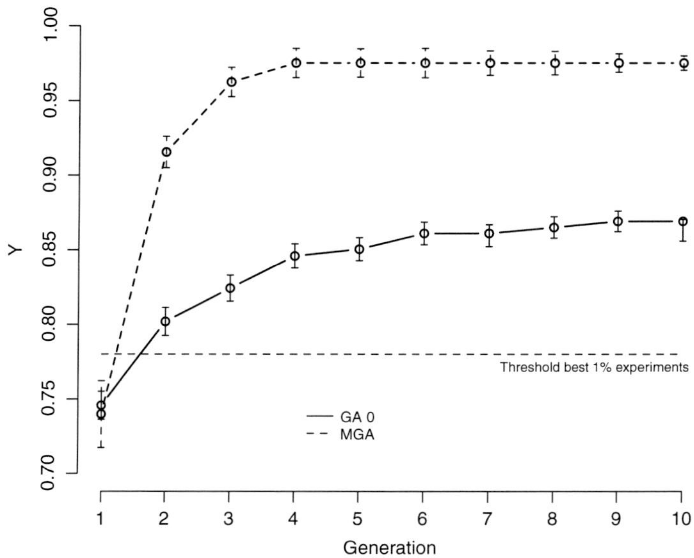

Fig. 5.14 The best response values at each generation achieved with the GA-Design and the MGA-Design

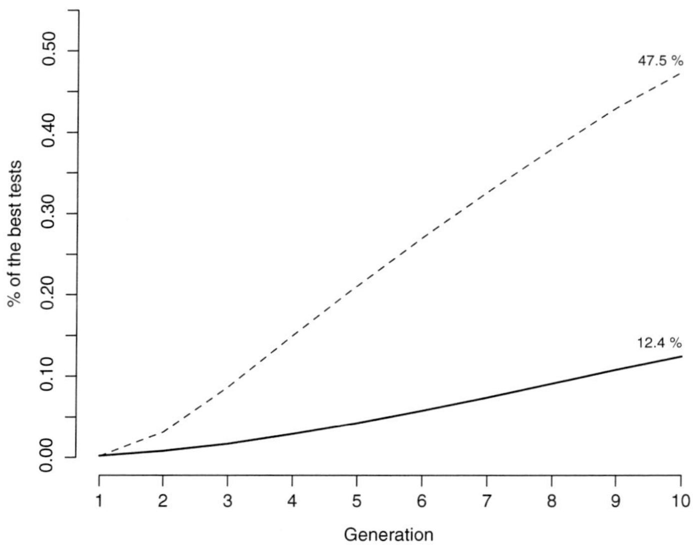

Fig. 5.15 The proportion of the best tests uncovered by the MGA-design in 0.01 right tail area of the response distribution (MGA, *dashed line*) compared with the proportion of the GA-Design (*solid line*)

response in the MGA-Design exhibits a strong increase from the first to the third generation and a constant behavior or a slow decrease after the fourth. The design finds the best solutions in the fourth generation and, since no composition can be considered more than once in all the generations, the average behavior starts to decrease. Therefore in this study the evolutionary design can find the best compositions in 4 generations, testing a very small number of experiments. This very good behavior of the MGA-design emerges also in comparison with the simple GA-Design reported in the Fig. 5.13. The performance of MGA with respect to GA is much higher, reaching the best compositions in very few generations.

Also the behavior of the best test in each generation exhibits a strong increase until the fourth generation, followed by a very slow decrease. The best composition in each generation is then uncovered at the fourth generation and takes a value much higher than the best composition found with the simple GA-design (see Fig. 5.14). Finally deriving the 99th quantile of the responses distribution, we observe a great increase of the proportion of the best compositions in the 1% right tail area of the distribution.

These results show that *modeling* can play a fundamental role in the evolutionary process making the search in high dimensional spaces much more efficient.

5.4.3 The Evolutionary Bayesian Network Design (EBN-Design)

In designing experiments the interaction network among the different factors should be identified and analyzed, since it might play an important role in affecting the response of the experimentation. This interaction network might be in fact the most, if not the only, relevant effect on the response. Getting insights into these networks, and uncovering their architecture and dynamics, can then be very valuable for designing experiments. A way to study these networks from data consists in modeling the dependence relationships among the experimental factors with the class of Bayesian networks (Lauritzen, 1996; Poli and Roverato, 1998; Cowell et al., 1999; Jensen, 2001; Borgelt and Kruse, 2002; Pelikan, 2005; Slanzi et al., 2008; Darwiche, 2009).

A Bayesian network consists of a set of nodes, which identify random variables $(X_i, i = 1, \ldots, n)$ with a finite set of states, and arcs, which identify the direct dependence relations between the variables. The dependence relation is described by the conditional probability values $P(X_i|X_j), i, j = 1, \ldots, n, i \neq j$, while the absence of a dependence relation between variables is described by the lack of a directed arc between nodes. The network is then described as a probabilistic graphical model that, using the combined capabilities of graph theory and probability theory, can describe and measure complex interaction structures.

For example, the variable set $(X_1, \ldots, X_{10}, Y)$ may be characterized by the dependence relation structure as presented in Fig. 5.16.

In this network the variables X_1, X_2, X_4 directly depend on X_5; X_6, X_9, X_{10} on X_2; X_3 and X_7 on X_1; X_8 on X_3 and the variable Y on X_6, X_9. Also, given the information in X_6 and in X_9, the variable Y is conditional independent of all the remaining variables of the system. The entire structure of the conditional dependence and independence relations can then be read from the topology of the network,

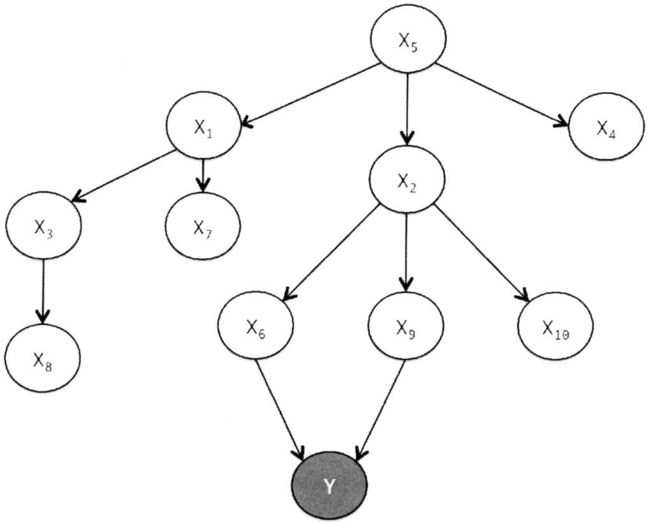

Fig. 5.16 Example of a Bayesian network

and can be represented by the joint probability distribution of the set of variables that define the problem. By using the probability multiplication law, the joint probability distribution of the variables can be decomposed as a product of $n-1$ conditional distributions and a marginal distribution, as follows:

$$P(\mathbf{X}) = P(X_1, \ldots, X_n) = \left[\prod_{i=2}^{n} P(X_i|X_1, \ldots, X_{i-1})\right] P(X_1).$$

In this framework the variable X_j may be said to be a descendant of the variable X_i if there is a path between X_j and X_i, otherwise X_j is said to be a non-descendant of X_i. The expression $pa(X_i)$ is used to represent the parent set of X_i, namely the set of variables on which X_i directly depends. Moreover, each variable X_i is conditionally independent of all its non-descendants in the graph given the set of its parents. This statement holds in any Bayesian network (BN) and it constitutes a fundamental property, also known in the literature as the Markov property. The network can then be factorized as the product of the variables probabilities conditional on their parents only:

$$P(\mathbf{X}) = P(X_1, \ldots, X_n) = \prod_{i=1}^{n} P(X_i|pa(X_i)).$$

The joint probability distribution, representing the interaction structure of the network in the Fig. 5.16 can then be factorized as

$$P(X_1, \ldots, X_{10}, Y) = P(X_1|X_5) \cdot P(X_2|X_5) \cdot P(X_3|X_1) \cdot P(X_4|X_5) \cdot P(X_5) \cdot P(X_6|X_2) \cdot P(X_7|X_1) \cdot P(X_8|X_3) \cdot P(X_9|X_2) \cdot P(X_{10}|X_2) \cdot P(Y|X_6, X_9).$$

In selecting a model to derive an experimental design, the BN can then be a useful way to estimate from data the dependence/independence relations between factors and their influence on the response of the experiment. Also, this estimated structure of dependence can be incorporated in the evolutionary approach and leads to the *Evolutionary Bayesian Network design*, EBN-Design (Slanzi et al., 2009a,b; Slanzi and Poli, 2009). In this approach, the experimental design is achieved according to the rules of the evolutionary paradigm, enriched by the information obtained by the estimated BN model. To build the EBN Design a first set of possible factor combinations is generated in a random way and the corresponding response Y is derived by conducting the experiments. A selection operator is then applied and according to the response Y a new set of factor combinations is chosen to build the next generation. On this first set of data a Bayesian network is then estimated by assessing and maximizing the posterior probability of the network. A well-known estimation procedure consists in deriving the "Bayesian score function" (Heckerman et al., 1995).

From this posterior probability distribution, a new set of factor compositions is then derived and a small set of the best compositions (the compositions with the highest values of Y), is selected and regarded as the second generation of experiments to be evaluated. The procedure continues through generations until a stopping rule is satisfied.

Example

In order to evaluate the performance of the EBN-Design, and make comparisons among different evolutionary algorithms, a simulation study has been conducted (Slanzi et al., 2009a,b; Slanzi and Poli, 2009). To facilitate the comparison, the same experimental problem described in Sect. 5.3.3, concerning biochemical mixture experiments is considered (De March et al., 2009a,b; Forlin et al., 2008, 2007). The EBN-Design starts with a population of 30 mixtures chosen in a random way in the experimental space. To each of these mixtures is assigned a response achieved by the same stochastic generator process used in the previous examples. Following the evolutionary process the selection operator is then applied to derive the next generation of mixtures, and on this data set a Bayesian network is estimated by maximizing the posterior probability distribution of the factors $\mathbf{X}$ and the response Y. Adopting this probability distribution a new set of mixtures is then generated and the best 30 factor compositions are selected and added to the previous set of mixtures. From this larger set the best 30 mixtures are then selected and adopted as a new generation to be tested. This evolutionary algorithm is repeated for 10 generations, and 500 simulations are conducted.

The main results of this study concern the average of the experimental response and the best value achieved in each generation. In the Fig. 5.17, we can notice that the behavior of the average is increasing monotonically until the 7th generation when the best compositions are achieved.

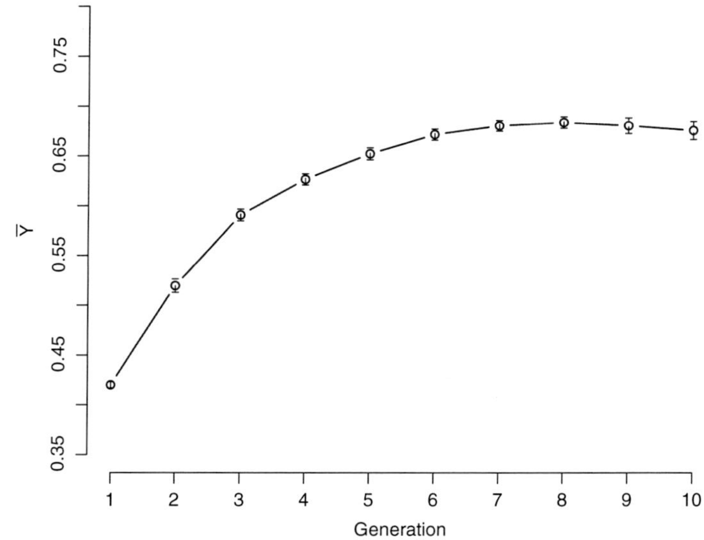

Fig. 5.17 The average response value at each generation achieved with the EBN-Design

This behavior of the EBN-design compares very favorably with the simple GA-design reported in the Fig. 5.5. Furthermore, the performance of the approach is very similar to the performance of the MGA-design reported in Fig. 5.13. The behavior of the best test in each generation (Fig. 5.18) exhibits a strong increase until the 8th generation, followed by a very slow decrease.

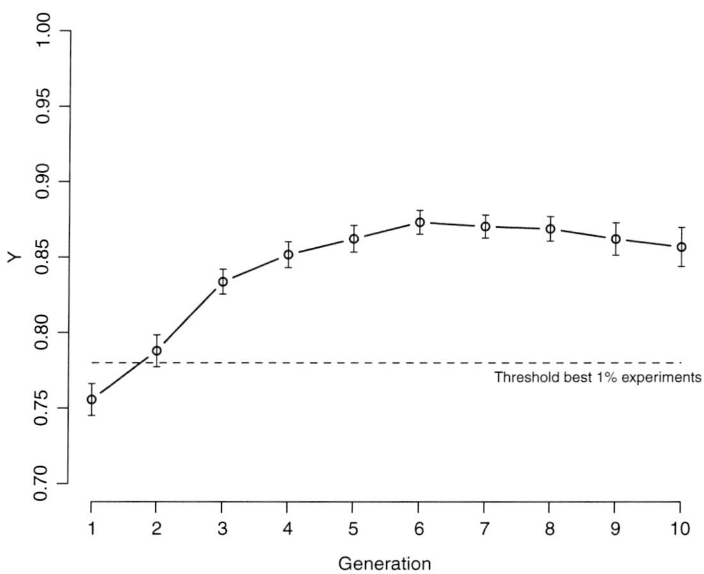

Fig. 5.18 The best response value at each generation achieved with the EBN-Design

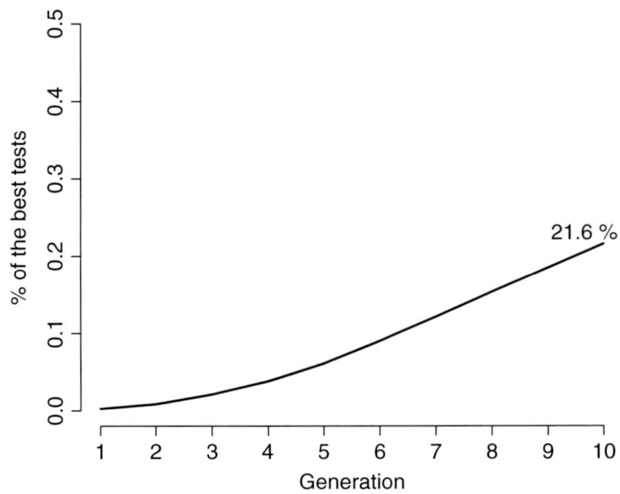

Fig. 5.19 The proportion of the best tests uncovered by the EBN-Design in 0.01 right tail area of the response distribution

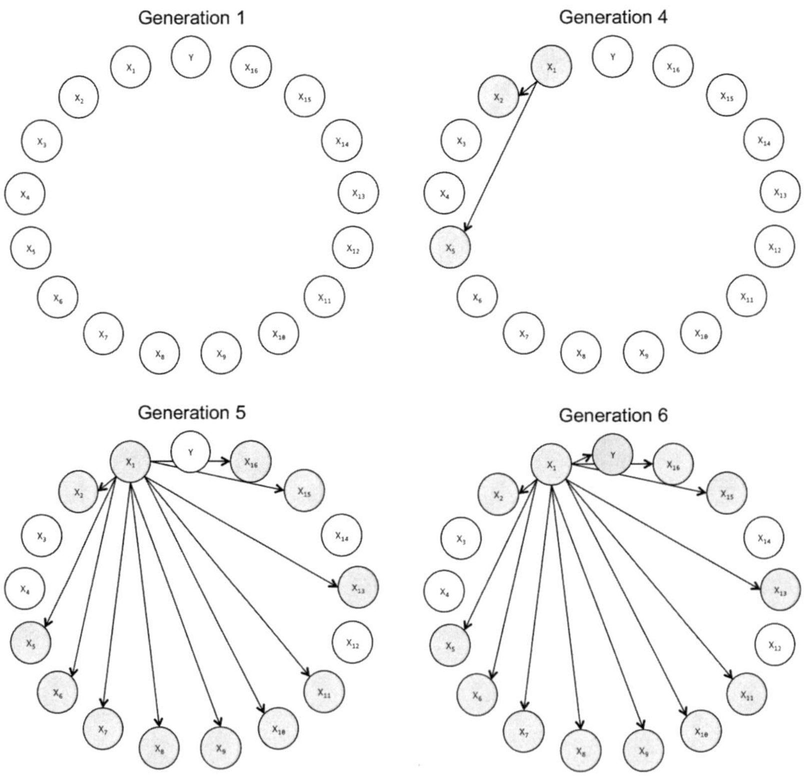

Fig. 5.20 The evolution through the generations of the EBN-design

Finally deriving the 99th quantile of the response distribution, we observe a great increase of the proportion of the best compositions in the 1% right tail area of the distribution (Fig. 5.19).

The main characteristic of the EBN-Design is the evolution of the dependence relationships among the factors of the compositions, i.e. the structure of the network. This evolution through the generations is reported in Fig. 5.20. At the beginning of the process, a random selection of the factor combinations is considered, so that no specific set of relevant interactions affecting the response is achieved. When the number of generation increases, the process starts to evolve the Bayesian network, and it detects the set of relevant factor interactions leading to the fitness increase. Finally, the EBN-Design finds the best set of solutions and the process defines the dependence structure among the variables. The EBN-Design can be considered as an efficient tool to derive an experimental design in high dimensional settings: by evaluating only a small percentage of the whole experimental space, the process is able to identify the factor components of the optimizing experimental mixture. Moreover the probabilistic model that guides the search for the optimum is expressive and easy to visualize and understand, leading to a minimal structure which explains the joint action of the factor components affecting the response.

Chapter 6
Outliers

Abstract Outliers, that is outlying observations, sometimes also known as aberrant observations, are being often studied in the literature closely related to missing data treatment and validation procedures. An interesting issue is concerned with the influence of outliers on the estimates of moments of the data distribution or indexes relevant for further data analysis and model building. The approach of robust statistics is oriented in such direction to ensure that good reliable estimates may be obtained even in the presence of gross errors or unusual measures originated by unexpected events. The approach we shall cope with here aims instead at discovering such outliers and either setting them apart or correcting them according to some properly fitted data model. The very complexity of such a problem prompted soon for employing general heuristic methods for outlier detection and size estimation for independent sample data. Owing to the dependence structure outlier analysis in time series proved to be much more difficult as observations have to be checked not only as regards their distance from the mean but as far as relationships among neighboring observations and correlation function are concerned. For this reason we shall give a brief account of evolutionary computing applications within independent data analysis framework while more detailed discussion will be devoted to outliers and influential observations in time series analysis.

6.1 Outliers in Independent Data

The analysis of a data set usually requires a preliminary step devoted to data cleaning from gross errors and data validation. It is well known that practically every data analysis technique often may lead to erroneous conclusions in the presence of even a single aberrant observation. This term (aberrant) applies to outlying observations, that is observations that markedly differ from the other ones. In some cases aberrant observations prove to be not strong enough to distort the analysis and conclusions significantly. Unfortunately more often aberrant observations are influential observations as well, that is they may impact the computed statistics and yield misleading results. A comprehensive review of statistical methods for the treatment of outliers in data sets is Barnett and Lewis (1994). In the next two sections we shall give some account of situations where data analysis is performed in the presence of aberrant

R. Baragona et al., *Evolutionary Statistical Procedures*, Statistics and Computing,
DOI 10.1007/978-3-642-16218-3_6, © Springer-Verlag Berlin Heidelberg 2011

observations and which results may be expected if this circumstance is overlooked. Robust statistics and outlier diagnostics are alternative approaches to the problem of obtaining reliable and accurate statistics from data sets that include aberrant observations. We concentrate on outlier diagnostics. For an introduction to robust statistics see, for instance, Huber (1981). In the sequel we shall refrain from calling aberrant the outlying observations and shall call them outliers. We assume that data analysis is to be performed on a sample set D randomly and independently drawn from a random variable Y associated to a probability space $(\Omega, \mathcal{A}, P)$ with generally unknown cumulative probability distribution function F. As a consequence, the sample data are identically and independently distributed and outliers, if any, have to be searched for amongst the subsets that according to some appropriate measure have an unusual large distance from the distribution center.

We have to notice at this point that for any given sample data subset we may assume that an appropriate distance measure may always be computed that allows us to decide if the subset either include multiple outliers or it is outlier free. Unless a rule to choose candidate outlier subsets may be defined in some obvious manner, trying all subsets is needed if we want multiple outliers to be discovered for certain. This circumstance implies that the multiple outliers diagnostics is a combinatorial problem which in general has

$$N = \sum_{i=1}^{\lfloor n/2 \rfloor} \binom{n}{i}$$

solutions, where n is the number of observations in the sample. This approach is the exhaustive solution enumeration. We try all subsets including a single observation, 2 observations, ..., $\lfloor n/2 \rfloor$ observations. This course of action leads naturally to the ultimate solution though it is computationally expensive and practically unfeasible unless n is smallest. So methods have been developed based on either simple *ad hoc* heuristic and distance measures or meta-heuristics and distance measures.

6.1.1 Exploratory Data Analysis for Multiple Outliers Detection

Barnett and Lewis (1994, p. 7) offer the definition of outlier as follows: *We shall define an outlier in a set of data to be an observation (or subset of observations) which appears to be inconsistent with the remainder of that set of data.* If, for instance, the random sample $\{y_1, y_2, \ldots, y_n\}$ is drawn from the random variable Y distributed according to F, let us consider the ordered sample (in ascending order) $\{y_{(1)}, y_{(2)}, \ldots, y_{(n)}\}$. The sample extremes are $y_{(1)}$ the lower one and $y_{(n)}$ the upper one. The extremes may or may not be outliers. Nevertheless, outliers have to be extreme values. This circumstance includes the case when some of the largest (or smallest) may be assumed as outlying observations as well. It may be the case, for instance, that for some positive integer $k << n$ $\{y_{(n-k)}, y_{(n-k+1)}, \ldots, y_{(n)}\}$ had to be considered a multiple outlier set.

The most obvious interpretation of outliers is to consider that a gross error happened in recording either manually or automatically by some malfunctioning of the recording machine. Another source of error in the data are unexpected events that may cause occasional fluctuations in data, for instance earthquakes, lightning, or unusual heavy rain. However, we do not know if and when such an error happened, so that we are forced to study every observation under the assumption that the data are distributed according to F. As a matter of fact any extreme value is to be judged too large (or too small) if the probability of larger (smaller) values under F is smaller than a pre-specified critical value. Just as a simple example, we generated 1000 independently identically distributed normal standard unit observations. The first one was modified by shifting the decimal point in such a way 6.353 was recorded instead of 0.6353. In Fig. 6.1 the histogram of the data is displayed and the standard unit normal probability density function was superimposed (dashed line). The outlier is apparent on the right side of the plot. However, it is not so apparent as an outlier if we assume the Cauchy distribution (solid line) as our hypothesized F. We may compute the p-values to assess a measure of distance of the potential outlying observation from the rest of the data set. In the former case the p-value is equal to 1.0558×10^{-10} and we may declare that the first observation is an outlier while in the latter case the p-value is equal to 0.0497 so that we may doubt about such a conclusion.

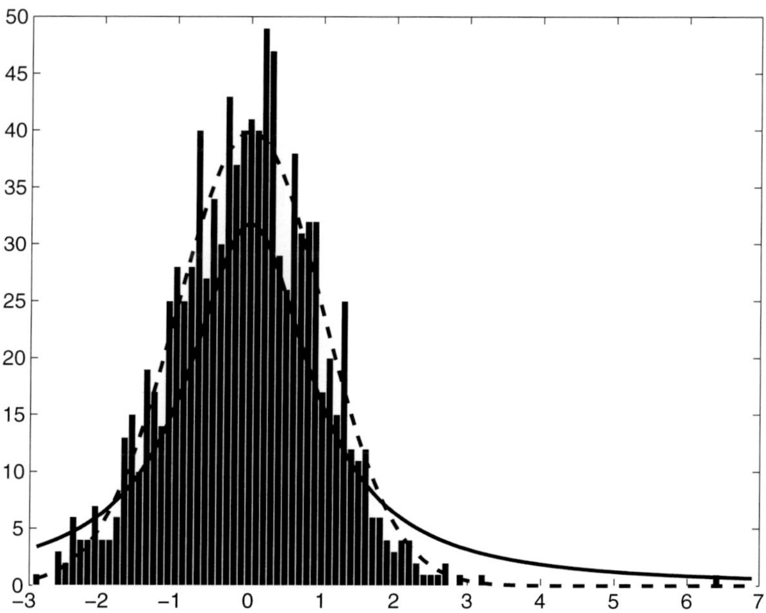

Fig. 6.1 Histogram of 1000 artificial data generated from a standard unit distribution (*dashed line*) with a gross error (*right hand side*). This appears as a contaminant if it is assumed as generated from a different (Cauchy for instance) distribution (*solid line*)

Sometimes a distinction is made between outliers and contaminants. The former ones are sample observations unexpectedly large or small but generated anyway from the distribution F. Contaminants are outliers which are actually drawn from a distribution F_1 different from F that in this case is assuming the meaning of a null hypothesis. Distinguishing the two types is a highly uncertain task and we shall not investigate this matter further. For instance, in the example displayed in Fig. 6.1 we could assume the outlier as a contaminant only if we consider our null hypothesis F the unit standard distribution.

In any case, the detection of outlier is related to a statistical model, which may be implicit or explicit, suggested by the data themselves or by prior knowledge and assumptions. If the model relates the data to other variables (as in regression models) the outlier evaluation is usually based on the residuals.

The deletion approach has been often suggested for dealing with outliers in a data set (see Cook and Weisberg, 1982, for instance). These methods start from a model which is fitted to all available data. Then computations are performed leaving out one observation at a time and recording the impact on some appropriate index chosen according to the context, for instance the residuals sum of square in regression analysis. However, if the data set include multiple outliers, then parameter estimates will be in general severely biased. As an alternative the forward search (FS) has been suggested for detecting multiple outliers in regression and general linear models (Atkinson and Riani, 2000, 2002). The FS uses robust methods, for example the least median of squares, to select an initial small outlier free subset of the data. The parameter estimates at the initial stages are not biased by the presence of outliers. Then an iterative procedure starts and proceeds iteratively by increasing in size the initial subset to include one by one the other observations. A criterion for progressing in the search is adopted that allows the potential outliers to be included only at the last steps. During the search several analytic and graphical diagnostic tools are used for monitoring the development of the iterative procedure. Basically the Mahalanobis distance is used under multivariate normality assumption, to be achieved possibly by preprocessing the data set according to a suitable Box-Cox-type transformation.

6.1.2 Genetic Algorithms for Detecting Outliers in an i.i.d. Data Set

Multidimensional data sets require complicated procedures to search for outliers. For the 1-dimensional, 2-dimensional and even the 3-dimensional case the data may be plotted and visual inspection helps in locating the set of outlying observations. Visual analysis is much more complicated for high dimensional data and dimensionality reduction techniques may be misleading because computations may be affected by the presence of the outliers themselves. So we have to deal with the combinatorial optimization problem outlined above.

An efficient search of such a large search space by evolutionary computing has been suggested by Crawford and Wainwright (1995). Ordered genetic algorithms are used for generating subsets of potential outlying observations. Some preliminary operations are to be performed necessarily for the algorithm to proceed properly.

1. Arrange the data set to be searched for outliers in the usual data matrix, that is observation $\times$ variables form. Let n be the number of observations and p the number of variables, that is the data are p-dimensional
2. Label each observations by simple enumeration, that is $1, 2, \ldots, n$. At this stage order does not matter
3. Define the solution encoding as a sequence of labels. In this case the order matters, as we assume that the first k labels define the potential outliers set. Each chromosome is a permutation of the labels $\{1, 2, \ldots, n\}$ and its length is $\ell = n$. For large data set, however, the chromosome length may be bounded by choosing a value ℓ such that $\ell < n$
4. Choose the GAs parameters, population size N, probability of mutation and crossover p_m and p_c, number of iterations I. Optionally, specify elitist strategy and a generational gap G, $0 < G < 1$
5. Choose an appropriate real positive measure to serve as fitness function
6. Build an initial population of order – based chromosomes. Each one of the N chromosomes in the population is a permutation of the observations integer labels $\{1, 2, \ldots, n\}$ possibly truncated to the first ℓ elements

Once the initialization has been performed, then the algorithm may start. The algorithm is iterative and proceeds through the following steps.

1. Evolve the initial population by applying the three genetic operators selection, mutation and crossover. Specialized operators are needed for order – based genetic algorithms
2. The new generation replaces the old population, then iterate steps 1 and 2 until the maximum number of iterations I is attained.

The data set Y includes n p-dimensional vectors $\{y_1, y_2, \ldots, y_n\}$ each numbered from 1 to n. The population size N is the number of permutations of the integer numbers $\{1, 2, \ldots, n\}$ (these permutations define ordered sets of vectors belonging to Y) we examine at each iteration. The ultimate goal of the iterative procedure is to get within I iteration a population that includes a permutation with the label of the k outlying observations in the first k places. Let $\{x_1, x_2, \ldots, x_N\}$ be the population at a given iteration $i < I$. Each of the x_j's is a (possibly truncated) permutation of length $\ell \leq n$. Each x_j is a solution in the sense that its first k entries are assumed to be the labels of the potential outlying observations.

The selected chromosomes are the next generation and are eligible to be included in the updated population. If neither elitist strategy nor generational gap are adopted, the new population replaces the old one completely and a new iteration may start. If the elitist strategy is assumed, complete replacement is conditioned to the appearance in the new generation of a chromosome whose fitness function is not less than the best fitness found in the past population. If this is not the case, then the chromosome with largest fitness function at iteration $i-1$ is included in the new generation at iteration i even if it was not selected and at the same time the worst chromosome in the new generation is deleted. A generational gap G is a number between 0 and 1 that specifies the number of times the selection is performed in each iteration as $N^* = G \times N$. This implies that $N \times (1 - G)$ chromosomes are allowed to survive from iteration $i - 1$ to iteration i. Notice, however, that genetic algorithms do not necessarily have the same population size in all generations and we may use devices that manage an increasing population size. We shall not consider here this feature further and assume a fixed population size.

It is assumed that the outliers correspond to the first labels in each permutation. In case of multiple outliers, their number is to be specified in some way. If k outliers are assumed, then the observations labeled by the k integer that come first in the permutation are taken as potential outliers. This kind of ordered chromosome encoding requires order crossover operators. Many have been proposed, for instance the partially-mapped (PMX), the order (OX), and cycle (CX) crossovers (Michalewicz, 1996b). We want to describe here the uniform order crossover (Kargupta et al., 1992, p. 50, section 3.2). The chromosomes are paired at random, and denote x_1 the first parent and x_2 the second one. The chromosomes x_1 and x_2 undergo the crossover with probability p_c. If so, the following steps are performed.

1. Generate uniformly randomly a binary mask of length equal to the chromosome length ℓ
2. For each 1 copy the allele value of the first parent to the first child in the same locus
3. Fill the rest of the first child loci by the genes of the first parent re-ordered as they appear in the second parent
4. Generate the second child by exchanging the roles of the first and second parents

In Table 6.1 a simple example is displayed to illustrate the procedure. In correspondence of the 1's the children inherit the parents allele exactly, in correspondence of the 0's the children inherit their respective parents alleles but ordered according to the other parent.

As an example of fitness function we may assume the following one. Let $\bar{y}$ be the p-dimensional mean of the data set Y and consider the population at some step $i < I$. Let d_m be the Euclidean norm of the vectors $y_m - \bar{y}$, $m = 1, \ldots, n$. Each chromosome x_j allows us to divide the set $\{1, 2, \ldots, n\}$ in two subsets, the subset A that includes the labels $x_{j_1}, \ldots, x_{j_k}$ of the potential outlying observations and the subset B which includes the remaining labels. The pooled Euclidean distance of the

Table 6.1 A simple example of uniform order crossover

	Labels permutations				
1st parent	3	2	5	4	1
2nd parent	1	2	3	4	5
mask	0	1	0	0	1
1st child	3	2	4	5	1
2nd child	3	2	4	1	5

observations in the outlier free subset is the smallest pooled distance that may be computed from $n - k$ observations.

In this case the fitness function may be defined

$$f(x_j) = \exp\left(-\sum_{m \in B} \|y_m - \bar{y}\|/c\right), \quad j = 1, \ldots, N,$$

where c is a positive constant which scales the fitness and avoids overflows/underflows.

The selection operator may be assumed the widely used roulette wheel rule. Let

$$F = \sum_{j=1}^{N} f(x_j).$$

A circle is divided in N spikes whose width is proportional to $f(x_j)/F$, $j = 1, \ldots, N$. So there are as many spikes as permutations. This kind of selection is called roulette wheel rule because in practice an uniform random number is generated each time we want to select a chromosome. The random number u points at a sector of a wheel because the angle of $u \times 360°$ may be computed and the sector which includes this angle may be easily located. In practice we select with replacement one of the chromosomes x_j's with probability $f(x_j)/F$.

A simple numerical example may help to clarify the method. Let Y denote a data set with 7 6-dimensional observations ($n = 7$, $p = 6$)

$$Y = \begin{pmatrix} 1 & 3 & 4 & 2 & 3 & 4 \\ 4 & 3 & 2 & 7 & 6 & 9 \\ 7 & 3 & 2 & 4 & 5 & 2 \\ 5 & 7 & 8 & 2 & 1 & 4 \\ 4 & 6 & 2 & 3 & 4 & 7 \\ 9 & 3 & 4 & 5 & 6 & 2 \\ 4 & 3 & -10 & 3 & 3 & -10 \end{pmatrix},$$

where each row vector is an observation whose label is the line number. For the sake of simplicity let us assume $k = 1$, that is there is only one outlier in the data set. Let $N = 5$, so that the population at some iteration $i < I$ includes 5 permutations of the integers $\{1, 2, 3, 4, 5, 6, 7\}$, for instance

$$P_i = \begin{pmatrix} 7 & 6 & 5 & 4 & 3 & 2 & 1 \\ 6 & 5 & 4 & 3 & 2 & 1 & 7 \\ 5 & 4 & 3 & 2 & 1 & 6 & 7 \\ 4 & 3 & 2 & 1 & 5 & 6 & 7 \\ 3 & 2 & 1 & 4 & 5 & 6 & 7 \end{pmatrix},$$

where each line is a chromosome, that is a potential solution. Solutions actually included in population P_i are the observations whose label comes first in each of the lines of P_i, that is $y_7 = (4, 3, -10, 3, 3, -10)$, $y_6 = (9, 3, 4, 5, 6, 2)$, $y_5 = (4, 6, 2, 3, 4, 7)$, $y_4 = (5, 7, 8, 2, 1, 4)$, and $y_3 = (7, 3, 2, 4, 5, 2)$.

Let us compute the fitness function for each of the chromosomes in P_i. We have

$$f_i = (0.4501, 0.1375, 0.1318, 0.1763, 0.1044),$$

where the normalizing constant $c = 10$ has been used. The largest fitness corresponds to the first chromosome within the population. Such a chromosome encodes the observation y_7 as a solution, that is, at iteration i, the outlier we are searching for has to be assumed the observation y_7. In Fig. 6.2 the wheel is divided in sectors, one for each chromosome, with width proportional to the normalized fitness function. The largest fitness is assigned to the sector which is exploded in the plot and actually corresponds to the outlier y_7.

For the fitness function that we have employed in the numerical example the mean has been assumed the multivariate mean. This is maybe the simplest choice. In practice, much more complicated problems may arise and different computations of the fitness function are required. For instance, outlier diagnostics in regression have been studied by Crawford et al. (1995) by using genetic algorithms. In this case the conditional mean computed from a regression model has been found appropriate as a basis for the fitness function computation. If a chromosome encodes a subset

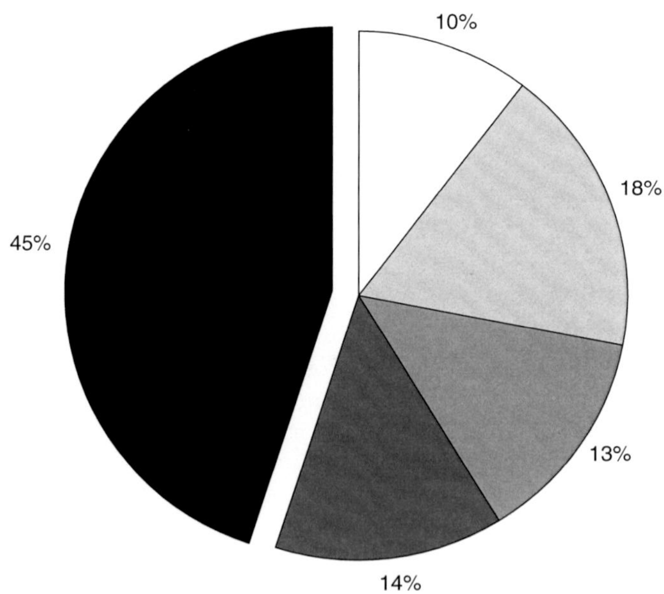

Fig. 6.2 Roulette wheel used for selection of chromosomes within a population of size $N = 5$. Each relative fitness is reported as percentage

A of observations as outliers, then computations are performed on the remaining subset B. Several formulas have been proposed to define a suitable fitness function, for instance the regression residual sum of squares, the Cook's squared distance for multiple-case diagnostics (Cook and Weisberg, 1982) and the determinantal ratio $\det(Y_B{}'Y_B)/\det(Y'Y)$, where Y_B is the data set with the observations in A removed (Andrews and Pregibon, 1978). The GAs were designed so as to maximize the aforementioned criteria and each criterion was the basis for a particular version of the algorithm. To determine the optimal number of outliers the GAs may be iterated by assuming several values of k up to $k = \lfloor \frac{n}{2} \rfloor$. To determine the optimal number of outliers, Crawford et al. (1995) propose to run the GA for any value of k up to $\lfloor \frac{n}{2} \rfloor$ and evaluate the reduction in the sum of squared residuals moving from k to $k + 1$ since we expect that such a reduction be inessential once the correct number of outliers has been reached. Simultaneous variable selection and outlier detection in regression models has been investigated by using GAs by Tolvi (2004).

6.2 Outliers in Time Series

In a time series some observations may be regarded as outlying ones if they are, in a sense, markedly different from the rest. The presence of such outlying observations may result from sampling errors or from the perturbed behavior of the observed phenomenon. If we hypothesize, for instance, that the data are generated by an autoregressive integrated moving-average (ARIMA) model, then we may assume as an outlier any observation that is unusually different from the value predicted by the model.

In the literature outliers are often studied in connection with the missing data problem and validation procedures. Another important interesting link has been found with the influential observations, that is observations that most impact the estimates of statistics of interest or model parameters. The study of influential observations has been usually performed in the framework of robust statistics. However outlier detection and size estimation is often chiefly of interest because we are not only able to correct the observed data but we may either compute some measure of their influence on the estimates or investigate the events that originated their occurrence and highlight interesting features of the phenomenon itself.

The main problem in this framework consists in supplying a clear unambiguous definition of outlier in time series. As a matter of fact observations are not independent. As a consequence an observation has to be examined not only as far as its value is concerned but as regards its date as well. A definition to be appropriate has to take into account the data that precede and follow the observation which may be possibly considered as an outlying one. Unlike independent data, time series outliers may not be searched for among the extreme values only. Indeed even an observation close to the mean of the series may actually be an outlying one if it is inconsistent with the neighboring observations. Moreover, two peculiar features of outliers, namely the masking and smearing effects (see, for instance, Bruce and Martin, 1989), make outlier detection often difficult in time series.

- Masking effect → The occurrence of large outliers may prevent diagnostics from detecting other close outlying observations.
- Smearing effect → The presence of some outliers may bias the diagnostics so as false identifications may occur.

Such special problems motivated the development of specifically oriented methods to cope with time series data.

Since the introductory paper by Fox (1972) outliers in time series have been an active research field and many approaches have been entertained and methods and procedures suggested. A brief account may be found in Barnett and Lewis (1994, chapter 10) and Box et al. (1994, chapter 12). A raw distinction may be done among three classes of techniques, ARIMA model building (Chang et al., 1988; Tsay, 1986, 1988), bilateral models based on the linear interpolator (Battaglia, 1988a; Maravall and Peña, 1989) and leave-k-out diagnostics (Bruce and Martin, 1989). The time series data set investigation is twofold, aimed at evaluating the outlier date and size and on the other hand at giving some appropriate measure of the outlier influence on the time series mean and correlation function and on model identification and parameter estimation procedures. Though this latter point is closely related to robust techniques, which attempt to minimize the effect of outliers, we focus on outlier diagnostics only.

Several difficulties are of course inherent to methods for outlier detection. If we resort to the fitting of either ARIMA, including the state – space formulation (Kohn and Ansley, 1983, for instance), or bilateral models to the data, outlying observations are anyway identified as those markedly different from their predicted value. Nevertheless both the appropriateness and the goodness-of-fit of the model impact the statistics that we may devise to assess the difference between observed and predicted values. The leave-k-out diagnostics are less affected by the model identification and estimation stages though it is likely that the correlation structure of the time series may be disrupted at such a degree that poor results may be expected. In order to avoid such drawbacks, methods for detecting outliers in time series using genetic algorithms have been developed (see Baragona et al., 2001a). The extension of forward search for detecting outliers in time series has been suggested by Riani (2004) with special attention to deal with the masking effect.

In what follows the contribution of evolutionary computing in overcoming the disadvantages of either approaches will be described. Notice that we confine ourselves to linear models, that is we are making the implicit assumption that time series data are generated by some linear structure. Outliers in non – linear time series are being currently studied though well established tools are not yet available and evolutionary computing applications are at their tentative proposals stage. Detection of outliers in univariate time series generated by a general state-dependent model (see Priestley, 1988) is considered by Battaglia and Orfei (2005) who propose identification and estimation methods for a single outlier in bilinear, self-exciting threshold autoregressive, and exponential autoregressive models. A similar development for outlier analysis in functional autoregressive models is introduced by Battaglia (2005). Chen (1997) considered detection of additive outliers in bilinear models. Finally, analogues to ARMA model based detection methods have been employed for discovering volatility outliers in ARCH and GARCH models. A review may be found in Gounder et al. (2007).

6.2.1 Univariate ARIMA Models

The ARIMA – based approach for studying outliers in time series assumes that the observed time series data are generated by an ARIMA model. The familiar procedure organized through the identification, estimation and diagnostic checking stages has been commonly applied since the paper by Chang et al. (1988) for multiple outlier detection and size estimation. The difference between the data and their predicted values provides us with the basic measure for deciding if an observation is an outlying one or not. Once a date is identified as an outlier occurrence its size is estimated by a function of the model parameters. Several outlier types are usually distinguished and we limit ourselves to those that are commonly considered in the literature, that is the additive outlier (AO), the innovation outlier (IO), the level shift (LS) and the transient change (TC) (see, for instance, Chen and Liu, 1993). The AO impact is limited to its occurrence time, while the IO and TC cause a perturbation in the observed time series which lasts for some time and may be assumed negligible afterwards. The LS corresponds to a permanent change in the mean of the time series.

Let $\{x_t,\ \text{integer } t\}$ be an outlier-free time series generated by an ARMA(p, q) model

$$\phi(B)x_t = \theta(B)a_t, \tag{6.1}$$

where $\phi(B) = 1-\phi_1 B - \cdots - \phi_p B^p, \theta(B) = 1-\theta_1 B - \cdots - \theta_q B^q$, $B^h x_t = x_{t-h}$, any integer h, $\mathbb{E}(x_t) = 0$, any t. Let $\{a_t,\ \text{integer } t\}$ be a white noise process with zero mean and constant variance σ_a^2. Further let us assume that the roots of the polynomials $\phi(B)$ and $\theta(B)$ be all outside the unit circle, so that the process $\{x_t\}$ turns out to be stationary and invertible.

The model for the AO (also known as type I) at time $t = T$ is

$$y_t = x_t + \delta_{t-T}\omega_0, \tag{6.2}$$

where $\{y_t,\ t = 1, \ldots, n\}$ is the observed time series, ω_0 the outlier size and δ is the Kronecker's delta, that is $\delta_{t-T} = 1$ if $t = T$ and equals zero otherwise. Only the observation at $t = T$ is affected by the outlier. This may happen, for instance, because of a gross error originated by an occasional malfunctioning of the recording device.

The model for the IO (also known as type II) at time $t = T$ is

$$y_t = \frac{\theta(B)}{\phi(B)}(a_t + \delta_{t-T}\omega_0). \tag{6.3}$$

In Model (6.3) the observation y_t is affected by an outlier at $t = T$. The outlier does not run out of influencing the observed time series as all subsequent observations are affected through the transfer function $\psi(B) = \phi(B)^{-1}\theta(B)$. The outlier size is ω_0 at $t = T$ while is equal to $\psi_\tau\omega_0$ at $t = T + \tau$ for $\tau = 1, 2, \ldots$. The impact of the outlier on the observed time series does not vanish, in general, though its absolute value decreases and is to be considered negligible in practice when $\tau > \tau_0$, for some positive integer τ_0. The only exception is the pure MA model. In this case, the outlier impact is non-zero only in the finite interval $[T, T + q]$, where q is the MA order. An IO may occur, for instance, from an occasional isolated shock that impacts the white noise process.

Model (6.1) under the aforementioned assumptions may be written in the following autoregressive form

$$\pi(B)x_t = \frac{\phi(B)}{\theta(B)}x_t = a_t, \tag{6.4}$$

where $\pi_0 = 1$ and the sequence $\{\pi_1, \pi_2, \ldots\}$ is quadratically convergent. Model (6.4) may be generalized to the ARIMA(p, d, q) model by substituting $\phi(B)$ with the generalized autoregressive operator $\phi(B)(1 - B)^d$, integer d. The time series $\{x_t\}$ is no longer assumed stationary, while a minimum positive integer d exists such that $(1 - B)^d x_t$ is stationary (that is, x_t is integrated of order d). It should be noted, however, that for integrated series the meaning and effects of innovational outliers are different from the stationary case, because the shocks are permanently incorporated into the series. For example, if $d = 1$, an IO produces ultimately a level shift (see Chen and Liu, 1993).

Let (6.2) hold. Then the size of an isolated AO in $t = T$ may be estimated by either least square or maximum likelihood methods. If the innovations are normally distributed, the two methods both yield the estimate

$$\hat{\omega_A} = \rho^2\pi(F)\pi(B)y_T, \tag{6.5}$$

where $\rho^2 = (1 + \pi_1^2 + \pi_2^2 + \ldots)^{-1}$ and $F^h x_t = x_{t+h}$. The estimate $\hat{\omega_A}$ is unbiased and its variance is equal to $\sigma_a^2\rho^2$.

The size of an isolated IO at $t = T$ may be estimated by computing the pseudo – residuals

$$e_t = \pi(B)y_t. \tag{6.6}$$

If the coefficients $\{\pi_1, \pi_2, \ldots\}$ are assumed known, then using (6.6) Model (6.3) may be written

$$e_t = \delta_{t-T}\omega_0 + a_t,$$

and both the least squares and, under the normality assumption, the maximum likelihood methods yield the estimate

$$\hat{\omega}_I = e_T, \tag{6.7}$$

that is the estimate of the size of an outlier of type II occurring at $t = T$ equals the pseudo – residual at $t = T$. The estimate $\hat{\omega_I}$ is unbiased and its variance is equal to σ_a^2.

The likelihood ratio criterion, under the normality assumption, provides us with suitable statistical tests to check the null hypothesis (H_0: the observation at $t = T$ is outlier-free) against the alternative hypotheses that the observation is affected by either an IO (H_1) or an AO (H_2) at $t = T$. We may obtain the following test statistics (see Chang et al., 1988)

- H_0 vs H_1, $\lambda_1(T) = \hat{\omega}_I/\sigma_a$,
- H_0 vs H_2, $\lambda_2(T) = \hat{\omega}_A/(\rho\sigma_a)$,
- H_1 vs H_2, $\lambda_{1.2}(T) = \frac{\rho^{-2}\hat{\omega}_A^2 - \hat{\omega}_I^2}{2\sigma_a^2(1-\rho^2)^{1/2}}$.

Under H_0 and assuming that the ARIMA model parameters are known, both test statistics $\lambda_1(T)$ and $\lambda_2(T)$ are normally distributed while $\lambda_{1.2}(T)$ is a product of two independent normal random variables. Detection of an outlier of either type depends on the comparison between the maxima of the absolute values of the test statistics $\lambda_1(t)$ and $\lambda_2(t)$ with a given threshold value c. The choice of c is chiefly based on simulation studies. As a practical rule, for time series of length $n < 200$ appropriate choices are $c = 3$ for high sensitivity and $c = 4$ for low sensitivity to the presence of outliers. Fox (1972) suggested distinguishing the outlier type, either IO or AO, whether the absolute value of $\lambda_1(T)$ or $\lambda_2(T)$ is the largest one provided that it exceeds the threshold c at the given time $t = T$. This may be used as an alternative procedure simpler than performing the test $\lambda_{1.2}(T)$.

An iterative procedure may be devised for multiple outlier detection by computing the test statistics at each time t in the interval $[t_0 + 1, n]$. The first t_0 observations are needed for initialization of the estimation algorithms. All dates t where either $|\lambda_1(t)|$ or $|\lambda_2(t)|$ or both exceed c are recorded and stored in a set H. We assume the presence of an AO in $t = T$ if $|\lambda_1(T)| = \max_{t \in H} |\lambda_1(t)|$ and $|\lambda_1(T)| > |\lambda_2(T)|$. Likewise, an IO is assumed in $t = T$ if $|\lambda_2(T)| = \max_{t \in H} |\lambda_2(t)|$ and $|\lambda_2(T)| > |\lambda_1(T)|$. The outlier size is estimated by either (6.7) or (6.5) and the outlying observation is corrected accordingly. Then the adjusted time series is ready for the next iteration. The procedure ends if either no more outliers are detected or a pre-specified number of iterations have been performed.

In practice the autoregressive parameters have to be estimated from the data, and the presence of outliers may produce a bias which in turn will bias the outlier magnitude estimates. Such a problem has been addressed by Battaglia (2006) who shows that the bias is of order $1/n$ and proposes simple bias-corrected estimates for both AO and IO outliers. In order to solve the same problem Chen and Liu (1993) proposed to modify the iterative procedure by re-estimating the model parameters at each stage and considering a final joint maximum likelihood estimation of model parameters and outliers magnitudes.

Equalities similar to (6.2) and (6.3) may be used to define the level shift and the transient change outlier models. In general, the presence of an outlier at time $t = T$ may be modeled as

$$y_t = x_t + \alpha(B)\delta_{t-T}\omega_0,$$

where different specifications are given to $\alpha(B)$ according to the outlier type (see Chen and Liu, 1993)

$$\begin{aligned} &\text{AO} \quad \alpha(B) = 1, \\ &\text{IO} \quad \alpha(B) = \psi(B), \\ &\text{LS} \quad \alpha(B) = \frac{1}{1-B}, \\ &\text{TC} \quad \alpha(B) = \frac{1}{1-\delta B}. \end{aligned} \tag{6.8}$$

In the definition of the IO the $\psi(B)$ polynomial is equal to $\phi(B)^{-1}\theta(B)$ where the $\phi(B)$ polynomial has all roots on or outside the unit circle. As regards the TC, δ is assumed a real number to be chosen in the interval (0, 1). Chen and Liu (1993, p. 285) recommend $\delta = 0.7$. The model for multiple outliers may be written using equalities (6.8)

$$y_t = x_t + \sum_{j=1}^{k} \alpha_j(B)\delta_{t-t_j}\omega_j,$$

where we assume that k outliers of size $\omega_1, \ldots, \omega_k$ occur at times $t_1, \ldots, t_k$ respectively, provided that all dates are different.

As an example, let us consider Series A from Box and Jenkins (1976, p. 525). This time series includes 197 observations recorded every two hours of a characteristic quantity of a chemical process. The data are displayed in Fig. 6.3, upper plot. Two models are suggested in Box and Jenkins (1976, p. 239). We may use for instance the first one, that is

$$(1 - B)x_t = (1 - \theta B)a_t.$$

We estimated this model by using the SCA package (Liu and Hudak, 1992, paragraphs UTSMODEL pp. 3.23–3.26 and UESTIM pp. 3.32–3.34) and obtained $\hat{\theta} = 0.7015$ (standard error 0.0511). The paragraph OUTLIER of the package SCA itself for multiple outliers detection and estimation yields a type II outlier in $t = 64$ ($\hat{\omega}_I = 1.13$, standard error 0.30) and a type I in $t = 43$ ($\hat{\omega}_A = -0.98$, standard error 0.27). The likelihood ratio statistics have been compared to the critical value $c = 3.5$ and only the statistics in $t = 64$ and $t = 43$ (absolute values) have been

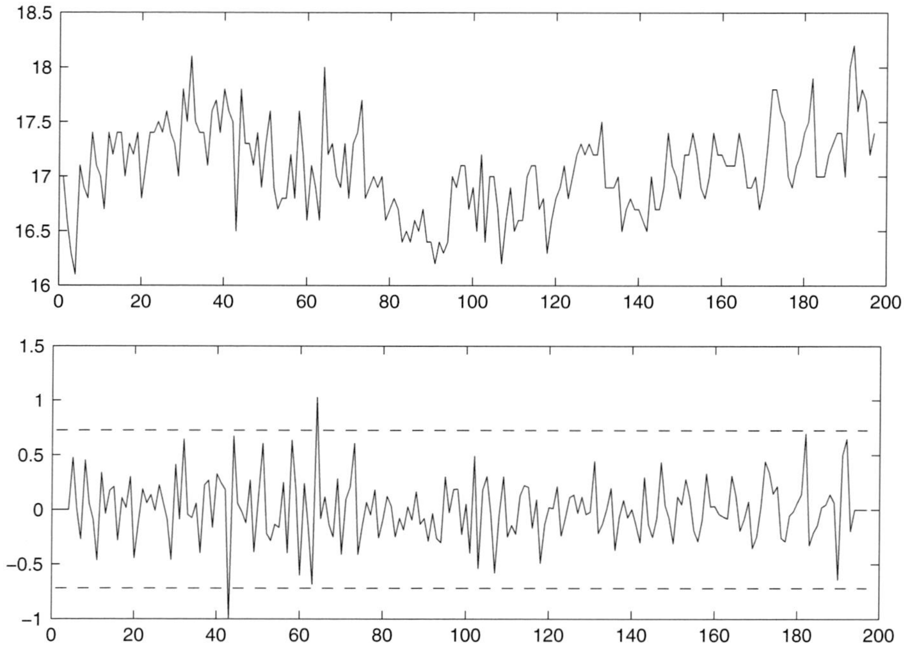

Fig. 6.3 Series A original data (*upper plot*) and linear interpolator errors (*lower plot*). In this latter plot *upper* and *lower* bounds denote the standard normal distribution 99% confidence interval

found to exceed this bound. The statistics for type II and type I were the largest ones respectively.

6.2.1.1 The Linear Interpolator

In time series framework linear interpolators have been defined and studied in connection with the problem of estimating a missing observation by means of a linear combination of neighboring data. Computation is done with the objective of minimizing the mean square error. The link between the outliers of additive type and the linear interpolator has been highlighted by Peña (1990). It may be shown that a missing data may be replaced by an arbitrary figure, the average of time series values for instance, and the least square error missing data estimate equals the estimated AO size. So introducing the linear interpolators is of interest not only as a mean for treating outlying observations but to deal with missing data as well.

Let $\{X_t, \text{ integer } t\}$ denote a random process stationary up to order two with mean zero and autocovariance function $R(h) = \mathbb{E}(X_t X_{t+h})$ independent of t, and spectral density function $f(\lambda)$, $-\pi < \lambda \leq \pi$, such that the integral of its reciprocal $1/f(\lambda)$ exists finite. The inverse autocovariance function $Ri(h)$ has been introduced by Cleveland (1972) as

$$Ri(h) = (2\pi)^{-2} \int_{-\pi}^{\pi} \{1/f(\lambda)\} \exp(i\lambda h) d\lambda.$$

Let $r(h) = R(h)/R(0)$ and $ri(h) = Ri(h)/Ri(0)$ denote the ordinary and inverse autocorrelation functions respectively. The inverse autocorrelation function owns the same properties of ordinary autocorrelation, i.e. it is definite positive, symmetric and $|ri(h)| \leq ri(0) = 1$.

It is well known (Grenander and Rosenblatt, 1957) that the inverse autocorrelations solve the following minimization problem with respect to the unknown real variables c_u, $u \neq 0$

$$\min \mathbb{E} \left(X_t - \sum_{u \neq 0} c_u X_{t-u} \right)^2,$$

that is $c_u = -ri(u)$, $u \neq 0$. The optimal linear filter

$$I_t^X = -\sum_{u \neq 0} ri(u) X_{t-u}$$

is a random process known as the linear interpolator of X_t. The difference

$$e_t^X = X_t - I_t^X$$

is the interpolation error. The process $\{e_t\}$ has mean zero, variance $\sigma_e^2 = \frac{1}{Ri(0)}$ and its autocorrelation function coincides with the inverse autocorrelation function $ri(h)$ of the process $\{X_t\}$.

For all non-negative integer pairs (m, s) we may consider the linear combination of the random variables

$$X_{t-m}, X_{t-m+1}, \ldots, X_{t-1}, X_{t+1}, \ldots, X_{t+s}$$

such that its difference $I_t^X(m, s)$ from X_t is smallest in quadratic mean. We have

$$I_t^X(m, s) = \sum_{u=-m}^{-1} k_u(m, s) X_{t+u} + \sum_{u=1}^{s} k_u(m, s) X_{t+u}$$

where the first (second) summation vanishes if $m = 0$ ($s = 0$). We call $I_t^X(m, s)$ the finite linear interpolator of X_t with horizon (m, s). As the random process X_t is assumed second order stationary then the coefficients $k_u(m, s)$ depend on m and s but do not depend on t. It may be shown (Bhansali, 1990) that the coefficients $k_u(m, s)$ may be written as a function of the inverse of the $(m + s + 1)$-dimensional variance-covariance matrix of the random process X_t. Moreover, if $m = s$, the difference between $-k_u(m, m)$ and $ri(u)$ converges to zero for any u as $m \to \infty$.

We may extend the definition of linear interpolator to include the case when the random process is covariance stationary but its mean is non-zero and time varying. Let $\{Y_t,\ \text{integer}\ t\}$ be defined as

$$Y_t = X_t + \omega_t,$$

where the ω_t's are some real constants and $\{X_t,\ \text{integer}\ t\}$ is the random process introduced so far. It is straightforward to show that $\mathbb{E}(Y_t) = \omega_t$ while $\operatorname{cov}(Y_t Y_{t+h}) = R(h)$ independent of t. We may define I_t^Y the linear interpolator of Y_t as the linear combination of Y_{t-u}, $u \neq 0$ and ω_{t-u}, any u, in such a way that we may approximate the random process $\{Y_t\}$ in mean square. Let

$$I_t^Y = \sum_{u \neq 0} g_u Y_{t-u} + \sum_{u=-\infty}^{\infty} p_u \omega_{t-u}$$

and

$$I_t^Y = I_t^X + \Delta_t.$$

Under the assumption that the sequence $\{\Delta_t\}$ minimizes the mean square error $\mathbb{E}\left(Y_t - I_t^Y\right)^2$ it follows that the equality $\Delta_t = \omega_t$ holds with probability 1. So we obtain the result

$$I_t^Y = I_t^X + \omega_t$$

and the interpolation error for Y_t may be written as

$$e_t^Y = Y_t - I_t^Y.$$

So we are allowed to exploit the linear interpolator and its finite counterpart properties even if the random process is not mean stationary. This circumstance makes the linear interpolator an useful device for outlier identification in time series.

Let $y = (y_1, \ldots, y_n)'$ denote the observed time series, that is a finite realization of a random process $\{Y_t\}$. If we want to check the presence of outliers in y by means of linear interpolators the first step is to estimate the inverse correlations. Various methods are possible (see e.g. Battaglia, 1988b). Note that linear interpolators and inverse correlations may be defined and easily estimated also for non stationary integrated series (see Baragona and Battaglia, 1995). Once the inverse correlation estimates $\widehat{ri}(u)$ are obtained, for a fixed $m \ll n$, the linear interpolator may be computed

$$i_t = -\sum_{u=1}^{m} \widehat{ri}(u)(y_{t-u} + y_{t+u}).$$

An outlier is assumed at time $t = q$ if

$$|y_q - i_q| > g\{\hat{R}i(0)\}^{-1/2},$$

where $\hat{R}i(0)$ is the interpolation error variance that may be conveniently estimated by the inverse variance. As the outlier detection depends on the pre-specified constant g, we may call y_q a g-outlying observation. The interpolation error $e_q = y_q - i_q$ may be shown to be equal to the estimate of an AO at time $t = q$. Moreover, in the ARIMA framework, estimates of the linear interpolator coefficients may be computed as functions of the ARIMA model parameter estimates. If the ARIMA model parameters are known, then the linear interpolator error exactly matches the AO estimate. This is a simple procedure to identify potential outliers. If the data are generated by a Gaussian stochastic process, then the interpolation errors are also Gaussian distributed and the Gaussian percentiles may be used for the constant g. However, seldom information about the random process probability distribution are available and the choice of g is usually done according to low, medium and high sensitivity whether the selected g-value is small, medium or large. The usual choices range from 2 to 4. An alternative would be using the Chebyshev inequality though often the g values turn out to be too large in practice. For instance, one has to select $g = 5$ to ensure a probability less than 4% that an interpolation error be so large only by chance.

In Fig. 6.3, lower plot, for instance, choosing $g = 2.58$ allows us to correctly identify $q = 43$ and $q = 64$ as potential outlier dates as the respective interpolation errors exceed the linear interpolator normal 99% bounds $m \pm 2.58s$, where m and s respectively are the mean and standard error of the residual series.

6.2.1.2 Sequences of Consecutive Outliers

The procedure described in Sect. 6.2.1 is known to be effective in the presence of isolated outliers. In case of level changes, that is the case when the mean value of the time series changes after some time point t_0, special approaches are needed. For example, a change in the level of the given time series may be dealt with by using multi-regime models in the class of the non-linear time series models. If non-linear models of this kind are not considered appropriate and it seems preferable to remain in the domain of linear models, then we may study the differenced series, that is $y_t = x_t - x_{t-1}$. A simple computation shows that a single level change in the original time series $\{x_t\}$ produces a isolated outlier in the differenced time series $\{y_t\}$. This latter time series may be investigated with the methods appropriate for isolated outliers in linear models. Nevertheless, it is often the case that outliers do not come neither in isolation nor in the form of a change in the level, but form a sequence occurring in consecutive dates without any interval of non outlying observations. The statistics computed for checking the outlier significance, such as the likelihood ratio statistics, are biased by the masking effect. The outliers which occur in the middle of the stretch of outlying observations are almost always unnoticed because they are often perfectly coherent with the neighboring observations. A sequence of consecutive outliers is called an outlier patch. It may happen that the sizes of the outlying observations in the patch are markedly different each other. Nevertheless still is present a masking effect that prevents the test statistics from correctly identifying some outliers in the patch.

As an example, we simulated 100 observations of an artificial time series $\{x_t\}$ generated by an AR(1) model with parameter $\phi = 0.6$ and standard unit white noise. The simulated time series has been contaminated by adding 3.75 to each and every observation $x_t, t = 51, \ldots, 55$ to yield the sequence $y = (y_1, y_2, \ldots, y_n)'$. The time series y is displayed in Fig. 6.4, upper plot. The circles mark the sequence of additive outliers. We assumed the correct identification and estimated $\hat{\phi} = 0.7042$ (standard error 0.1209) the autoregressive parameter and constant term 0.0523 (standard error 0.0715). The lower plot shows the linear interpolation error. It is apparent that the difference between the observations y_{50} and y_{51} produces a jump in the interpolation error series and so does the difference between the observations y_{55} and y_{56}. The paragraph OUTLIER from the package SCA detects a type II outlier at $t = 51$ ($\hat{\omega}_I = 4.2819$, standard error 1.2) and an outlier of the type I at $t = 56$ ($\hat{\omega}_A = -2.7088$, standard error 0.87). This outcome may be easily explained. The likelihood ratio test is found significant for the observation at $t = 51$ which is markedly incoherent in comparison with most of the observations in the time series.

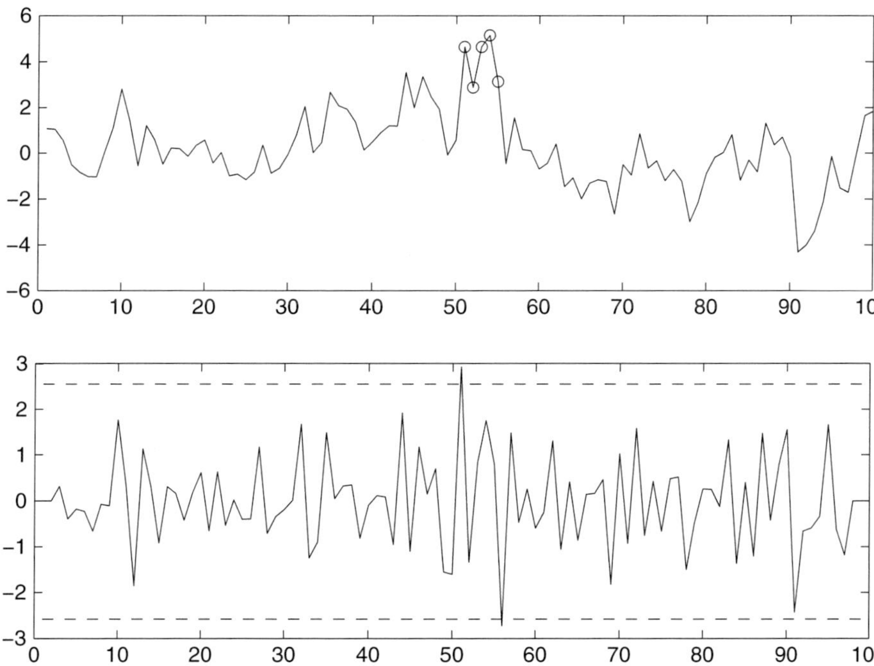

Fig. 6.4 Artificial time series generated by an AR(1) model with a patch added at the time interval [51, 55] (*upper plot*) and its linear interpolation error sequence (*lower plot*). The latter plot includes (*dashed lines*) the normal *upper* and *lower* bounds at 1% significance level

The observations after $t = 51$ are markedly different from the remaining ones as well and this behavior is assumed typical of an innovation (type II) outlier. On the other hand, the observation at $t = 56$ does not conform to the preceding ones, but it is not followed by any other outlying observations, so that the likelihood ratio test finds the appropriate classification as an outlier of the additive type (type I). Summing up, the procedure detects the correct location but the wrong type of the outlier in $t = 51$, the observations from $t = 52$ to $t = 55$ are not identified though actually they are type I outliers, and a wrong detection is performed as regards the observation at $t = 56$.

A procedure specially designed for the detection of sequences of consecutive outliers has been proposed by Bruce and Martin (1989) based on a deletion approach. Several sequences of observations are tentatively assumed as potential patches and an ARIMA model is identified and estimated by treating such patches as missing data.

Let $y = (y_1, \ldots, y_n)'$ denote the observed time series where the presence of an outlier patch is suspected at some dates. An ARIMA model is preliminary identified and estimated using all available observations y. Let σ_a^2 be the computed residual variance. Let a potential patch be assumed with t as starting time and k as its length. The positive integers t and k suffice to uniquely identify a patch, that is we tentatively assume the presence of the set of outlying observations $\{y_t, y_{t+1}, \ldots, y_{t+k-1}\}$. By treating the dates in the interval $[t, t+k-1]$ as missing data locations an ARIMA model may be estimated and let $\sigma_a^2(t, k)$ be the *leave-k-out* residual variance. Then under mild assumptions the statistic

$$DV(t, k) = \frac{n}{2} \frac{\sigma_a^2}{\sigma_a^2(t, k)}$$

may be shown to be distributed as a χ_1^2 if no outlier is present. Given a significance level α the null hypothesis that the sequence $\{y_t, \ldots, y_{t+k-1}\}$ includes regular observations is to be rejected if $DV(t, k) > z_\alpha$ where z_α is the $(1-\alpha)100$th percentile of the χ_1^2 distribution.

The test based on the leave-k-out statistic $DV(t, k)$ may be used iteratively to detect the presence of a patch and to assess its initial time t and its length k. For $k = 1, 2, \ldots$ a window of length k is applied $n-k+1$ times to the time series y and each time the observations $\{y_t, \ldots, y_{t+k-1}\}$ are deleted and $DV(t, k)$ is computed. The initial times are $t = 1$ at the first step, $t = 2$ at the second one, and $t = n-k+1$ at the last one. The presence of a patch starting at t and of length k is accepted if $DV(t, k)$ is the largest statistic value which exceeds the critical value at the prespecified significance level α.

Complications may arise, of course, namely

1. Two patches are near each other, or an isolated outlier is present in the neighbor of a patch so that the masking effect may lead to overlook one of the two disturbances

2. The statistics $DV(t, 1)$ and $DV(t, k)$ are often similar so that an isolated outlier in t may happen to be identified whilst there is actually a patch which starts at time t and ends at time $t + k - 1$.

Such drawbacks call for trying iteratively simultaneously both t and k. The outlier or the sequence with largest test statistic over the complete set of pairs (t, k) is assumed as an outlier and the time series y is adjusted accordingly. The procedure is replicated until no more outliers are found.

The time series y (number of observations $n = 100$) displayed in Fig. 6.4, upper plot, may be useful to illustrate the leave-k-out procedure. We may hypothesize the possible largest patch length equal to 6. Then the statistic $DV(t, k)$ has been computed for $k = 1, \ldots, 6$ and $t = 1, \ldots, 100 - k + 1$. From the complete time series y the following model has been estimated

$$y_t = 0.0523 + 0.7042 y_{t-1} + a_t, \qquad \sigma_a^2 = 1.435.$$

In Fig. 6.5 the values computed for the statistic DV(t,k) are displayed for some selected values of k of special interest. These latter are those at the edges of the patch, because values in the middle produce small values of the test statistic by the masking effect. The largest value is obtained by assuming that the time series is perturbed by a patch with starting time $t = 51$ and length $k = 5$. Comparable values are obtained only by assuming the hypothesis of either an isolated outlier in $t = 51$ or a patch of length $k = 4$ or $k = 6$ starting in $t = 51$.

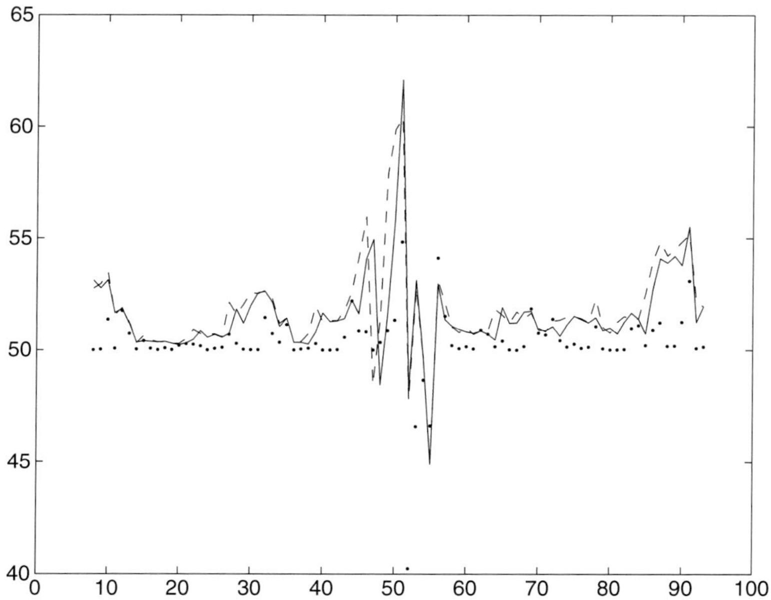

Fig. 6.5 Statistics $DV(t, k)$ varying t and assuming $k = 1$ (*dotted line*), $k = 5$ (*solid line*), and $k = 6$ (*dashed line*)

Table 6.2 Statistics $DV(t, k)$ at time when the patch actually starts ($t = 51$) and at another locations ($t = 49, 91$) where the diagnostic statistics are found large

k	1	2	3	4	5	6
$DV(49, k)$	50.8680	53.3669	55.1679	48.5711	51.5734	57.8988
$DV(51, k)$	54.8340	48.4048	51.4162	57.7022	62.0878	60.3998
$DV(91, k)$	53.0947	53.7992	54.1227	54.4375	55.5151	55.1645

In Table 6.2 the statistics $DV(t, k)$ are displayed only for the dates t where largest values were obtained for at least one value of k. As far as the true outlier timing $t = 51$ is concerned, the maxima of $DV(t, k)$ varying k have been attained almost always. Exceptions are $k = 2$ where the largest value is obtained for $t = 91$ and $k = 3$ where the largest value corresponds to $t = 49$. In this example both masking and smearing effects are apparent. The statistic $DV(t, k)$ is small at $t = 52, 53$ because of the masking effects due to the neighboring observations. On the other hand the smearing effect causes the large value of the test statistic at $t = 56$. The cleaned times series shows no more outliers but a disturbance at $t = 91$ which may be either an isolated outlier or a patch of length $k = 5$.

An alternative method for patch detection which requires less computational effort may be based on finite linear interpolators. Let $i_t(m, s)$, m, s non-negative integers much less than n, denote the finite linear interpolator with horizon (m, s) computed from the observed time series y.

For all pairs (m, s) the finite interpolator errors

$$e_t(m, s) = y_t - i_t(m, s)$$

are defined. However, only the interpolators for the pairs (m, m), $(0, m)$ and $(m, 0)$ have to be computed. The detection of a patch may proceed as follows. A constant g is chosen and each and every date t is checked to decide the presence/absence of an outlying observation. The interpolator $i_t(m, m)$ is known to have smaller variance than both $i_t(0, m)$ and $i_t(m, 0)$, so that it is likely to be more sensible to detect potential outliers. If a detection occurs far apart any other one we may assume the presence of an isolated outlier. If there are several detections in a close neighbor, that is within a small time span, then the presence of a patch may be suspected. The interpolator $i_t(m, 0)$ is an AR(m) model and is able to locate the starting date of a sequence of potential outliers. On the other hand, the interpolator $i_t(0, m)$ is a forward AR(m) model (the backshift operator B is replaced by F, where $Fy_t = y_{t+1}$) and is able to locate the end of a potential patch. More details may be found in Battaglia and Baragona (1992).

The time series displayed in Fig. 6.4 may serve as an example. The lower plot is the linear interpolation error which exceeds the upper bounds for $g = 2.58$ at $t = 51$ and $t = 56$. The two potential outliers are close together and call for checking the presence of a sequence of outlying observations. The backward and forward interpolation errors are displayed in Fig. 6.6. The backward one $e_t(2, 0) = y_t - i_t(2, 0)$ exceeds the upper bound at $t = 51$ and may locate the starting of a patch.

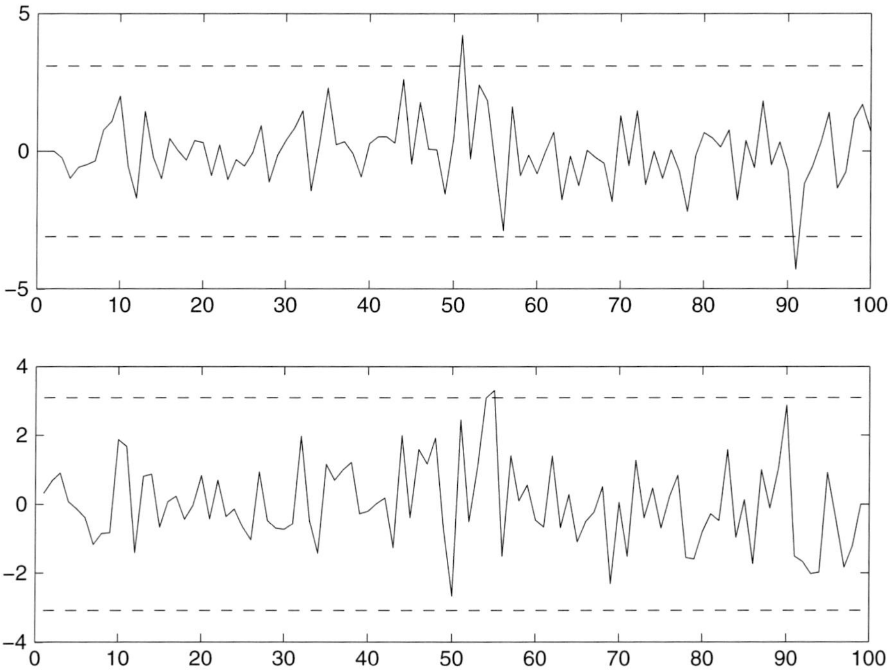

Fig. 6.6 Residual error sequence (*upper plot*) from a linear interpolator $i_t(2, 0)$ to mark the starting of the patch at $t = 51$ and residual error sequence from a linear interpolator $i_t(0, 2)$ (*lower plot*) to mark the ending of the patch at $t = 55$ for the artificial time series generated by an AR(1) model. *Dashed lines* are normal bounds at 1% significance level

The end of the patch may then be located at $t = 55$ where the forward interpolation error $e_t(0, 2) = y_t - i_t(0, 2)$ exceeds the upper bound. Notice that the bilateral interpolation error sequence alone fails to locate the patch and may lead to erroneous detection as

1. Though the outlier at $t = 51$ is correctly detected, it is not recognized as the first of an outlier sequence
2. The patch is completely overlooked
3. A false detection occurs as regards the observation at $t = 56$.

The consideration of the three linear interpolators $i_t(2, 2)$, $i_t(2, 0)$ and $i_t(0, 2)$ allows instead the patch to be detected exactly.

6.2.2 Multivariate Time Series Outlier Models

Let $z_t = [z_{1t}, ..., z_{st}]'$ be a discrete parameter s components vector second order stationary time series, with mean zero for each component and covariance matrix Γ_u, for integer lag u. We assume as usual in this Section that $\{z_t\}$ is generated by a linear process

$$z_t = \Psi(B)a_t \tag{6.9}$$

where (Reinsel, 1993) $\Psi(B) = I + \sum_{j=1}^{\infty} \Psi_j B^j$, and $a_t = [a_{1t}, ..., a_{st}]'$ is a zero mean Gaussian white noise with covariance matrix Σ. The process (6.9) is said to be invertible if $\det(\Psi(z)) \neq 0$ if $|z| < 1$. In this case let $\Pi(B) = \Psi(B)^{-1}$ so that (6.9) may be written

$$\Pi(B)z_t = a_t, \tag{6.10}$$

where $\Pi(B) = -\sum_{j=0}^{\infty} \Pi_j B^j$, $\Pi_0 = -I$. Then it may be shown that the optimum vector linear interpolator is

$$I_t = \sum_{u \neq 0} (-\Gamma i_0^{-1} \Gamma i_u) z_{t-u},$$

where Γi_u is the lag u inverse covariance matrix. Let $e_t = [e_{1t}, ..., e_{st}]'$ denote the interpolation error, that is the difference between z_t and the optimum vector linear interpolator

$$e_t = z_t - I_t.$$

The following orthogonality relationship may be shown to hold

$$\sum_{u=-\infty}^{\infty} \Gamma_u \Gamma i'_{u+j} = \delta_j I, \tag{6.11}$$

where δ_j denotes the Kronecker's delta and I the $s \times s$ identity matrix. Properties and detailed assumptions may be found in Bhansali (1990).

If k disturbances $\omega_t = [\omega_{1t}, ..., \omega_{st}]'$ happen to be located at time points $t = t_1, ..., t_k$, then the mean value of z_t will be different from zero, at least for some components. Given n observations $\{z_1, ..., z_n\}$, the outlier configuration may be described by means of the pattern design matrix X. For the sake of simplicity we introduce X under the assumption that all outliers are of the additive type. Details for other outlier types will be given later. Let i_j be the number of the contaminated component series at time t_j, $j = 1, ..., k$, and let $h = i_1 + ... + i_k$. The integer h represents the number of the scalar outliers, and $h = ks$ at most, if all outliers were global. For any pair (t, r), $t = 1, ..., n$, $r = 1, ..., s$, consider the row $(t-1)s + r$ of X. All entries in such row are zero unless an outlier is present at time t for the component series of index r. In this case, if i denotes such scalar outlier, the entry in column i and row $(t-1)s + r$ will be unity. The $n \times hs$ matrix X contains, in binary form, all information about the given (additive) outlier pattern.

Let $z = [z'_1, ..., z'_n]'$ be the vector obtained by stacking the s component observations at each time point, and let Γ denote the $ns \times ns$ block Toeplitz matrix with Γ_{i-j} as the (i, j)th block. Assume, at this moment, that both Γ and X are known.

Then, on assuming Gaussianity, the natural logarithm of the likelihood for z may be written, by omitting all constant terms,

$$\ell = -\frac{1}{2}(z - X\omega)'\Gamma^{-1}(z - X\omega). \tag{6.12}$$

Maximization of (6.12) with respect to ω yields

$$\hat{\omega} = (X'\Gamma^{-1}X)^{-1}X'\Gamma^{-1}z. \tag{6.13}$$

The approximation $\Gamma^{-1} \approx \Gamma i$ may be derived from (6.11), where Γi denotes the $ns \times ns$ block Toeplitz matrix with Γi_{i-j} as the (i, j)th block. Then, the maximum likelihood estimate (6.13) of ω takes the form

$$\hat{\omega} = (X'\Gamma iX)^{-1}X'(I \otimes \Gamma i_0)e, \tag{6.14}$$

where $e = [e'_1, ..., e'_n]'$ are the interpolation errors and $\otimes$ denotes the Kronecker's product. Equality (6.14) establishes in the multivariate framework the relationship between the additive outlier and the linear interpolator. For a fixed pre-specified truncation point m, the formula suggested by Battaglia (1984) may be used for the computation of the inverse covariance matrices

$$\Gamma i_u = \sum_{j=0}^{m-u} \Pi'_j \Sigma^{-1} \Pi_{u+j}, \qquad 0 \le u \le m, \tag{6.15}$$

where the truncated version of (6.10) is assumed for the definition of the matrices Π_j. For negative lag integer values, the relationship $\Gamma i_u = \Gamma i'_{-u}$ should be used. The natural logarithm of the maximized likelihood is obtained, by replacing, in (6.12), ω with (6.14) and Γ^{-1} with Γi

$$\ell = \frac{1}{2}\{X'(I \otimes \Gamma i_0)e\}'(X'\Gamma iX)^{-1}X'(I \otimes \Gamma i_0)e, \tag{6.16}$$

where all constant terms are omitted.

In practice inverse covariance matrices Γi_u have to be estimated. This may be done by first estimating the matrices Π and Σ fitting a vector autoregressive model, or alternatively by estimating first the ordinary autocovariance matrices Γ_u and then using the orthogonality relationship (6.11).

An extension of the univariate ARIMA based outlier detection procedure to multivariate series was proposed by Tsay et al. (2000). A vector ARIMA model is fitted to the observed time series, the maximum likelihood vector estimates of $\hat{\omega}$ (in the Gaussian case) are computed for the four outlier types AO, IO, LS and TC, and the significance of such estimates is evaluated through finite sample critical values generated by simulation. The algorithm proceeds iteratively as in the univariate case. If an outlier is detected at time q, all components of the series are assumed as perturbed at that time.

More recently, new methods for multivariate outlier detection have been proposed, based on the computation of univariate linear combinations of the multivariate series, and application of the univariate outlier detection techniques. The coefficients of the linear combination may be selected according to the projection pursuit techniques, in order to maximize the kurtosis (Galeano et al., 2006) or by independent component analysis (Baragona and Battaglia, 2007).

6.3 Genetic Algorithms for Multiple Outlier Detection

The iterative procedure for multiple outlier detection and estimation in time series does not guarantee that all outliers are properly identified as no objective function is specified that has to be globally optimized. Furthermore if an observation is detected incorrectly as an outlying one at some iteration no reverse action may be entertained and such an error is likely to completely bias the next iterations. The best course of action could consist in examining all possible subsets of the integers in $[t_0 + 1, n]$ and computing the likelihood function of the time series data taking each one into account. This is an unfeasible procedure even for moderate n as the number of subsets grows largest soon. Furthermore computations are cumbersome because the data are not independent and the full covariance matrix enters the likelihood function.

As for independent data, general heuristics allow us to evaluate only a limited number of subsets as potential outliers. The temporal dependence, however, prevents us from using the ordered GAs so that a different encoding has to be adopted.

We assume that there exists a maximum number of outliers K, say, as outliers are to be considered rare events and only a limited number, 5% of observations, for instance, may occur. The number of subsets is large, but it becomes even larger if we want to distinguish the outlier type as well. By assuming m outlier types then the number of subsets of potential outlier configurations is equal to

$$mn + m^2\binom{n}{2} + m^3\binom{n}{3} + \ldots + m^K\binom{n}{K}.$$

We may define some GAs for searching such a large solution space to provide us with the optimal (or at least near optimal) solution. As ordered encoding does not seem appropriate, we may use a binary encoding, that is we may define a binary string of length $\ell = n - t_0$ and assume 1 if there is an outlying observation and 0 otherwise. Each bit is associated a time point t. If, in addition, we want to distinguish outlier type as well, we may use m binary string, each string for each type, under the constraint that in any time point there is only a single 1.

Let, for instance, the time series $y=(y_1, y_2, \ldots, y_n)'$ have $n = 30$ observations, and let outliers (any type) be located at $t = 9, 20, 21, 22$. Then, the binary encoding may look as follows

000000001000000000011100000000

Consider instead the case where we want to distinguish between the AO and IO types. If there is a IO at $t = 9$ and there are AO at $t = 20, 21, 22$, then we may use the binary encoding in two lines

000000000000000000011100000000
000000001000000000000000000000

For meta heuristics to work in a reasonable time, the objective function has to be chosen so that it may be properly and quickly computed. We may attempt to minimize the residual sum of squares computed from some autoregressive moving average model fitted to the data as an approximation to the likelihood function. An identification stage, in necessarily automatic way, has to be performed, however, which requires in most cases a considerable computational effort. Then, a valid course of action consists in exploiting the relationship between the linear interpolator and the AO (see Peña, 1990, p. 237). Similar guidelines with extension to IO were suggested by Choy (2001). Only the inverse covariance function (Cleveland, 1972) is needed which may be easily estimated from the data. Let us consider, for the sake of simplicity, only the AO type. Let k outliers be located at $t = t_1, \ldots, t_k$. Let us define the $n \times k$ "design matrix" X, where $X_{j,h} = 1$ if $j = t_h$ (that is, the hth outlying observation is located at time $t = j$) and 0 otherwise. Let $y=(y_1, \ldots, y_n)'$ be the observed time series and x the unobserved outlier – free realization. Then, the relationship

$$y = x + X\omega$$

holds, where $\omega = (\omega_1, \ldots, \omega_k)'$ is the outlier size array. The likelihood to be maximized is approximately, under Gaussianity assumption,

$$\ell\,(X, \omega; y) = (2\pi)^{-\frac{n}{2}} \sqrt{\det(\Gamma i)} \exp\left\{-\frac{1}{2}\,(y - X\omega)'\,\Gamma i\,(y - X\omega)\right\}. \qquad (6.17)$$

The matrix Γi of the inverse autocovariances may be estimated from the data by using robust techniques (see Glendinning, 2000). Holding Γi fixed speeds the computation, but robustness of the estimates may be inadequate in some circumstances. However, Baragona et al. (2001a) considered the case when the estimate of Γi is iteratively adjusted. The Toeplitz property of the matrix Γi is exploited in order to make the computation to become not too demanding. In addition, the procedure is extended to cover the case where IO may occur as well. Some adjustment on the GAs parameters may allow the number of iterations to be reduced (see Aytug and Koehler, 2000, for instance). The probability of mutation and the size of the population seem to be the most important parameters to take under control if we want to obtain at least a near optimal solution in the shortest time.

6.3.1 Detecting Multiple Outliers in Univariate Time Series

Let $\xi = (\xi_1, \ldots, \xi_\ell)'$ denote a chromosome, that is a string of characters of assigned length ℓ that can be evaluated by some suitable fitness function. A natural choice consists in setting the length ℓ of the chromosome equal to n, where n is the number of observations of the time series. This choice allows us to interpret each locus as a time point where an outlier may occur. Assignment of allelic values is to be made as simpler as possible, though obviously other choices may be done. A gene ξ_j takes the value zero, if the locus is an outlier-free time point, the value 1 if the observation at this time point is an outlier of the additive type, and the value 2 if it is an innovation outlier.

However, it is customary to assume that a maximum number of outliers $h_{\max} \ll n$ may be found in the series. This poses a problem of chromosome legality, because all chromosomes which have less than $n - h_{\max}$ genes equal to zero are not legal, and a validation stage has to be performed at each new generation. Alternative encodings, which avoid such a problem, may be considered. For example, a chromosome may be formed by $h_{\max}$ genes each of which is an integer ranging from 1 to n and denotes the position of an outlier. If the gene values are not all different, the resulting configuration has less than $h_{\max}$ outliers. For example, a chromosome with all genes equal to 20 corresponds to a series with only one outlier at time 20. However, in that case the one to one correspondence is lost, since many chromosomes encode the same outlier configuration. Both encoding systems are able to represent the whole set of possible outlier arrangements, but in the binary encoding case the total number of different chromosomes is 2^n, while in the integer encoding is $n^{h_{\max}}$. The comparison between these two numbers may suggest which encoding system is more efficient.

Particular care is needed in the choice of the fitness function. A suitable fitness function to be used for detecting outliers in multivariate time series in a GAs framework may be built on the log-likelihood (6.17). Two problems have to be solved, however.

1. The function (6.17) increases as the number of outliers increases, so that it cannot be optimized with respect to the number of outliers.
2. In general (6.17) is not a positive function, whilst this is a property required to properly define a fitness function.

The first problem may be fixed for example by adopting the asymptotic information criterion (AIC) (Akaike, 1977). So, the function which has actually to be minimized is

$$\ell^* = -2\ell + 2h, \tag{6.18}$$

where h denotes the numbers of outliers. Positive values may be obtained by using a monotone transform of (6.18) which yields only real positive values and is as larger as closer to the optimal solution, for instance

$$\ell^* = \exp\{(2\ell - 2h)/c\}. \tag{6.19}$$

The positive constant c is introduced to scale the fitness and to avoid the occurrence of overflow during computation. Criteria other than the AIC may be adopted, and so other transforms that are believed to be more appropriate may be chosen. A slightly more general choice is using a penalized likelihood function instead of the AIC:

$$\ell_\alpha^* = \exp\{(2\ell - \alpha h)/c\}, \tag{6.20}$$

where α is an arbitrarily selected constant. We stress that on changing α the optimum outlier configuration may change, therefore the choice of α may crucially modify the results of the GA application. Baragona et al. (2001a) suggest a way of choosing α using a Bayesian argument in terms of the a priori probability of outlying observations.

Finally, it may be observed that the proposed method is a hybrid genetic algorithm, because the fitness function is obtained through maximum likelihood. Therefore this method integrates the random search in the space of solutions with an analytical derivation of the optimal outlier magnitudes.

6.3.2 Genetic Algorithms for Detecting Multiple Outliers in Multivariate Time Series

For the multivariate case the fitness definition may follow the same guidelines as for univariate series, adopting a penalized likelihood form (6.20) where ℓ is given by the maximized multivariate likelihood (6.16). The function ℓ_α^* as defined by (6.20) depends on both the integer h and the matrix X which appears in (6.16) explicitly. The integer parameter h varies from 0 to the maximum pre-specified allowed number of scalar outlying observations $h_{\max}$. Let k_y denote the number of outlier types. The matrix X takes values on a discrete set, H say. The set H has $1 + \sum_{i=1}^{h_{\max}} \binom{ns}{i} k_y^i$ elements, the no-outlier case included, so that it is very large, unless either n or $h_{\max}$ are quite small. As H is a discrete set, the optimization techniques which require that the function to be maximized fulfills some regularity conditions, continuity, differentiability, and convexity, for instance, do not apply. On the other hand, H is often such a large set that the complete enumeration of its elements is not feasible, and most available searching algorithms are likely to yield some local optimum as a result. So simple GAs seem a suitable choice for finding the maximum of (6.20) as a stochastic searching technique which does not require any particular assumption about the function to optimize.

The function ℓ_α^* in (6.20) is assumed, in the present framework, to depend only on the matrix X. In fact, the integer h is straightly determined from X. The other parameters in (6.16) are to be considered fixed, so that their computation has to be done only once. The method described in Chan and Wei (1992) is employed which yields robust trimmed estimates of the covariance matrices. Then, the matrices Π_j

are estimated by using the Yule-Walker equations, and (6.15) provides the estimate of the inverse covariance matrices.

The definition of the outlier pattern design matrix X may be extended to cover other types of disturbance than the AO. For example, an IO in the component series r at time t is coded into the matrix X as follows. Let such IO be the ith scalar outlier. The coefficients of the pure MA representation of the vector time series z_t are needed which may be computed from the recursive matrix equation (see Reinsel, 1993, p. 27)

$$\Psi_u = \Pi_u + \sum_{j=1}^{u-1} \Pi_j \Psi_{u-j}, \qquad u = 1, 2, \ldots,$$

where the summation vanishes if $u \leq 1$. The coefficient Ψ_u is an $s \times s$ matrix and let

$$\Psi_u = \begin{pmatrix} \psi_{11}^{(u)} & \psi_{12}^{(u)} & \cdots & \psi_{1s}^{(u)} \\ \psi_{21}^{(u)} & \psi_{22}^{(u)} & \cdots & \psi_{2s}^{(u)} \\ \vdots & \vdots & \ddots & \vdots \\ \psi_{s1}^{(u)} & \psi_{s2}^{(u)} & \cdots & \psi_{ss}^{(u)} \end{pmatrix}.$$

As n data are available, and assuming an IO at time t, the coefficient matrices $\Psi_1, \ldots, \Psi_{n-t}$ only are of practical use. Moreover, if the entries in matrices Ψ_u's are decreasing in absolute value, we may want to use only matrices $\Psi_1, \ldots, \Psi_q$ for a suitable truncation point q. Let the positive integer $q \geq 0$ be either user-defined or set to $n - t$. Then, in the column i of X, after the unity has been inserted in row $(t-1)s + r$, the entries in column i and rows $ts + 1, \ldots, (t+q)s$ are to be filled with the coefficients $\psi_{jr}^{(u)}$, $j = 1, \ldots, s$, $u = 1, \ldots, q$, according to the ordering

$$\left(\psi_{1r}^{(1)}, \ldots, \psi_{sr}^{(1)}, \psi_{1r}^{(2)}, \ldots, \psi_{sr}^{(2)}, \ldots, \psi_{1r}^{(q)}, \ldots, \psi_{sr}^{(q)}\right)'.$$

In a similar way other disturbance types may be further defined by extending to the multivariate case the definitions (6.8) (Tsay et al., 2000). If the ith scalar outlier occurs as a LS at time t for the component series r, then the entries in column i and rows $(t-1)s + r, ts + r, (t+1)s + r, \ldots$ of X are set to 1. For a TC at time t, the column i of X contain, in the rows $(t-1)s + r, ts + r, (t+1)s + r, \ldots$, the values δ^j, $j = 0, 1, 2 \ldots$, where $0 < \delta < 1$. The figure $\delta = 0.7$ has been suggested (Chen and Liu, 1993).

In what follows a simple genetic algorithm is described that is able to handle the search for multiple outliers and determining their type simultaneously. A binary encoding is used as it seems both natural and simple, though the chromosome length may grow largest in the presence of a large number of observations. Different encoding, integer for instance, may be used that allow smaller chromosomes to be handled, but in the multivariate case the definition of suitable genetic operators would be more difficult.

6.3.2.1 Encoding

The encoding establishes a one-to-one correspondence between any matrix $X \in H$ and a binary chromosome. This latter may be represented as a stack of $k_y s$ binary sequences, each of length n, the number of observations of the vector time series. So, the chromosome is actually assumed as a binary matrix where each row is concerned with an outlier type in a component series, and each column represents a time point. For any given component series, an obvious constraint is that, at each time point, no more than a single 1 has to be present through the k_y rows.

Consider, for instance, a bivariate time series of length $n = 40$, let $k_y = 4$, and suppose that the proposal outlier pattern includes a global (so as to say, in each component series) AO at time $t = 30$, a partial IO for the second component only at time $t = 20$, and, in addition, a global level shift (LS) at time 10, and a partial transient change (TC) for the first component at time $t = 25$. Then, as the order is assumed AO, IO, LS, and TC, the chromosome is as follows

1st	AO	0000000000000000000000000000010000000000
component	IO	0000000000000000000000000000000000000000
series	LS	0000000001000000000000000000000000000000
	TC	0000000000000000000000001000000000000000
2nd	AO	0000000000000000000000000000010000000000
component	IO	0000000000000000000100000000000000000000
series	LS	0000000001000000000000000000000000000000
	TC	0000000000000000000000000000000000000000

If one wants to consider, as it may found in many applications, only the AO and IO outlier types, then it suffices to drop the last two rows concerned with every component series in each chromosome. In this case, each chromosome has $2s$ rows instead of $4s$. Note that in this way it is possible to restrict the effect of each outlier to selected components. This would be impossible at the identification stage with the vector ARIMA based methods.

An alternative could be concatenating the $k_y s$ binary strings of each individual so that a chromosome with $k_y sn$ binary digits is considered. This, however, does not reduce the complexity of the problem, and does not allow the four outlier types to be treated independently, specially as far as the crossover operator is concerned. With this encoding also a validation stage at each new generation is required, since only one outlier type at the time for each component is allowed, and no more than $h_{\max}$ genes equal to one in each component are legal.

6.3.2.2 Selection

The population includes ν individuals, each of which may be decoded in such a way that the fitness function may be computed. We noted already that (6.20) meets the requirements for a properly defined fitness function. The "roulette wheel" rule generates ν individuals by selecting, ν times with replacement, an individual from the current population with probability proportional to its fitness function. If the fitness function values were calculated as $f_1, f_2, \ldots, f_\nu$, then the probability for the individual i to be selected equals $f_i/(f_1 + f_2 + \cdots + f_\nu)$. The chromosome of the selected individual is copied into that of a newly created one. These new individuals replace the old ones completely, according to the choice $G = 1$ for the generation gap. The only exception to this total replacement is concerned with using the "elitist strategy." In this case, the replacement involves the whole population if the best individual is selected by the "roulette wheel." The total replacement involves only $\nu - 1$ individuals of the past population if the best individual happens not to be selected. Then, the last individual of the next population is given the chromosome of such best individual.

6.3.2.3 Crossover

Given a pre-specified crossover probability p_c, the pairs that may be considered for applying this operator are $n_p = [p_c\nu/2]$. For n_p times, two different individuals are chosen uniformly randomly in the population, and their chromosomes are compared row by row. An integer ℓ_t is selected from the uniform distribution over the integers from 1 to $\ell - 1$. The first row of the first chromosome, from the gene in $t = \ell_t + 1$ through the last one, in $t = \ell$, is exchanged with the genes from $\ell_t + 1$ to ℓ of the first row of the chromosome of the other individual in the pair. This operation is repeated for each row, and the "cutting point" may vary from a row to another. Then, k_y new chromosomes result, that substitute the original chromosomes of the two individuals in the pair.

For example, let only the AO and IO outlier types ($k_y = 2$) be considered. The chromosomes of two individuals chosen at random are supposed to be as follows

individual	1st	AO	00000000000000000000|00000000010000000000
1	series	IO	0000000001|000000000000000000000000000000
	2nd	AO	000000000000000000000000000001|0000000000
	series	IO	0000000000000000000000000|000000000000000
individual	1st	AO	00000000010000000000|00000000000000000000
2	series	IO	0000000000|000000000000001000000000000000
	2nd	AO	000000000000000000000000000000|1000000000
	series	IO	0000000001000000000000000|000000000000000

The first individual encodes in its chromosome a global AO in $t = 30$ and an IO only in the first component in $t = 10$. The second individual encodes in its chromosome only partial outliers. In the first component, an AO in $t = 10$ and an IO in $t = 25$. In the second component, there are an AO in $t = 31$ and an IO in $t = 10$.

Let the "cutting points" be 20, 10, 30, 25 for each of the four rows respectively. Note that the "cutting point" are the same for both individuals in the corresponding rows. A vertical line indicates these values in the binary strings for the first and the second individual. The crossover changes the chromosomes of the two individuals to obtain the new chromosomes

individual	1st	AO	00000000000000000000|00000000000000000000
1	series	IO	0000000001|000000000000001000000000000000
	2nd	AO	000000000000000000000000000001|1000000000
	series	IO	0000000000000000000000000|000000000000000
individual	1st	AO	00000000010000000000|00000000010000000000
2	series	IO	0000000000|000000000000000000000000000000
	2nd	AO	000000000000000000000000000000|0000000000
	series	IO	0000000001000000000000000|000000000000000

Now the first individual has two IO in the first component only, whilst the second component has two consecutive AO. The second individual has two AO, well far apart, in the first component, and a single IO in the second component. The global outlier disappears, whilst there are now two partial AO close together. This latter pattern may often occur in practice, and is likely to be produced by crossover.

6.3.2.4 Mutation

Each individual is examined, and each gene of its chromosome is given a probability p_m to change its value from 0 to 1 or vice versa. For example, let the second individual considered in the preceding subsection undergoes a unique mutation in the first row of the second component at $t = 30$. Its chromosome becomes

individual	1st	AO	0000000001000000000000000000010000000000
2	series	IO	0000000000000000000000000000000000000000
	2nd	AO	0000000000000000000000000000010000000000
	series	IO	0000000001000000000000000000000000000000

so as to recover the global AO in $t = 30$.

6.3.3 An Example of Application to Real Data

The well-known gas furnace data (Box and Jenkins, 1976) were examined for outliers using the GA procedure. The plot of the time series is displayed in Fig. 6.7. The first component of this bivariate time series is the gas rate in cubic feet per minute, the second one the percentage of CO_2 in outlet gas, measured in 9-s time intervals. There are $n = 296$ observations.

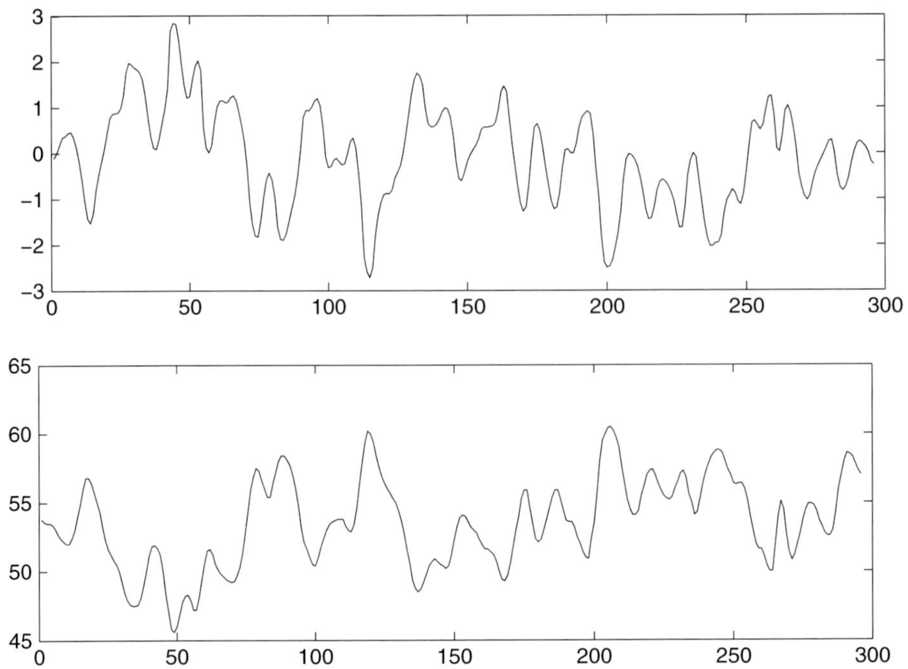

Fig. 6.7 The gas furnace data, Series J from Box and Jenkins (1976)

The VARIMA-based procedure for outlier detection and estimation differs from the GAs-based approach essentially in two ways. Firstly, in this latter approach the implicit assumption is made that the time series model is the "truncated" vector linear interpolator (Battaglia, 1984; Bhansali, 1990).

$$z_t = \sum_{u=-m}^{m} (-\Gamma i_0^{-1} \Gamma i_u) z_{t-u} + e_t.$$

Tsay, Peña and Pankratz assume, instead, a VARIMA model to represent the time series data. Secondly, in the GAs framework, the candidate outliers are never examined separately, but comparison is made amongst different complete outlier patterns. The one which yields the maximum of the fitness function in the last iteration is taken as the final solution. The Tsay, Peña and Pankratz's identification procedure considers, instead, every single time location t in turn, and several tests, against the null hypothesis that the observation at time t is not an outlying one, are performed. These tests may indicate the outlier type as well by comparing the p-values of the test statistics and choosing the type that corresponds to the smallest p-value. Once an outlier is identified, its magnitude is estimated and is removed from the time series. The adjusted time series is considered as a new one, and the identification procedure is iterated.

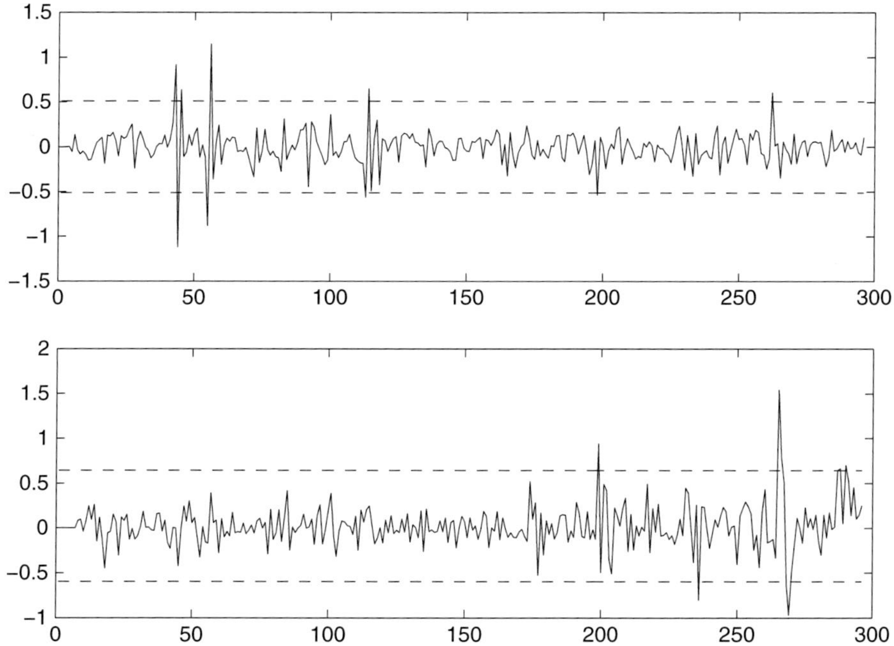

Fig. 6.8 Residuals computed from the gas furnace data by using a transfer function model (*solid lines*). The *dashed lines* are the normal bounds at 1% significance level

We also took into account the transfer function model reported in Tsay, Peña and Pankratz and obtained by using the joint estimation and detection procedure of Chen and Liu (1993). The residuals are displayed in Fig. 6.8. The normal bounds at 1% significance level are plotted for comparison and outline the presence of several outliers in both components at the dates where the model residuals are either larger than the upper bound or smaller the the lower bound. This circumstance is to be assumed only as a preliminary diagnostic for deciding if more detailed investigation of outliers in the time series has to be performed.

Likewise, the residuals computed from a vector autoregressive model of order 6 and the linear interpolation errors from a linear interpolator with $m = 4$ computed for the series J are displayed in Figs. 6.9 and 6.10 respectively. The bounds computed as for Fig. 6.10 are plotted as dashed lines to show the locations of large residual absolute values.

In Table 6.3 the time points are reported where graphical inspection of residuals in Figs. 6.8, 6.9, and 6.10 shows large residual absolute values. Thresholds are assumed $m \pm 2.58s$ for each series, corresponding to the dashed straight lines, where m and s stand for the mean value and residual variance respectively. It seems natural to search for potential outliers referring to the normal probability distribution as a first approximation. The significance 1% level has been considered.

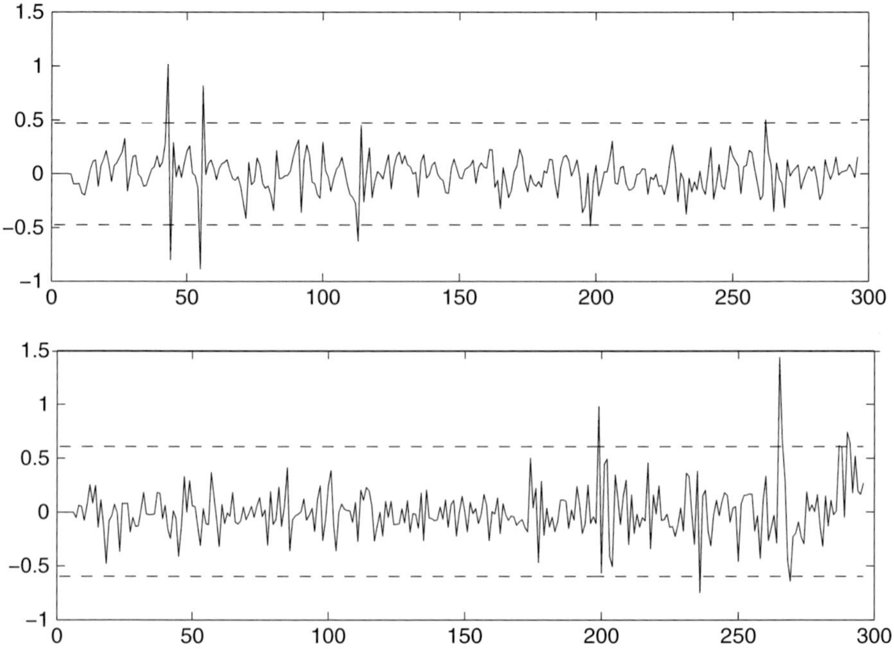

Fig. 6.9 Residuals computed from the gas furnace data by using a vector autoregression of order 6 (*solid lines*). The *dashed lines* are the normal bounds at 1% significance level

Table 6.3 Preliminary identification of dates when potential outliers may be located with comparison to the 1% unit standard normal distribution lower and upper bounds, that is 0.005 on left tail and 0.995 on right tail percentiles

Model	Series	Dates when model residuals exceed normal 99% lower/upper bounds								
Transfer	1st	**43**	44	45	**55**	56	**113**	114	198	262
Function	2nd	**199**	236	265	266	268	269	288	290	
VAR(6)	1st	**43**	44	**55**	56	**113**	198	262		
	2nd	**199**	236	265	266	269	287	290	291	
Lin.Int.	1st	42	**43**	54	**55**	112	**113**	261		
$m = 4$	2nd	198	**199**	234	235	263	264	288		

Large absolute values residuals common to all three models are reported in boldface in Table 6.3. These are locations that are to be carefully investigated to check the occurrence of outlying observations. The potential outliers occur within the first half of the time series time span in the first component series whilst in the second component series potential outliers are present in the second half of the data. As noted already by Tsay, Peña and Pankratz the transfer function model and the multivariate model share a similar structure and as a consequence the residual variances are close. The residual linear interpolator error variance is less than that computed from the other two models as it is expected when comparing one-sided and bilateral models. According to the outlier estimates of innovative and additive

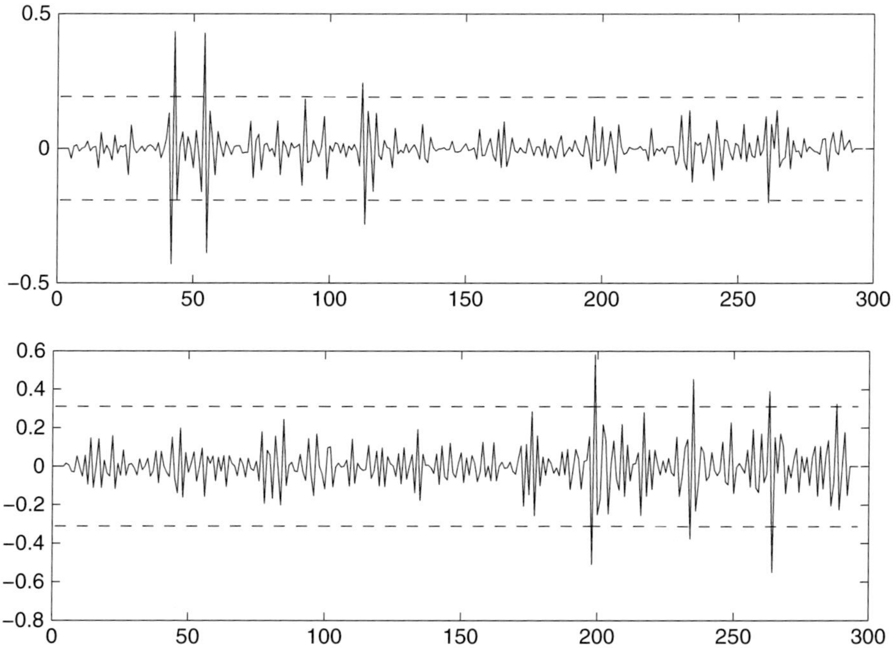

Fig. 6.10 Interpolation errors computed from the gas furnace data by using a linear interpolator with $m = 4$ (*solid lines*) and the normal bounds at 1% significance level

type, the VAR(6) model is to be assumed to give evidence to IO's while the linear interpolator points at dates where possibly AO's will be found. The transfer function model shows a greater number of potential outliers than the multivariate models. This circumstance too has to be expected because some of the outlying observations may be better explained by the dynamic multivariate structure.

It is of interest to compare the results obtained from GAs application with those presented, for this same data set, in Tsay et al. (2000). Computations for the GAs-based procedure has been done by assuming

- 5% the percentage of the data excluded for trimmed mean and covariance calculation (Chan and Wei, 1992, pp. 152–153), that is the 2.5% of the smallest and the 2.5% of the largest observations do not enter computations,
- $m = 18$ the truncation point of the linear interpolator,
- $q = 18$ the number of matrix weights in the truncated linear model (6.9)
- 20 the maximum allowable number of outlier time locations,
- $p_c = 0.9$ and $p_m = 0.01$ the crossover and mutation probabilities respectively,
- 101 the population size, that is a single generation in a GA iteration includes 101 potential solutions,
- 1000 GAs generations.

Table 6.4 Outliers in series J. Identification and estimation results from iterative VARIMA-based and GAs-based procedures (standard errors of the estimates are enclosed in parentheses)

VARIMA-based procedure				GAs-based procedure			
Time	Component	Outlier type	Size estimate	Time	Component	Outlier type	Size estimate
43	1st	TC	0.4732	12	1st	LS	−0.1495
			(0.1696)				(0.0666)
43	2nd	TC	−0.0520	12	2nd	LS	0.3202
			(0.3223)				(0.2220)
55	1st	TC	−0.6261	43	1st	AO	0.3675
			(0.1690)				(0.1491)
55	2nd	TC	−0.4868	54	1st	AO	0.5673
			(0.3236)				(0.1491)
82	1st	LS	−0.0562	74	1st	IO	−0.5254
			(0.3236)				(0.2528)
91	1st	TC	0.3136	95	1st	IO	0.5103
			(0.1696)				(0.2528)
113	1st	TC	−0.5071	112	1st	IO	−0.5739
			(0.1699)				(0.2527)
113	2nd	TC	0.0018	201	2nd	LS	0.5391
			(0.3226)				(0.2107)
197	1st	TC	0.1738	218	2nd	LS	−0.4648
			(0.1699)				(0.2245)
199	1st	LS	−0.3440	268	2nd	TC	0.7906
			(0.0866)				(0.3228)
199	2nd	LS	1.1956	285	2nd	LS	0.6050
			(0.2605)				(0.3248)
236	1st	LS	0.0549	288	1st	LS	0.2192
			(0.0904)				(0.1148)
236	2nd	LS	−0.1507	289	2nd	AO	0.7291
			(0.2740)				(0.3461)
262	1st	IO	−0.0143	290	2nd	LS	1.8661
			(0.2541)				(0.4523)
265	1st	IO	0.1538	291	2nd	IO	0.6666
			(0.2557)				(0.3921)
265	2nd	IO	0.9663	293	2nd	TC	0.8771
			(0.3780)				(0.3635)
287	1st	LS	0.2843	294	2nd	IO	0.5892
			(0.1635)				(0.4169)
287	2nd	LS	1.0422				
			(0.3074)				
288	1st	LS	0.1515				
			(0.1634)				
288	2nd	LS	1.1609				
			(0.3036)				

The best solution found in the final population, that is the chromosome for which the largest fitness function has been computed, yielded both the identified outliers and their size estimates. The fitness function (6.19) has been computed with $c = 100$. As the VARIMA-based method is concerned, for an equal comparison we assumed the outlier identification reported by Tsay, Peña and Pankratz, but estimates have been computed in both cases using the same algorithm based on the inverse correlations. Difference in the estimated values are rather small, however, according to the relationships that allows the vector time series inverse covariances to be expressed as a function of a VARIMA model parameters (see Battaglia, 1984). The AIC for both models after accommodation for outliers has been obtained AIC $= -166.6653$ for the VARIMA-based and AIC $= -167.6176$ for the GAs-based procedure. This slight improvement is entirely due to parsimony in outlier identification, as in the former case 20 scalar outliers are detected while in the latter case the procedure identifies 17 scalar outliers (an outlier in both components counts as 2 scalar outliers). As a matter of fact, the log-likelihoods equal 103.3325 and 100.8088 respectively but in the presence of a different number of outlying observations detected. In Table 6.4 estimated outlier size and standard errors are displayed computed from the VARIMA-based and GAs-based procedures.

The two approaches yield rather different dates for identified outliers. The only matching regards the LS outlier at $t = 288$ but the GAs-based procedure identifies a partial outlier in the first component only, while the VARIMA-based procedure identifies a global outlier in both components. In other cases outliers are detected at different but close dates. The Tsay, Peña and Pankratz's procedure, for instance, is reported to find a TC at $t = 55$, significant for the first component. The GA procedure find an IO in $t = 54$ for the first component only. In this case, confusion may arise from the fact that the IO and the TC exhibit similar behavior. Another example is the TC detected by the VARIMA-based procedure at time $t = 113$, significant for the first component. The GA procedure found an IO in $t = 112$ for the first component. In the latter case, the timing and type choice was influenced by the difference between the two consecutive observations, in $t = 112$ and $t = 113$, whilst, in the former one, the behavior of the perturbation after $t = 113$ was emphasized.

Chapter 7
Cluster Analysis

Abstract Meta heuristic methods have been often applied to partitioning problems. On one hand this proceeded from the fact that heuristic methods have always been applied to such problems since their earliest formulations. On the other hand, meta heuristic found a promising field of application because cluster analysis has two characteristic features that make it specially suitable for designing algorithms in this framework. The solution space is large, and grows fast with the problem dimension. The solutions form a discrete set that cannot be explored by the gradient – based methods or whatever method that is grounded on the exploitation of the properties of analytic functions. A large lot of algorithms based on genetic evolutionary computation have been proposed and have been found excellent solvers of partitioning problems. In this chapter we shall recall the usual classification of cluster algorithms and explain which class may be successfully handled by genetic evolutionary computation techniques. While most chapter is devoted to crisp partition problem, the fuzzy partition problem will be discussed as well. Then, the theoretical framework offered by the mixture distributions will be examined related to evolutionary computing estimation techniques. Also we will account for the genetic algorithms-based approach to the CART technique for classification. Applications of genetic algorithms for clustering time series will be described. Finally, the multiobjective clustering and implementation in the genetic algorithms framework will be outlined. Some examples and comparisons will illustrate the evolutionary computing methods for cluster analysis.

7.1 The Partitioning Problem

Let n objects be given each of which is characterized, and, as far as we are concerned here, coincides with p attributes that may be conveniently defined by real numbers. That is, we have the usual $n \times p$ data matrix where each line may be called an observation related to one of the n objects and each column corresponds to a variable. We assume that such a data set has a structure so that objects may be grouped into clusters. The objects that belong to a cluster are to be considered similar, while objects that belong to different clusters are to be considered dissimilar. Further, we assume that a similarity (or dissimilarity) measure between each and every pair of objects

R. Baragona et al., *Evolutionary Statistical Procedures*, Statistics and Computing, DOI 10.1007/978-3-642-16218-3_7, © Springer-Verlag Berlin Heidelberg 2011

may be computed from their variable values. Furthermore, an optimality criterion is intended to be devised such that in accordance with the chosen similarity measure its optimum value is achieved if the internal cluster cohesion and the external cluster dissimilarity are both maximized.

Then, the partitioning problem consists in grouping the objects so that the resulting cluster structure satisfies the chosen optimality criterion. Every object belongs to a cluster and if none is similar it is assumed to form a cluster on its own.

If the number of clusters g is assumed known the number of partitions of n objects may be computed (Liu, 1968)

$$N(n, g) = \frac{1}{g!} \sum_{j=1}^{g} (-1)^{g-j} \binom{g}{j} j^n ,$$

while if the number of clusters is unknown, and g is only a pre – specified upper bound, then the number of possible solutions is equal to

$$N(n, [1, g]) = \sum_{s=1}^{g} \frac{1}{s!} \sum_{j=1}^{s} (-1)^{s-j} \binom{s}{j} j^n .$$

This number grows fast with n. Unless n is very small the exhaustive search based on the enumeration of all partitions to choose the best one, according to some optimality criterion, is unfeasible. For moderate n algorithms are available that ensure finding the optimal partition in practice. If n is large most algorithms are likely to find a partition that is sub – optimal but may be quite poor sometimes. This circumstance explains on one hand the so many proposal algorithms for finding an optimal partition and on the other hand the need of meta heuristic stochastic algorithms that are able to search efficiently so large a discrete solution space.

If an object may belong to only one cluster, then we are performing a hard (or crisp) partition. Otherwise, if an object is allowed to belong to more than one cluster, possibly by defining some degree of belonging, we usually say that we are seeking for a fuzzy partition.

Methods for cluster analysis are the object of a large literature and are an active research field specially in connection with data mining techniques. General references are for instance Kaufman and Rousseeuw (2005) and Berkhin (2002), this latter for a review of the many clustering techniques that have found applications in data mining.

7.1.1 Classification

For the moment we may assume that, as it is often the case, clusters are defined and their number is given. We may call classes such ready-made clusters and each and every objects in a set $\mathcal{O}$ is assigned to its class without ambiguity. Let g denote the number of clusters, and let C_s be the set of objects that belong to cluster s, $s = 1, \ldots, g$. With the convention that an object is identified by its variable values, we may let the $p \times 1$ column vector x_i denote the object i, where

$$x_i = \begin{pmatrix} x_{i1} \\ x_{i2} \\ \vdots \\ x_{ip} \end{pmatrix}, \tag{7.1}$$

and x_{ij} denote the observed value of variable j on object i, $j = 1, \ldots, p$ and $i = 1, \ldots, n$. The observed values, that is the observations, are usually arranged in the data matrix with n rows (each row is an observation taken on an object) and p columns (each column is a variable)

$$X = \begin{pmatrix} (x_1)' \\ (x_2)' \\ \vdots \\ (x_n)' \end{pmatrix}. \tag{7.2}$$

A class is often defined by assuming that the variables have to take certain values, or values for each variables have to belong to some given interval. A convenient way for defining classes often consists in assuming a set of class identifiers, that is g $p \times 1$ column vectors

$$\bar{x}^{(h)} = \begin{pmatrix} \bar{x}_{h1} \\ \bar{x}_{h2} \\ \vdots \\ \bar{x}_{hp} \end{pmatrix} \qquad h = 1, \ldots, g, \tag{7.3}$$

that may or may not coincide with p-dimensional observations taken on objects in the set $\mathcal{O}$. The dissimilarity between x_i and $\bar{x}^{(h)}$ will be denoted by $d_{i\bar{h}}$. Then, the object x_i belongs to the class C_h if

$$d_{i\bar{h}} < \bar{d} \tag{7.4}$$

for some given positive real constant $\bar{d}$. For a given classification, it naturally arises the problem of allocating a new observation to a class. The discriminant analysis offers methods for designing suitable rules to allow an object to be properly assigned to a given class. Such methods often are comprised in the domain of supervised classification.

If classes are not available that may identify clusters, then we have to handle the unsupervised classification problem. Cluster analysis is often used as a synonymous for unsupervised classification. In this case we assume that the cluster structure, if any, has to be estimated from the data. Almost always the data matrix X offers all the information needed to compute the $n \times n$ dissimilarity matrix,

$$D = \begin{pmatrix} d_{11} & d_{12} & \cdots & d_{1n} \\ d_{21} & d_{22} & \cdots & d_{2n} \\ \vdots & \vdots & \ddots & \vdots \\ d_{n1} & d_{n2} & \cdots & d_{nn} \end{pmatrix}, \tag{7.5}$$

where

$$d_{ij} = d(x_i, x_j) \tag{7.6}$$

for some suitable real valued positive function d. The function d is defined in such a way $d(x_i, x_i) = 0 \; \forall i$.

A special class of dissimilarity measures, called dissimilarity coefficients (Gordon, 1981, p. 14), are often a convenient choice as they satisfy the following useful properties

1. $d_{ij} \geq 0 \; \forall (x_i, x_j) \in \mathcal{O}$
2. $d_{ii} = 0 \; \forall x_i \in \mathcal{O}$
3. $d_{ij} = d_{ji} \; \forall (x_i, x_j) \in \mathcal{O}$.

Some dissimilarity coefficients have the metric property that

$$d_{ij} + d_{ih} \geq d_{jh} \quad \forall (x_i, x_j, x_h) \in \mathcal{O}.$$

The dissimilarity coefficients that own the metric property are generally known as distance measures. The Euclidean distance is a well known example of a dissimilarity coefficient that satisfies the metric property. It is a special case of the Minkowski metrics

$$d_{ij}^{(\lambda)} = \left\{ \sum_{h=1}^{p} |x_{ih} - x_{jh}|^{\lambda} \right\}^{1/\lambda} \qquad \lambda > 0, \, (x_i, x_j) \in \mathcal{O}$$

by taking $\lambda = 2$.

If we are seeking for a hard partition, then a number of clusters g and g subsets $C_1, \ldots, C_g$ of $\mathcal{O}$ have to be found such that both

$$\mathcal{O} = C_1 \cup \ldots \cup C_g \tag{7.7}$$

and

$$C_s \cap C_r = \emptyset, \;\; s, r = 1, \ldots, n, \;\; r \neq s \tag{7.8}$$

hold. In this section we shall confine ourselves to hard partitioning for unsupervised classification.

Example 7.1.1 Iris Plants data base

The data have been downloaded from Asuncion and Newman (2007). The data set refers to $n = 150$ iris specimens (the objects) from the three classes setosa, versicolor and virginica. Each class includes 50 objects. Measurements are $p = 4$, namely sepal length in cm, sepal width in cm, petal length in cm and petal width in cm. The number of partitions that may be formed assuming $g = 3$ clusters is $N(150, 3) = 6.1665 \times 10^{70}$. The class setosa is known to be linearly separable from the other two while these latter are not linearly separable.

For illustrating the distance matrix computation (7.5) we use only the following sample of 9 objects, 3 for each class. Data are displayed in Table 7.1.

Table 7.1 The 4 measurements for some of the objects in the iris data set

Class	Label	Sepal length	Sepal width	Petal length	Petal width
Setosa	48	5.1000	3.5000	1.4000	0.2000
Setosa	49	4.9000	3.0000	1.4000	0.2000
Setosa	50	4.7000	3.2000	1.3000	0.2000
Versicolor	98	7.0000	3.2000	4.7000	1.4000
Versicolor	99	6.4000	3.2000	4.5000	1.5000
Versicolor	100	6.9000	3.1000	4.9000	1.5000
Virginica	148	6.3000	3.3000	6.0000	2.5000
Virginica	149	5.8000	2.7000	5.1000	1.9000
Virginica	150	7.1000	3.0000	5.9000	2.1000

The Euclidean distance has been computed for each pair of objects. The distance matrix is a 9-dimensional square matrix. Only the lower half of the matrix D is reported because the matrix is symmetric. Notice that all diagonal entries are equal to zero.

$$D = \begin{pmatrix} 0 & & & & & & & & \\ 0.5385 & 0 & & & & & & & \\ 0.5099 & 0.3000 & 0 & & & & & & \\ 4.0037 & 4.0963 & 4.2767 & 0 & & & & & \\ 3.6166 & 3.6865 & 3.8497 & 0.6403 & 0 & & & & \\ 4.1641 & 4.2367 & 4.4159 & 0.2646 & 0.6481 & 0 & & & \\ 5.2849 & 5.3385 & 5.4727 & 1.8439 & 1.8083 & 1.6155 & 0 & & \\ 4.2083 & 4.1809 & 4.3347 & 1.4491 & 1.0630 & 1.2530 & 1.3342 & 0 & \\ 5.3019 & 5.3572 & 5.5290 & 1.4071 & 1.6882 & 1.1874 & 0.9487 & 1.5684 & 0 \end{pmatrix}.$$

In general the distances between objects in the same class are markedly smaller than those between objects in different classes.

7.1.2 Algorithms for Clustering Data

Cluster analysis algorithms in general may be distinguished according to a useful classification in hierarchical and non-hierarchical algorithms. The first ones detect cluster sets ordered according to different levels. Ordering may be either descending or ascending according to the number of clusters that are present in each level. Agglomerative and divisive methods are to be distinguished. The former ones proceed along a bottom-up direction, that is the first level consists in assuming that each and every object forms a cluster on its own, then in subsequent levels an increasing number of objects are included in the same cluster until, at the final level, all items form a single cluster. The latter methods proceed top-down. At the beginning it is assumed that a single cluster exists which includes all objects. Intermediate levels are iteratively operated in such a way clusters split to yield an increasing number of clusters. At the final level each and every object forms a cluster on its own. It is commonplace to illustrate the hierarchical procedures by means of a graphical device called dendrogram where aggregating or splitting corresponds to merging or branching off the branches of a tree. The second class, non-hierarchical algorithms, are required to produce a unique partition of objects that either maximize or minimize a numerical criterion. The non-hierarchical algorithms are often referred to as optimization techniques that not necessarily form a hierarchical classification of the data. Most algorithms in this class assume that the number of clusters is known. However several optimization criteria are available which include the number of clusters within the set of variables that enter the optimization criterion. A useful reference as regards clustering algorithms is Hartigan (1975). See also Berkhin (2002) and references therein.

7.1.2.1 A Basic Relationship for the Dispersion Matrix of the Data

Let X be the matrix of the data (7.2), each row characterizing and corresponding to one of n objects that form the set $\mathcal{O}$. Assume g clusters and let $\{C_1, \ldots, C_g\}$ be a known partition of the set $\mathcal{O}$ such that (7.7) and (7.8) hold. For the whole set $\mathcal{O}$ the $p \times p$ total dispersion matrix T may be computed with entry in each row i and column j

$$T_{ij} = \sum_{h=1}^{n} (x_{hi} - \bar{x}_i) \left(x_{hj} - \bar{x}_j\right), \tag{7.9}$$

where

$$\bar{x}_i = \frac{1}{n} \sum_{h=1}^{n} x_{hi}, \quad i = 1, \ldots, p,$$

is the ith variable average. In matrix form, (7.9) reads

$$T = \sum_{h=1}^{n} (x_h - \bar{x})(x_h - \bar{x})', \tag{7.10}$$

where $\bar{x} = (\bar{x}_1, \ldots, \bar{x}_p)'$. Likewise, let $\bar{x}^{(h)}$ in (7.3) be the vector of the within-cluster variable averages with entries

$$\bar{x}_{hj} = \frac{1}{n_h} \sum_{x_s \in C_h} x_{sj}, \quad j = 1, \ldots, p,$$

where

$$n_h = |C_h|, \quad h = 1, \ldots, g$$

is the number of objects in cluster C_h. The $p \times p$ dispersion matrix W_h within any cluster C_h has entries

$$W_{ij}^{(h)} = \sum_{x_s \in C_h} (x_{si} - \bar{x}_{hi})\left(x_{sj} - \bar{x}_{hj}\right), \quad i, j = 1, \ldots, p.$$

In matrix form,

$$W_h = \sum_{x_s \in C_h} \left(x_s - \bar{x}^{(h)}\right)\left(x_s - \bar{x}^{(h)}\right)'. \tag{7.11}$$

We may consider the pooled within-group dispersion by summing matrices (7.11) across all clusters and obtain the within-group dispersion matrix

$$W = \sum_{h=1}^{g} W_h. \tag{7.12}$$

The matrix W accounts for the variability internal to the g clusters. Then consider the inter-cluster variability defined as the $p \times p$ between-group dispersion matrix

$$B = \sum_{h=1}^{g} n_h \left(\bar{x}^{(h)} - \bar{x}\right)\left(\bar{x}^{(h)} - \bar{x}\right)', \tag{7.13}$$

where n_h is the number of objects that belong to cluster C_h. According to the cluster definition, internal cohesion is larger as smaller the diagonal entries of W, while external dissimilarity is larger as larger the diagonal entries of B. Other measures based on (7.12) and (7.13) may be defined. It may be proven that the following basic relationship

$$T = W + B \tag{7.14}$$

holds. Many clustering criteria are based on (7.14). Moreover, as T is fixed given the data matrix X, most criteria may be established only in terms of either W or B because minimization of a monotone non-decreasing function of W is often equivalent to maximization of the same function of B. Well known criteria are, for instance,

- minimizing trace(W) (it is equivalent to maximizing trace(B)),
- minimizing det(W) (it is equivalent to maximizing det(T)/det(W)),
- maximizing trace(BW^{-1}) (Friedman and Rubin, 1967),
- maximizing the variance ratio criterion $\frac{\text{trace}(B)}{g-1} \big/ \frac{\text{trace}(W)}{n-g}$ (Calinski and Harabasz, 1974).

This latter criterion includes the number of cluster g as a parameter and it is a possible choice as an objective function if the number of cluster is unknown.

Example 7.1.2.1 Cars data

The cars data are concerned with 38 1978–1979 model cars and originally have been collected from *Consumer Reports*. Each car (the object) is identified by the nationality of manufacturer and the car name. For each object 6 measurements are included in the data set. The gas mileage in miles per gallon (MPG) is reported as measured by Consumers' Union on a test track. Other measurements about each car in this data set are weight, drive ratio, horsepower, displacement of the car (in cubic inches) and the number of cylinders, and all these were reported by the manufacturer. The data set used for this example has been downloaded from Statlib (2008). A cluster analysis of MPG, Weight, and Drive Ratio for cars reveals three main clusters, which we might identify as large sedans (Ford LTD, Chevrolet Caprice Classic, etc.), compact cars (Datsun 210, Chevrolet Chevette, etc.), and upscale, but smaller, sedans (BMW 320i, Audi 5000, etc.). We retained the three measurements MPG, Weight and Drive ratio only to give a practical example of (7.14). We assumed $g = 3$ clusters according to the aforementioned partition. The total number of partitions in three clusters are 2.2514×10^{17}. The cluster sizes are 12, 19 and 7 respectively. As we assumed $p = 3$ measurements the matrices T, W and B are 3-dimensional square matrices. The total dispersion matrix, the pooled within-group and between-group dispersion matrices may be computed as

$$T = \begin{pmatrix} 1586.0908 & -154.6417 & 52.3211 \\ -154.6417 & 18.4876 & -9.3131 \\ 52.3211 & -9.3131 & 9.9149 \end{pmatrix},$$

$$W = \begin{pmatrix} 191.1579 & -11.8022 & 4.4025 \\ -11.8022 & 2.9753 & -3.1395 \\ 4.4025 & -3.1395 & 6.4567 \end{pmatrix},$$

$$B = \begin{pmatrix} 1394.9329 & -142.8395 & 47.9186 \\ -142.8395 & 15.5123 & -6.1737 \\ 47.9186 & -6.1737 & 3.4581 \end{pmatrix},$$

and it may be checked readily that (7.14) is fulfilled.

Table 7.2 Trace and determinant of total and within-group dispersion matrices of the cars data

	W_1	W_2	W_3	W	T
Trace	16.8721	179.4628	4.255	200.5899	1614.5
Determinant	16.378	137.2584	0.2135	1157.4	16156

Table 7.2 displays the trace and determinant of total and within-class scatter matrices. Both trace and determinant of a dispersion matrix may be interpreted as generalized variance measures. The trace accounts for the dispersion of the measurements (the variables) by summing the dispersions computed for each variable separately, while the determinant includes also the interactions among the variables. This latter however involves a much larger computational burden. The basic relationship (7.14) is reproduced as far as the trace is concerned while the determinant is not a linear function of matrix entries so that in general $\det(T)$ is not the sum of $\det(W)$ and $\det(B)$. We may note that both trace and determinant of the pooled within-class scatter matrix is a small percentage of trace and determinant of the total dispersion matrix, namely 12.42 and 7.16% respectively. This result supports the validity of the partition in the three clusters. We may notice that the smallest trace and determinant of the within-scatter matrices has been computed for cluster 3, while we have obtained larger figures for cluster 1 and even larger for cluster 2. This latter is to be considered less compact than the other two, namely the measurements for cluster 2 though close yet are rather far apart. The objects in cluster 1 are more similar each other and so are the objects in cluster 3.

The criteria that combine the matrices T, W and B yield

- $\det(T)/\det(W) = 13.9592$,
- $\text{trace}(BW^{-1}) = 9.5779$,
- VRC = 123.3527.

These criteria may be regarded as examples of indexes of internal validity. We shall give more details about the indexes of internal validity in Sect. 7.1.3.1. Such criteria may serve to decide among several partitions which is to be considered the best one. Nonetheless, in their own these indexes cannot lead to a meaningful interpretation. An attempt may be done to compare the criteria computed for the known partition with the corresponding figures computed for a random partition. This latter may provide us with a baseline to evaluate the effectiveness of the chosen measurements or of the clustering criterion. We may consider the partition in 3 clusters obtained from the data set by assuming the same cluster sizes and choosing the group membership at random. This experiment yielded $\det(T)/\det(W) = 1.0633$, $\text{trace}(BW^{-1}) = 0.0628$, and VRC $= 0.8588$. Comparison of these latter figures with those obtained from the current partition may suggest that the measurements are to be considered truly useful to define a clustering structure and that maximizing $\det(T)/\det(W)$, $\text{trace}(BW^{-1})$ or the VRC may serve as a valid criterion to find a proper partition.

7.1.2.2 Agglomerative Methods

The basic algorithm for implementing agglomerative methods requires that a distance be defined which is meaningful between both clusters and objects. The algorithm starts by assuming that each and every object is the unique element of a cluster, that is $g = n$, $x_i \in C_i^{(1)}$ and $|C_i^{(1)}| = 1$, $i = 1, \ldots, n$. The superscript is used to specify the level of the set of clusters formed by the algorithm. The next step consists in choosing the closest pair of clusters and merging them to obtain a new cluster, that is $C_r^{(2)} = C_i^{(1)} \cup C_j^{(1)}$. Lance and Williams (1967) define a recurrence formula which is useful to evaluate the distance between a new proposal cluster $C_i \cup C_j$ and an existing one C_r and synthesize several distances that have been suggested in the literature. We have

$$d(C_i \cup C_j, C_r) = \alpha_i d(C_i, C_r) + \alpha_j d(C_j, C_r) + \beta d(C_i, C_j) + \gamma |d(C_i, C_r) - d(C_j, C_r)|,$$

where $\alpha_i, \alpha_j, \beta, \gamma$ are parameters that may be specified according to the methods we want to implement. For example the well known single linkage technique also known as nearest neighbor (see e.g. Gower and Ross, 1969) is obtained by setting $\alpha_i = \alpha_j = 1/2$, $\beta = 0$ and $\gamma = -1/2$. The algorithm ends as soon as all objects are included in a single cluster, that is $g = 1$ and $C_1 = \mathcal{O}$. It is of interest choosing a partition in a level that is optimal according to some criterion. This choice often relies on the analyst's judgement though several rules have been suggested to choose in automatic way or to give reliable guidelines in order to help to make the most convenient choice.

Example 7.1.2.2 Single linkage cluster of the Cars data

Let us consider the data illustrated in Sect. 7.1.2.1 and use the single linkage agglomerative method to cluster the data. We have $n = 38$ objects with $p = 3$ measurements each, namely MPG, Weight, and Drive Ratio. We obtain the partition displayed as the dendrogram in Fig. 7.1. It is apparent that the data split in two clusters that merge at a very large distance. In top-down direction, the first cluster includes 7 upscale, but smaller, sedans, including BMW 320i (37) and Audi 5000 (9), and 12 large sedans, including Ford LTD (18) and Chevrolet Caprice Classic (17), and the second cluster includes 19 compact cars, including Datsun 210 (33) and Chevrolet Chevette (5).

7.1.2.3 Divisive Methods

The basic algorithm that characterizes this class of methods proceeds along the top-down direction. In the first level all objects are included in a single cluster. In the second level the algorithm seeks for a partition using the distance matrix D (7.5) under some conditions such as (7.4). The procedure is replicated in each and every second-level partition so that, in the third level, partitions are present that result from further division of the partitions found in the second level. The algorithm ends as

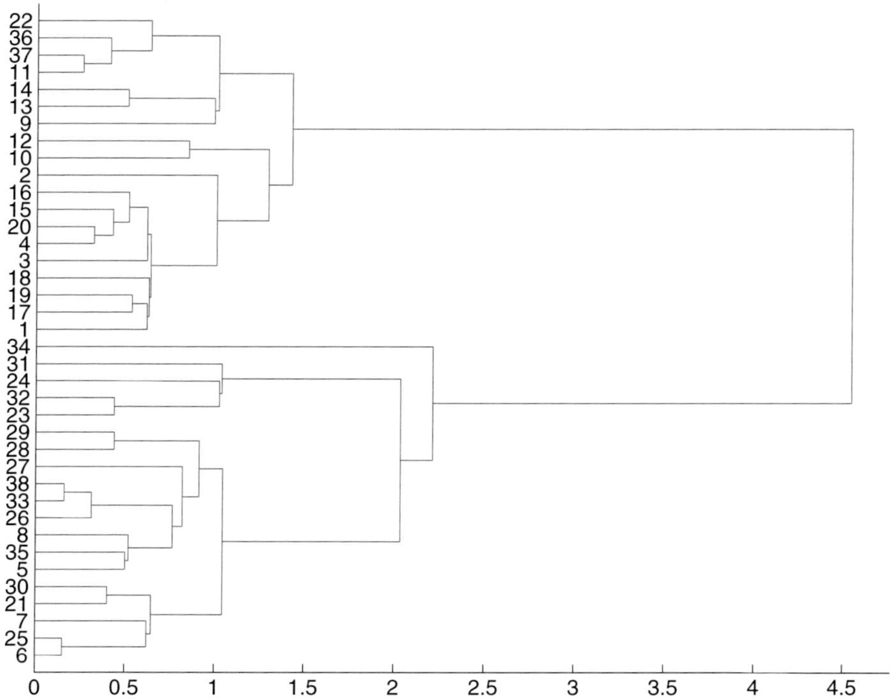

Fig. 7.1 Dendrogram of the cars data according to the single linkage method

soon as each and every object forms a one-element partition. At each step $i-1$ the set $C_j^{(i-1)}$ is split into r subsets $\{C_{j_1}^{(i)}, \ldots, C_{j_r}^{(i)}\}$ to optimize some pre-specified crierion. For example, the method of Edwards and Cavalli-Sforza (1965) assumes $r = 2$ at each level, that is all clusters that form the partition at each level are split in two. The objects that enter the two new partitions are chosen in such a way that trace(W) is minimized, where the matrix W is computed from the objects included in the parent partition only. The method requires a considerable computational burden even at the first level because the possible partitions of n objects into two clusters are $2^{n-1} - 1$, a large number even for moderate n. Bisection by hyperplanes computed by the singular value decomposition has been suggested in applications such as document collections (Boley, 1998). Other devices may be useful to reduce the computation time. Application of GAs to implement the divisive method will be presented later.

Example 7.1.2.3 Italian regions activity rate and value-added pro-capite

Figures of working people compared to the resident population are referred to as activity rate. For the 20 regions in Italy the activity rate and the pro-capite value-added in 2005 have been used as measurements for classification purpose. The data have been downloaded from ISTAT (2008). With only $n = 20$ objects the binary divisive method is viable. In the first step all $2^{19} - 1 = 524287$ partitions in two clusters have been considered and for each one trace(W) has been computed. The best partition has been assumed that with the smallest trace(W). Then a second step has been performed to split in two clusters each one of the two clusters obtained in the first step. In this second step the number of partitions for which trace(W) had to be computed has been considerably smaller than in the first step. In fact, the best partition yielded by the first step of the procedure included a cluster with 12 objects and a cluster with 8 objects, so that the further binary partitions were $2^{11} - 1 = 2047$ in the first case and $2^7 - 1 = 127$ in the second one. The dendrogram is displayed in Fig. 7.2. The first partition in two clusters splits the Italy regions in 12 northern and 8 southern regions, approximately north and south of Rome. The wealthier northern regions are split in two further and the regions in the north-east that are characterized by larger activity rate and value-added cluster together. The two clusters of the southern regions are rather mixed and do not offer easy interpretation. Obviously trace(W) decreases from 208.0759 in the first step to 62.0798 in the second one. Notice however that the partition in 4 clusters should be preferred according to the VRC criterion as for 2 clusters we have VRC = 99.2393 while for the partition in 4 clusters we obtain the slight larger figure 111.0983.

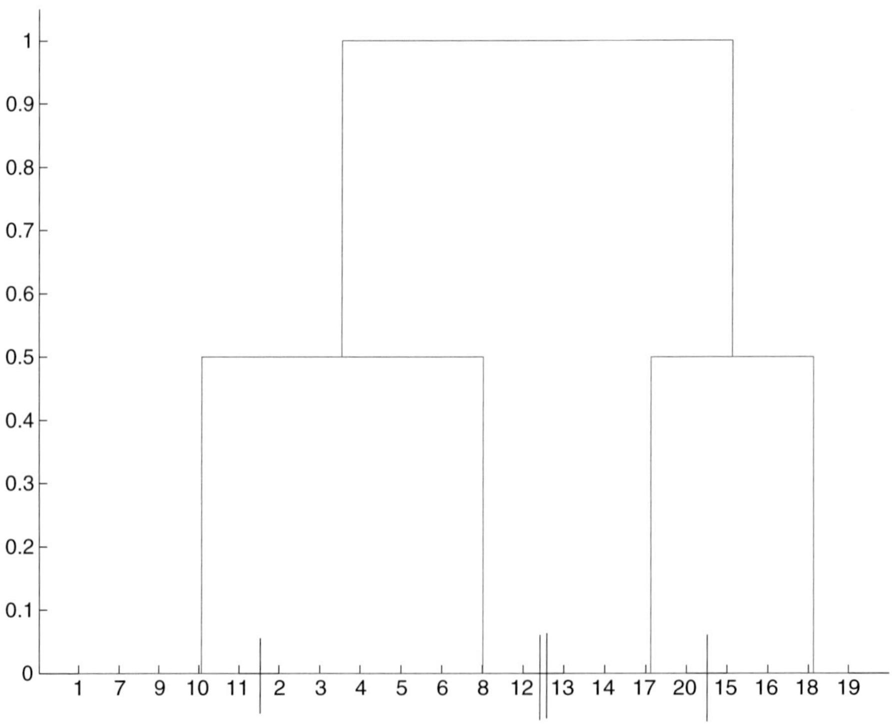

Fig. 7.2 Dendrogram of the Italy regions data according to the binary divisive method

7.1.2.4 Non-hierarchical Methods

Non-hierarchical methods seek for a unique partition that optimizes a pre-specified criterion. Unlike the hierarchical methods, the partitions found in each iteration have little value in their own and are to be considered only approximations of the final partition. Usually the number of clusters is assumed known. However, several algorithms that implement non-hierarchical methods assume the number of clusters as an unknown parameter to be included in the objective function specification.

The k-means algorithm (see e.g. Hartigan and Wong, 1979) constitutes maybe the most employed implementation of non-hierarchical methods. For any given $k > 1$ each of k clusters of n objects is represented by the mean of its objects. The algorithm starts with k vectors $\{x_0^{(1)}, \ldots, x_0^{(k)}\}$, called centers or centroids, and a preliminary partition is obtained by grouping together the objects according to their distance from the vectors $x_0^{(j)}$'s. If $d(x_i, x_0^{(s)})$ is the smallest among the distances $d(x_i, x_0^{(j)})$, $j = 1, \ldots, k$, then x_i is assumed to be included in cluster C_s. This computation is replicated for each and every object, that is for $i = 1, \ldots, n$. This step initializes the algorithm. Then iterations follow and from iteration t to iteration $t + 1$ two steps are performed.

- A set of k centroids $\{x_t^{(1)}, x_t^{(2)}, \ldots, x_t^{(k)}\}$ is available. A partition of the objects in k clusters is computed by assigning each and every object to the nearest centroid.
- The cluster means $\{\bar{x}_1, \ldots, \bar{x}_k\}$ are computed and the centroids are updated by setting $x_{t+1}^{(1)} = \bar{x}_1, x_{t+1}^{(2)} = \bar{x}_2, \ldots, x_{t+1}^{(k)} = \bar{x}_k$.

Iterations stop as soon as stable clusters are obtained.

The k-means algorithm requires that the number of clusters be pre-specified. If the number of clusters is unknown, then the algorithm has to be applied for $k = 1, \ldots, g$, where it is believed that the set $\mathcal{O}$ may be reasonably partitioned in at most g clusters.

A distance (7.6) and an optimality criterion have to be specified. The method in general depends on the initial centers and different initial choices may lead to different partitions and different values of the objective function. This means that the k-means algorithm is likely to yield sub-optimal partitions whilst the global optimum will be left essentially unknown, unless either n or g or both are very small. Several variants of the basic algorithm have been suggested to overcome critical drawbacks. The GAs-based algorithm will be discussed later.

Some methods employ k-medoid algorithms instead of k-means, that is a cluster is represented by one of its point. The main advantages of these methods consist in that any object type is allowed, not only those that may be represented by numerical variables, and outliers have only limited impact on computations. Moreover, such methods have been used for clustering sets of spatial data (Ng and Han, 1994).

Example 7.2.4.1 Diabetes data

For this example we shall use the Diabetes data set downloaded from SI (2008). The Diabetes data consists of $p = 3$ measurements: the area under a plasma glucose curve (degree of glucose intolerance), the area under a plasma insulin curve (insulin response to oral glucose), and steady-state plasma glucose response (SSPG, insulin resistance) for $n = 145$ subjects. The subjects are clinically classified into $g = 3$ groups, chemical diabetes, overt diabetes and normal. The shape of the data set in three dimensions is that of a "boomerang with two wings and a fat middle." The parts differ in that one of the "wings" is almost planar, the other is linear with some curvature, the "fat middle" is nearly spherical. We have used the k-means algorithm assuming 3 clusters and the following options.

- Squared Euclidean distances.
- To initialize the algorithm k observations have been chosen at random from the data set.

Several runs of the k-means algorithm showed that two different solutions are yielded depending on the centroid set used for initialization. The existence of a global maximum and a local one of the objective function is the natural explanation. We report in Table 7.3 the initial and final centroid coordinates in two runs of the algorithm. The same final coordinates are obtained from many other samples of initial centroid sets.

Table 7.3 Initial and final centroids in two runs of the k-means algorithm for the diabetes data

		Initial centroid			Final centroid		
Run	Centroid	Glucose	Insulin	SSPG	Glucose	Insulin	SSPG
1	1	93	472	285	241.7	1152.9	75.7
	2	83	351	81	91.4	359.3	166.7
	3	100	367	182	107.4	531.5	323.7
2	1	105	319	143	93.4	375.5	166.2
	2	93	391	221	241.7	1152.9	75.7
	3	90	327	192	105	525.6	376

The final centroid coordinates obtained in the two runs are very close and for a cluster the centers are coincident. The initial coordinates are similar as well, though not so close as the final ones. However, the solution yielded by the algorithm in the first run may be considered better than that obtained in the second run, as the misclassification rate has been 15.86% in the former case and 17.93% in the latter.

7.1.3 Indexes of Cluster Validity

A partition may be evaluated according to several criteria. For problems that involve low dimensional data the graphical display of objects and clusters provides us with a meaningful insight into the structure of the data. For high dimensional data still two or three dimensional plots may be used by resorting to methods for dimensionality reduction, multidimensional scaling for instance. Though some information will be lost the visual inspection of the graphical display may turn very useful as regards the evaluation of the quality of the clustering procedure.

Nevertheless, the need of a single index to assess the cluster validity is apparent if we have to provide a clustering algorithm with an objective function to guide the search for some optimal partition. Indexes that serve this purpose are the indexes for internal cluster validity. Further, we may need to compare two partitions in order to judge if they are similar. In simulation experiments the true partition, that is the partition that has been assumed to generate the data set, is available, and the quality of a clustering algorithm may be conveniently summarized by a table of correspondence or by a single index. In this case we may compute indexes of external validity. Many such indexes, both for internal and external validation, are available in the literature. We shall describe here two such indexes that have been commonly employed both in theoretical studies and practical applications and proved to be reliable and effective for cluster evaluation. The index of internal validity we shall describe is the Davies–Bouldin (DB) index, of external validity the corrected Rand index.

7.1.3.1 The Davies–Bouldin index

The objective function for a partitioning problem should preferably include the number of clusters as an additional parameter to be estimated within the optimization procedure. An useful measure of cluster validity which incorporates this feature is the Davies–Bouldin (DB) index (Davies and Bouldin, 1979). A comprehensive account of the DB index and comparison with several cluster validation indexes may be found in Bezdek and Pal (1998).

Let the matrix X, as defined by (7.2), denote the observed data. The DB index is a function of the ratio of the total within – class scatter measure $TWSM$ to the total inter – class separation measure $TISM$. Let k clusters, $k > 1$, be available and, for $i = 1, \ldots, k$, let the within ith cluster scatter be defined

$$S_{i,q} = \left(\frac{1}{|C_i|} \sum_{x_h \in C_i} \|x_h - \bar{x}^{(i)}\|_2^q \right)^{1/q},$$

where

$$\|x_h - \bar{x}^{(i)}\|_2 = \sqrt{\sum_{j=1}^{p} (x_{hj} - \bar{x}_{ij})^2},$$

and q is a pre-specified positive integer. Let the distance between cluster C_i and C_j, $i, j = 1, \ldots, k$, be defined

$$d_{ij,t} = \left\{ \sum_{r=1}^{p} |\bar{x}_{ir} - \bar{x}_{jr}|^t \right\}^{1/t} = \|\bar{x}^{(i)} - \bar{x}^{(j)}\|_t,$$

where t is a positive integer that may be selected independently of q.

The Minkowski distance of order q and t generalizes the Euclidean distance which is used in the definitions of *TWSM* and *TISM* though retaining the essential of the principle behind the objective of obtaining simultaneously maximum cohesion within cluster and maximum intra-cluster separation. Accordingly, we are searching for a cluster partition such that the $S_{i,q}$'s are minimized while the $d_{ij,t}$'s are maximized. For each cluster i, let

$$R_{i,qt} = \max_{j,\, j \neq i} \left\{ \frac{S_{i,q} + S_{j,q}}{d_{ij,t}} \right\}.$$

Then, the DB index (to be minimized) is defined

$$\text{DB} = \frac{1}{k} \sum_{i=1}^{k} R_{i,qt}.$$

The assumption $k > 1$ ensures that DB is well defined. In general, provided that the partition that is being considered includes neatly separated clusters, the minimum of the DB index is achieved in correspondence of the correct number of clusters $k = g$. The DB index may be included within an automatic detection procedure easily and it has been suggested as a valid choice for genetic algorithms – based procedures. It has to be noticed that if the DB index is assumed as objective function, then its reciprocal $1/\text{DB}$ has to be assumed as fitness function as the optimal partition corresponds to the smallest DB value.

Example 7.1.3.1 Indexes of cluster validity of Iris Plants partitions

Let us consider the data set Iris Plants introduced in Sect. 7.1.1. The k-means algorithm has been used to obtain a partition of the data set for each given number of cluster g, $g = 2, \ldots, 8$. For each given g the algorithm has been run 30 times to take into account the dependence of the results yielded by the k-means algorithm from the initial values which have been chosen at random within the observed objects. The most frequent partition has been assumed as final result for each given g. Then for each one of the chosen partitions we computed the misclassification rate and 4 internal indexes of cluster validity, namely the DB index, the Dunn's index (Dunn, 1974) and the VRC and $\det(W)$ criteria introduced in Sect. 7.1.2.1. This latter has been used according to the modified version suggested by Marriott (1982), that is the optimal partition is to be considered the one for which $g^2 \det(W)$ attains its minimum. In fact, the comparison among the internal indexes of cluster validity has to take into account primarily the ability of the criterion in choosing the correct number of clusters as it does not make sense any comparison between values from

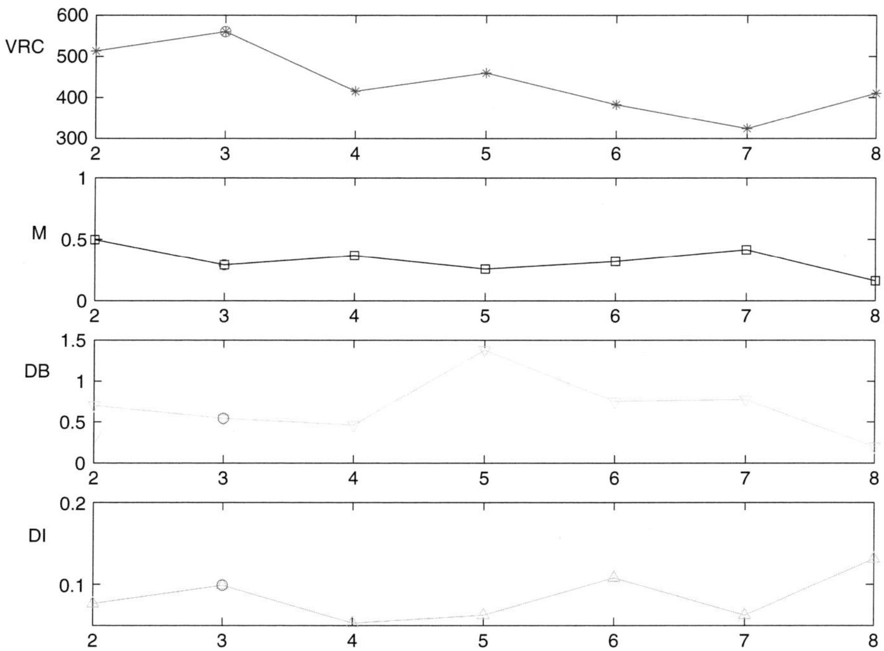

Fig. 7.3 Internal indexes of cluster validity for the partitions computed by the k-means algorithm varying the pre-specified number of cluster. Circles indicate the number of clusters to choose

different indexes. In Fig. 7.3 the misclassification rate and the internal indexes of cluster validity are plotted against the number of clusters. The misclassification rate attains its minimum 10.67% for the partition in 3 clusters as expected. More objects are misclassified if the wrong number of clusters is assumed. We expect that the internal indexes attain their optimal value for $g = 3$. The optimal value may be either the maximum or the minimum of the computed index values according to the definition of each index, namely

- VRC: maximize,
- $g^2\det(W)$ (M): minimize,
- DB: minimize,
- Dunn's index (DI): maximize.

Both VRC and DB indexes attain correctly their optimal value (the maximum and minimum respectively) at $g = 3$. The other two indexes both display a trough in correspondence of $g = 3$ and the parsimony principle could suggest this latter as the chosen number of clusters. Nevertheless for these two latter indexes the overall minimum and maximum are attained $g = 8$ and $g = 6$ respectively. The misclassification rate is equal to 50% in the latter and 48.67% in the former case so such solutions seem very poor ones. Notice, however, that no index of cluster validity is able to give the best performance in all situations so that we simply assume that the indexes VRC and DB are appropriate for the Iris Plants data set while the indexes M and DI may lead to the wrong choice in this context.

7.1.3.2 The Corrected Rand Index

The Rand index (Rand, 1971) is a popular device for comparing partitions. It is useful as well if we want to check the effectiveness of a clustering procedure by comparing the actual partition with the estimated partition. A simulation study by Milligan and Cooper (1986) supports the usage of the Rand index.

Given partitions U and V of the same set $\mathcal{O}$ of objects, let a be the number of pairs of elements that are placed in the same cluster in U and in the same cluster in V, b the number of pairs of elements that are in different clusters in U and in different clusters in V, c the number of pairs of elements that are placed in the same cluster in U and in different clusters in V, and d the number of pairs of elements that are in different clusters in U and in the same cluster in V. For n elements, the total number of pairs is $\binom{n}{2}$. We have

$$a + b + c + d = \binom{n}{2}.$$

The number of agreements may be assumed equal to $a + b$, while the number of disagreements equals $c + d$. An useful device to compare the two partitions is Table 7.4 where we assume that U consists in $g^{(U)}$ clusters $\{C_1^{(U)}, \ldots, C_{g^{(U)}}^{(U)}\}$ and V consists in $g^{(V)}$ clusters $\{C_1^{(V)}, \ldots, C_{g^{(V)}}^{(V)}\}$. Let the cluster labels $\{1, \ldots, g^{(U)}\}$ identify the columns and the cluster labels $\{1, \ldots, g^{(V)}\}$ identify the rows of the table. Then the cell (i, j) contains the number of objects in $\mathcal{O}$ that belong to cluster $C_j^{(U)}$ according to partition U while belong to $C_i^{(V)}$ according to partition V. The number of agreements and disagreements between partitions U and V may be easily computed from Table 7.4.

The Rand index is $R = (a + b)/(a + b + c + d)$, and takes values in the interval $(0, 1)$. The index equals 1 if the two partitions U and V are identical, zero if U and V disagree on any pair of elements. A more appropriate descriptive measure should include some correction for chance as the Rand index does not necessarily

Table 7.4 Comparison of partitions U (clusters in columns) and V (clusters in rows), the cells contain the number of objects classified according to either partitions

$V \setminus U$	1	$\cdots$	j	$\cdots$	$g^{(U)}$
1	n_{11}	$\cdots$	n_{1j}	$\cdots$	$n_{1g^{(U)}}$
$\vdots$	$\vdots$	$\ddots$	$\vdots$	$\ddots$	$\vdots$
i	n_{i1}	$\cdots$	n_{ij}	$\cdots$	$n_{ig^{(U)}}$
$\vdots$	$\vdots$	$\ddots$	$\vdots$	$\ddots$	$\vdots$
$g^{(V)}$	$n_{g^{(V)}1}$	$\cdots$	$n_{g^{(V)}j}$	$\cdots$	$n_{g^{(V)}g^{(U)}}$

equal zero if both partitions U and V are purely random. The Hubert and Arabie (1985) adjusted Rand index assumes the generalized hypergeometric distribution as the (null) model for randomness. The corrected Rand index is normalized by subtracting its expected value and dividing by the difference between its maximum value and its expected value. The index again takes values in the interval (0, 1), and partitions may be considered in agreement if the index approaches 1, while if the two partitions disagree the index will be close to zero. In some cases the index may take small negative values, in general if the two partitions are very different. Let n_{ij} denote the entry in row i and column j within Table 7.4, and let $n_{i.}$ and $n_{.j}$ denote the row-wise and column-wise sums respectively. Then, the corrected Rand index R^* may be written

$$R^* = \frac{\sum_{i,j}\binom{n_{ij}}{2} - \mathbb{E}\left\{\sum_{i,j}\binom{n_{ij}}{2}\right\}}{\frac{1}{2}\left\{\sum_i\binom{n_{i.}}{2} + \sum_j\binom{n_{.j}}{2}\right\} - \mathbb{E}\left\{\sum_{i,j}\binom{n_{ij}}{2}\right\}},$$

where $\mathbb{E}$ means expectation and

$$\mathbb{E}\left\{\sum_{i,j}\binom{n_{ij}}{2}\right\} = \frac{\left\{\sum_i\binom{n_{i.}}{2}\sum_j\binom{n_{.j}}{2}\right\}}{\binom{n}{2}}.$$

The following equalities hold

$$a = \sum_{i,j}\binom{n_{ij}}{2},$$

$$b = \sum_{i}\binom{n_{i.}}{2} - \sum_{i,j}\binom{n_{ij}}{2},$$

$$c = \sum_{j}\binom{n_{.j}}{2} - \sum_{i,j}\binom{n_{ij}}{2},$$

and

$$d = \binom{n}{2} - c - b - a.$$

It is known that the index R overestimates the agreement measure between the two partitions, while the index R^* includes a correct baseline.

Example 7.1.3.2 The European Jobs data

The data are the percentage employed in different industries in Europe countries during 1979. The job categories are agriculture, mining, manufacturing, power supplies, construction, service industries, finance, social and personal services, and transport and communications. It is important to note that these data were collected during the Cold War. Thus it seems natural to expect the data to split into two main clusters i.e. countries of the communist East Bloc and countries of capitalist Western Europe. Nonetheless, Yugoslavia and Turkey are expected to stand alone in a singleton each because both display peculiar though different characteristics. The former was unaligned and shared some characteristics of both main groups while the latter is probably more properly classified as an Asian nation since only a small percentage of its land area lies on the European continent. The data have been downloaded from Statlib (2008). The data set has $n = 26$ objects and $p = 9$ measurements each. We considered two reference partitions, the first one with $g = 3$ clusters with Yugoslavia and Turkey both in the third cluster, the second one with $g = 4$ and Yugoslavia and Turkey in separate singletons. In the former case the number of partitions is $N(26, 3) = 4.2361 \times 10^{11}$, in the latter $N(26, 4) = 1.8723 \times 10^{14}$.

We used four hierarchical agglomerative methods, namely the single linkage, complete linkage, average linkage and Ward's method, and a non-hierarchical method, that is the k-means algorithm. In Table 7.5 results are reported for $g = 3$ and $g = 4$ concerned with the agreement between the reference partition and the partitions yielded by the 5 methods. The external indexes of cluster validity have been the misclassification rate (MR), the corrected Rand index (R) and the Jaccard's (Jaccard, 1901) index (J). Unlike the preceding sections, the MR is displayed as the ratio of the misclassified objects to the number of objects and no percentage figures are computed. The R and J indexes both are greater than zero and less than unity, where zero stands for complete disagreement and one for complete agreement. The Ward's method yields the best partition when compared with the reference partition in 3 clusters. Unlike the reference partition, the estimated partition is composed of a small cluster of 3 objects, as Greece joins Yugoslavia and Turkey in the classification. There are differences concerned with the two main clusters as well. Portugal and Spain join the countries in the East Bloc while East Germany joins the Western Europe countries. Similar results are given by both the complete linkage method and the k-means algorithm. In this case, however, Ireland too joins the East Bloc. The reference partition with 4 clusters finds the best agreement with the partition estimated by the average linkage method. According to such estimated 4 clusters partition, Turkey forms a singleton while Greece and Yugoslavia are assigned to

Table 7.5 Comparison between reference partition and estimated partition for the European jobs data

	Index\method	Single	Complete	Average	Ward	k-means
$g = 3$	MR	0.3462	0.1923	0.3462	0.1538	0.1923
	R	0.2123	0.4183	0.2123	0.5178	0.4183
	J	0.5203	0.5079	0.5203	0.5806	0.5079
$g = 4$	MR	0.1923[a]	0.4615	0.2308	0.4615	0.5000
	R	0.4535[a]	0.1784	0.4181	0.1763	0.1569
	J	0.5165[a]	0.2722	0.5053	0.2471	0.2299

[a] For the estimated partition g has been set to 6

the same cluster. As regards the larger clusters, again East Germany is assigned to the cluster that includes the Western Europe countries excepted Ireland, Portugal and Spain that join the East Bloc countries. The single linkage method yields appreciable results only if 6 clusters are allowed. In this case Greece, Spain, Turkey and Yugoslavia form 4 singletons while the two main clusters include most of the East Bloc and Western Europe countries respectively excepted East Germany that is found in the Western Europe cluster and Ireland and Portugal that are included in the East Bloc countries.

7.2 Genetic Clustering Algorithms

A large amount of GAs-based procedures has been developed to solve cluster analysis problems incorporating several different features, for instance large data sets, cluster constraints and special data structures (Murthy and Chowdhury, 1996, for instance). Genetic algorithms may be viewed in this context as function optimizers in the sense that they perform a search for the optimal solution in whatever space a positive real valued function may be defined. The set of candidate solutions has to be allowed to include at any step any feasible solution and no constraint is usually introduced to leave parts of the solution fixed once and for all. Multi-objective clustering has been suggested by Ferligoj and Batagelj (1992) and GAs-based multi-objective cluster analysis has been introduced by Bandyopadhyay et al. (2007). In principle the hierarchical algorithms framework does not fit the requirement typical of genetic algorithms, as of almost all meta heuristics, to move freely around the solutions space. For this reason genetic clustering has been developed essentially in the non hierarchical framework. However, the GAs-based implementation of a hierarchical divisive method will be considered. As regards non hierarchical methods, we shall consider in detail the two common alternatives. The first one exploits the idea which supports the quick cluster algorithm, the second one develops along the guidelines of the k-means algorithm and its variants.

7.2.1 A Genetic Divisive Algorithm

GAs seem specially useful for handling divisive clustering iterative algorithm which are designed in such a way at each iteration each cluster that includes more than 2 objects is to be split into two new clusters. This case is attractive because a simple binary coding which is both natural and easy to interpret may be used for each splitting task. Let a data matrix X be available defined as in (7.2). An observation is a row of X which identifies an object in a given set $\mathcal{O}$. A row of X is the transpose of the p-dimensional vector (7.1). Let the algorithm start with all observations included in a single cluster $C_1^{(0)}$ and let $g^{(0)} = 1$ be the initial number of clusters. In the generic iteration t there will be $g^{(t)}$ clusters with cluster labels the positive integers

$\{1, \ldots, g^{(t)}\}$. A cluster will be denoted $C_k^{(t)}$ where the superscript identifies the iteration and the subscript the cluster label.

Let s be the population size, N the number of iterations, p_c and p_m the probabilities of crossover and mutation respectively and let $f = \text{trace}(B)$ denote the fitness function, where the matrix B is the between-cluster scatter (7.13). The first step of the algorithm consists in splitting $C_1^{(0)}$ into the two clusters $C_1^{(1)}$ and $C_2^{(1)}$ in such a way f is maximized. The genetic algorithm we use for this task may be described as follows.

- *Encoding*. Let $n_1^{(0)}$ denote the number of objects in $C_1^{(0)}$. Then a binary chromosome of length $n_1^{(0)}$ is generated where the ith gene is either 0 or 1 whether we want the ith object to be assigned to the cluster $C_1^{(1)}$ or $C_2^{(1)}$ respectively.
- *Initial population*. We generate uniformly randomly s binary strings. The all-zero and all-unity strings are discarded and new strings are generated for replacement. Each binary string represents a chromosome that may be decoded to identify two new clusters.
- *Genetic algorithm*. The three usual step of the GA are performed N times.

1. *Selection*. The fitness function of each chromosome is computed and the next population is formed by sampling with replacement from the current population. According to the roulette wheel rule the selection probability for a chromosome is proportional to its fitness value. The elitist strategy is applied, that is the best chromosome in the current population is included in the next population if no better one is selected. In this latter case the worst chromosome in the next population is deleted to keep unchanged the population size s.
2. *Crossover*. $\lfloor s/2 \rfloor$ chromosome pairs are chosen and the paired chromosomes may exchange part of their genes with probability p_c. The single point crossover may be used. The offsprings replace their parents provided that neither is the all-zero or the all-one string. In this latter case the parents pass to the next generation unchanged.
3. *Mutation*. Any bit of any binary string may flip with probability p_m. If a mutation yields the all-one or the all-zero string then the chromosome pass unchanged to the next population.

Note that in this context a chromosome is a binary string and a chromosome gene is a bit. Moreover the binary string that defines the chromosome does not encode any integer or real number as its meaning is completely different from usual binary encoding. In the present case the chromosome meaning stems from the one-to-one mapping between the observations labels and the gene locations.

The iteration of the divisive genetic algorithm may be described as the passage from step t to step $t + 1$ as follows.

- Set $g^{(t+1)} = g^{(t)}$,
- For $k = 1 : g^{(t)}$

- If the set $C_k^{(t)}$ includes less than 2 objects, next k,
- Else perform the divisive GA on the set $C_k^{(t)}$ to obtain $C_{k_1}^{(t+1)}$ and $C_{k_2}^{(t+1)}$, and set $g^{(t+1)} = g^{(t+1)} + 1$

• Next k.

Then algorithm stops as soon as there are no more clusters to split, that is when the partition of the set $\mathcal{O}$ in n clusters each including a single observation is attained. The we may examine the partitions obtained at each step t and choose the one that fulfils some appropriate criterion, for instance a desired number of clusters.

Example 7.2.1.1 Genetic divisive algorithm for Italian regions data

In Sect. 7.1.2.3 a hierarchical divisive method has been applied where the optimal cluster structure has been found by the complete enumeration of all possible partitions into two clusters. Finding the best split in two clusters requires 524287 evaluations of the within-cluster scatter matrix W. Such computational burden ensures that the optimal partition is found that corresponds to the minimum of trace(W). The GAs may allow us to obtain the optimal partition by performing only a limited number of evaluations of trace(W). We run the divisive GA 5 times and obtained the optimal partition with less than 200 iterations in 3 cases and with less than 5000 iterations in the remaining two cases. We used a population size $s = 40$ so that the number of evaluations of trace(W) required to attain the optimal partition has been 200,000 at most and no more than 8000 in three cases. In Fig. 7.4 the fitness function evolution in 5 runs is plotted against the number of iterations. The fitness function is computed as trace(T) − trace(W) so that the GA has to maximize the fitness function to attain the optimal partition. For the present example the minimum of trace(W) is equal to 208.0759 while the trace of the total scatter matrix T is trace$(T) = 1355.3$. So the maximum of the fitness function is 1147.2241. This latter figure is the maximum value of trace(B) where B is the between-cluster scatter matrix. We may notice that in 3 cases the convergence is very quick and the fitness function exhibits a steep ascent behavior. If such quick convergence does not occur the fitness function increases rather slowly.

7.2.2 Quick Partition Genetic Algorithms

The quick partition algorithm (Hartigan, 1975) starts with the list of n objects. Computations are performed on the dissimilarity matrix D. If there are storage problems, that is if n is very large, the data matrix X may be used conveniently as input to the algorithm while dissimilarities may be computed any time they are needed with obvious additional computation cost. The skeleton of the algorithm is as follows.

1. Let $i = 1$, $s = 1$ and $x_i \in C_s$
2. While $i < n$ let $i = i + 1$, otherwise stop

   • For $j = 1 : s$,

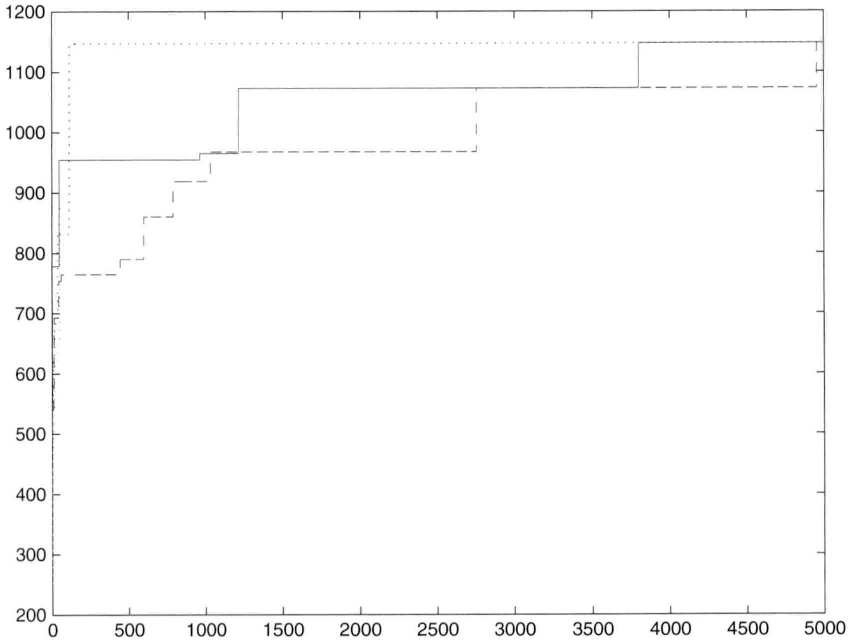

Fig. 7.4 Fitness function for the genetic divisive algorithm in 5 different runs. The *dotted* lines correspond to the cases of fast convergence to the maximum while the *solid* and *dashed* lines refer to the cases where the evolution towards the maximum is slower

- If, for each $r : x_r \in C_j$, $d_{i,r} < \bar{d}$ then $x_i \in C_j$, $|C_j| = |C_j| + 1$ and exit, otherwise next j

3. If x_i is not assigned to any existing cluster, then $s = s + 1$ and a new cluster C_s is initialized with $x_i \in C_s$.

This algorithm is very fast but depends heavily on the order of objects. A solution could be to consider all permutations, but this would involve too much computation, practically unfeasible even for small size problems. Some devices may be useful, such as several restarting of the algorithm by using random permutations. This device may be conveniently handled by ordered genetic algorithms. Let us briefly explain how these kind of GAs work. Let $1, \ldots, n$ be the labels of the objects in the given set $\mathcal{O}$. In this context a permutation is itself a potential solution of the problem, because the quick partition algorithm generates a unique partition given the initial permutation and the problem-dependent constant $\bar{d}$. Then, the initial population is a subset of the set of all permutations of the natural numbers $1, \ldots, n$. Given the size N of the population, the chromosomes in the population are N permutations. Usually they are randomly generated and it seems convenient to impose that all permutations are different each other.

The decoding of the chromosomes is performed by the quick partition algorithm. For each chromosome the number of clusters and the assignment of objects to clusters are well defined after decoding. The partition that is obtained as a result has to be evaluated by an index of internal cluster validity. A transform of the index may be used to meet the requirements for it to represent a suitable fitness function. The initial population is assumed as the current one, and, through a pre-specified number of iterations N, the following steps are executed.

7.2.2.1 Selection

The well known roulette wheel rule may be used for selecting the chromosomes that in the next generation are to be maintained in the population. The probability for a chromosome to remain in the population is proportional to its fitness function. A chromosome may well be selected more than once, while other chromosomes may disappear, if we want the size s of the population to be constant. The elitist strategy has to be adopted to prevent the possible loss of the best chromosome in the past population. This latter circumstance has to be avoided if each and every chromosome selected for the next generation has a fitness function smaller than the best chromosome in the past generation. If this latter is not selected, yet it is taken to replace the chromosome with smallest fitness. Such reproduction strategy implies complete replacement (or generational gap 1), that is all the s selected chromosomes replace the old chromosomes

7.2.2.2 Crossover

Let p_c denote the crossover rate, that is the probability that a couple of chromosomes undergo the crossover procedure. In the applications, for ordered GAs, p_c usually ranges in the interval [0.6, 0.9]. We may choose among several mating strategies. Selecting pairs of chromosomes at random may imply that a chromosome is allowed to enter more than a couple for possible crossover. If we want each and every chromosome to undergo crossover, then the alternative strategy may be chosen that consists in splitting the population in two, so having two sets of chromosomes of size $s/2$. Obvious corrections apply if s is odd. Then chromosomes of first and second set are paired at random.

For ordered GAs problems may occur if the usual crossover devices, such as the one cutting point crossover, are adopted, because these crossover devices do not guarantee that the offsprings are permutations as their parents are. Several crossover devices have been proposed for the special purpose of obtaining permutations as offsprings from pairs of permutations. Instances are the ordering crossover (OX) (Davis, 1985) and the partially matched crossover (PMX) (Goldberg and Lingle, 1985). We shall describe the PMX. Comparisons with OX and other reordering operators and some theoretical issues are addressed in Goldberg (1989b) and Jones and Beltramo (1991).

To perform the PMX, two chromosomes are randomly selected within the current population. Moreover, two crossing sites, where the two chromosome strings will be cut, are randomly chosen in the range from 1 to n. Then, the object labels included between these two cut points are exchanged. This procedure cannot be expected to yield two new permutations necessarily. For instance, it may happen that the new chromosomes contain some labels twice while some other labels may be missing. To solve this problem, the mapping defined by the exchange itself turns out useful. If a label occurs twice, the one outside the sub-string between the crossing sites is replaced by its image given by the correspondence induced by the map. For example, let $n = 9$ and the cutting points for the two permutations that are undergoing the crossover be selected 4 and 7 (let the cut points be denoted with "|")

$$123|4567|89$$
$$452|1876|93$$

The exchange of the labels between the two cut points will give

$$123|1876|89$$
$$452|4567|93$$

but, in the first chromosome, labels 1 and 8 are each included twice, and so are labels 4 and 5 in the second one. The mapping $\{1, 4\}$ and $\{8, 5\}$ allows the problem to be solved, so yielding the following two chromosomes, that are "legal" permutations,

$$423|1876|59$$
$$182|4567|93$$

It has to be noted that such a procedure has to be iterated if the situation is more complicated. Consider, for instance, the chromosomes

$$123|4567|89$$
$$472|1856|39$$

that, after the crossover, become

$$123|1856|89$$
$$472|4567|39$$

The mapping, when applied as before, yields the two chromosomes

$$423|1856|59$$
$$162|4567|39$$

that are not yet legal permutations. The mapping, however, may be used again. The iteration gives

423|1856|69
152|4567|39

and finally yields

423|1856|79
182|4567|39

It is very unlikely that this kind of iterative mapping application be unable to deliver a pair of 'legal' offsprings.

7.2.2.3 Mutation

The third step of the GAs is mutation, for which the selection of a mutation rate p_m, usually small, is required. The figures found in the applications usually vary from 0.001 to 0.1. Mutation is allowed to occur at rate p_m per gene. This operator ensures that the population maintains some diversity, as any gene may mutate at any iteration. As a matter of fact, selection and crossover do not create new genes, so it may happen that if a gene in a locus comes to assume the same value for all chromosomes it will not change anymore in next generations. The smallest change that may intervene in ordered GAs consists in the exchange of two genes. So, each label in each chromosome is considered in turn, and, with probability p_m, the mutation is performed by swapping the current label with another one selected at random. For example, let $k = 9$, and consider the chromosome

1234|5|6789.

If, for the gene 5, an uniform random number u in the interval (0, 1) is generated such that $u < p_m$, then 5 mutates. One of the remaining labels is selected at random, say 8. It results the new permutation

1234|8|67|5|9,

which replaces the previous one.

Example 7.2.2.1 Protein Localization Sites data

This is the E.coli data set that may be downloaded from Asuncion and Newman (2007). The number of instances is $n = 336$ and the number of (predictive) attributes is $p = 7$. The predicted attribute is the localization site of protein and is used as the class label. The predictive attributes are as follows.

- mcg: McGeoch's method for signal sequence recognition.
- gvh: von Heijne's method for signal sequence recognition.
- lip: von Heijne's Signal Peptidase II consensus sequence score. Binary attribute.

- chg: Presence of charge on N-terminus of predicted lipoproteins. Binary attribute.
- aac: score of discriminant analysis of the amino acid content of outer membrane and periplasmic proteins.
- alm1: score of the ALOM membrane spanning region prediction program.
- alm2: score of ALOM program after excluding putative cleavable signal regions from the sequence.

The class is the localization site. We list the 8 known clusters and the number of objects that belong to each one.

cp	(cytoplasm)	143
im	(inner membrane without signal sequence)	77
pp	(perisplasm)	52
imU	(inner membrane, uncleavable signal sequence)	35
om	(outer membrane)	20
omL	(outer membrane lipoprotein)	5
imL	(inner membrane lipoprotein)	2
imS	(inner membrane, cleavable signal sequence)	2

The number of partitions in $g = 8$ clusters is very large as $N(336, 8) = 6.8032 \times 10^{298}$. We used the genetic quick partition algorithm described in Sect. 7.2.2 to recover the data set known partition. Usually GAs maximize a real positive valued fitness function, so we define for convenience for the object pair (x_i, x_j) a similarity index $v_{ij} = 1/d_{ij}, \quad i \neq j$, where d_{ij} is the squared Euclidean distance. Then the fitness function may be defined as the k-min cluster criterion (Sahni and Gonzalez, 1976)

$$f(C_1, C_2, \dots, C_g; g) = \sum_{\omega=1}^{g} \sum_{i,j \in C_\omega, i \neq j} v_{ij},$$

where g is the number of clusters and $\{C_1, C_2, \dots, C_g\}$ denotes the partition that may be decoded from the current chromosome. Application of this criterion to cluster of time series will be discussed in Sect. 7.6.1. The GA parameters have been chosen as follows.

- Population size $s = 10$,
- Crossover probability $p_c = 0.8$,
- Mutation probability $p_m = 0.01$,
- Maximum number of GA iterations 100,
- Threshold 2.

The last parameter is specially important in this algorithm because the threshold controls the aggregation of the objects. If the threshold is large then it will be more difficult for two objects to belong to the same cluster. The value appropriate for the threshold depends on the definition of the distance and on the average of the computed similarities. The similarity sequence computed for each and every pair of objects has mean value equal to 8.3091. This latter may give only a guideline

Table 7.6 Comparison between known and estimated partitions for the E.coli data. Estimated group labels are listed in the first column and the known group labels in the first row

Cluster	1	2	3	4	5	6	7	8	Total
1	0	1	1	1	0	0	0	0	3
2	137	4	7	0	0	0	0	0	148
3	3	1	42	0	19	0	0	1	66
4	0	65	1	33	0	0	0	1	100
5	1	6	0	0	0	0	0	0	7
6	0	0	0	0	0	5	1	0	6
7	0	0	0	1	1	0	1	0	3
8	2	0	0	0	0	0	0	0	2
9	0	0	1	0	0	0	0	0	1
Total	143	77	52	35	20	5	2	2	336

for a first approximation and running the algorithm with some trial thresholds is advisable as the distribution is rather disperse (standard deviation 20.5185).

The largest fitness function value has been obtained at iteration 41. The best estimated partition has $g = 9$ clusters. Table 7.6 allows the known and estimated partitions to be compared. The largest cluster is recovered almost entirely while the pairs of clusters $(3, 5)$ and $(2, 4)$ of moderate size are not discriminated. Notwithstanding, the corrected Rand index is rather large and equal to 0.6937. Using alternative dissimilarity indexes (city block, Mahalanobis distance, correlation) does not improve this result.

7.2.3 Centroid Evolution Algorithms

The k-means algorithm yields reliable and accurate solutions to most partitioning problems and in general it is as fast as the quick partition algorithm. However, it suffers of a similar problem as the quick partition algorithm. This latter depends heavily on the choice of the initial permutation of the objects in the set, while the k-means algorithm depends heavily on the choice of the starting centers that represent each and every cluster in the initial partition. Further, the number of clusters has to be set in advance. In the quick partition algorithm the number of clusters may well be left unknown, but the key-constant $\bar{d}$ has to be chosen anyway which is essential as regards the determination of the number of clusters. As for quick partition algorithm, random restart may soften the dependence of the final optimal partition by the initial settings. Evolutionary algorithms may simultaneously seek for number of clusters and cluster centers so that some suitable objective function be optimized.

We shall describe the algorithm Genetic Clustering for Unknown K (GCUK) (Bandyopadhyay and Maulik, 2002) which exemplifies well this class of evolutionary clustering algorithms. GCUK refers directly to the k-means algorithm, though a number of features are added and special devices are adopted to allow the number of groups to vary. A suitable interval $[g_{\min}, g_{\max}]$, where $g_{\min} > 1$ and $g_{\max} \leq n$

has to be pre-specified. The chromosome has fixed length $g_{\max}$. The characteristic features of GCUK may be summarized as follows:

- *Encoding*. Any solution is coded as a string of $g_{\max}$ symbols. These latter may be either center coordinates or the character # that in this context reads "don't care". The genes of the first type are vectors of p floating-point numbers each of which represents a cluster. The genes of the second type account for empty clusters. Their introduction is essential to ensure the algorithm to search for both the number of clusters and the assignment of objects to clusters at the same time. As $g > 1$ the number of symbols # cannot be greater than $g_{\max} - 2$. However, chromosomes possibly may not include any "don't care" symbol at all. In general, the chromosome will contain, arranged in any order, g centers and $g_{\max} - g$ symbols #.
- *Fitness function*. Each chromosome is associated, as a measure of adaptation to the environment, the Davies-Bouldin index (DB). DB is a function of the ratio of the sum of the internal cluster dispersion and the cluster separation and depends on the number of clusters. So DB is a suitable objective function for the case of unknown number of clusters. The algorithm yields as optimal partition that which corresponds to the minimum DB. As evolutionary algorithms usually maximize the fitness function, this latter is defined equal to 1/DB.
- *Initial population*. The size s of the population has to be pre-specified. Then, in the initial population for $i = 1, 2, \ldots, s$ an integer g_i is generated uniformly randomly in $[g_{\min}, g_{\max}]$. In the data set $\mathcal{O}$ g_i objects are chosen at random. Each one of these g_i objects are assigned to a gene selected at random within the chromosome. The genes that are left unassigned are set to the symbol #.

The genetic operators implemented by GCUK are the roulette wheel parent selection, the single point crossover and mutation.

- *Selection*. Each chromosome is examined and its fitness function is evaluated. The probability that any chromosome will be inserted in the new generation is proportional to its fitness (roulette wheel parent selection). The old population is entirely replaced by the chromosomes selected to form the new one.
- *Crossover*. With a fixed probability p_c, two parent chromosomes are selected for generating two children chromosomes. A positive integer number is randomly chosen in $[1, g_{\max}]$. Then, the genes from the right side of the chosen number are exchanged between the parent chromosomes. Notice that in this context a gene is either an array of real numbers (the coordinates of a centroid) or a symbol #.
- *Mutation*. Each and every centroid coordinate mutates with probability p_m. Let ν denote a coordinate. Then, if a mutation occurs, ν becomes either $\nu \pm 2\delta\nu$ if $\nu \neq 0$ or $\pm 2\delta$ if $\nu = 0$. δ is a number generated from the uniform distribution in $[0, 1]$. The $+$ or $-$ sign occurs with equal probability.

Example 7.2.3.1 The Wisconsin breast cancer data

This breast cancer database was obtained from the University of Wisconsin Hospitals, Madison from Dr. William H. Wolberg. There are 699 cases classified 458 as benign and 241 as malignant ($g = 2$). The number of variables is $p = 9$ and in 16 cases some values are missing. Using list-wise deletion makes a data set of $n = 683$ cases be available, 444 benign and 239 malignant. The number of possible partitions in two clusters is $N(699, 2) = 1.315 \times 10^{210}$. The 9 variables are as follows.

1. Clump Thickness
2. Uniformity of Cell Size
3. Uniformity of Cell Shape
4. Marginal Adhesion
5. Single Epithelial Cell Size
6. Bare Nuclei
7. Bland Chromatin
8. Normal Nucleoli
9. Mitoses

The data may be downloaded from the URL http://www.ailab.si/orange/ (Demsar et al., 2004).

We run the GCUK-clustering algorithm using the following GA parameters.

- 50 population size
- 100 number of iterations
- 2 and 10 the minimum and maximum number of clusters
- 0.8 crossover probability
- 0.001 mutation probability

For computing the Davies-Bouldin index we set $q = 1$ and $t = 1$ for the sake of simplicity.

The GA estimate of the number of clusters has been $g = 2$. Estimated partition conformity to the known partition is summarized in Table 7.7. Only 28 cases out of 683 are misclassified. The recovery of the known clusters is satisfactory as suggested as well by the large values of the Rand and Jaccard indexes of external cluster validity.

Table 7.7 Results obtained from the GCUK algorithm using the Davies-Bouldin index (DB). Estimated partition is evaluated by the misclassification rate, the corrected Rand index and the Jaccard coefficient

DB	Fitness function	Misscl.rate	Rand	Jaccard
0.2689	3.7187	4.1%	0.8409	0.8664

7.2.4 The Grouping Genetic Algorithm

The grouping genetic algorithm proposed by Falkenauer (1998) forms the basis of the algorithm GGA developed by Baragona et al. (2001b). The fitness function is provided by the Calinski and Harabasz (1974) variance ratio criterion displayed at the end of Sect. 7.1.2.1. Let X be the $n \times p$ data matrix (7.2) where each row corresponds to an observations. The chromosome for encoding a candidate solution is a string of integer values of length $n + g$ where n is the number of observations and g is the number of clusters. Two distinct substrings have to be distinguished in each chromosome, the first one of length n and the second one of variable length g. In the former each gene, which may take an integer value between 1 and g, relates to a specific object and denotes the cluster to which the object itself belongs. The latter encodes the clusters labels as a sequence of g integer numbers. The population is evolved by applying the genetic operators selection, crossover, mutation and inversion. This latter operator has been introduced by Holland (1975) and several implementations have been suggested by Goldberg (1989b) specially in ordered genetic algorithms. The variable length chromosome encoding requires that a specialized crossover operator has to be implemented. The genetic operators, except mutation, are applied only to the last substring of a chromosome, that is the group-part substring. The parameters to be pre-specified are the population size s, the probabilities of crossover p_c, mutation p_m and inversion p_i, the maximum number of clusters $g_{\max}$ and the maximum number of iterations N. The population is initialized by generating a number g from a uniform distribution in $[1, g_{\max}]$ for each chromosome. Then each object is assigned to a group by generating at random a number from a uniform distribution in $[1, g]$.

The GGA operators are defined as follows.

1. *Selection*. The selection is performed by using the roulette wheel rule and the new population entirely replaces the past one. To improve the genetic algorithm performance and ensure asymptotic convergence the elitist strategy is applied. If the best chromosome in the past generation has been neither selected nor produced by the evolutionary operators and no better chromosome is included in the next generation, then such best chromosome replaces the worst chromosome in the next generation so that the population size remains fixed.
2. *Crossover*. The Bin Packing Crossover (BPX) proposed by Falkenauer (1998) is adapted to the fitness function in order to accelerate the convergence towards the solution. The objects occurring twice are put aside and each is re-assigned to the group whose centroid is the nearest one in terms of the squared Euclidean distance. The BPX is performed on each pair of chromosomes with probability p_c.
3. *Mutation*. A mutation occurs when an object moves from one cluster to another. Therefore, in practice, any gene of the first substring of each chromosome undergoes mutation with probability p_m by changing its value to another one chosen randomly among values within the second substring.

4. *Inversion*. For each chromosome in the population, inversion may take place with pre-specified probability p_i as follows. Two cutting points are randomly chosen in $[1, g]$, c_1 and c_2, say, where $c_1 \leq c_2$. The genes between the two cutting points are taken in reverse order.

Example 7.2.4.1 Thyroid gland data

Five laboratory tests are used to try to predict whether a patient's thyroid is to be classified 'normal', hypo and hyper functioning. The diagnosis (the class label) was based on a complete medical record, including anamnesis, scan etc. There are a total of $n = 215$ observations and the number of variables is $p = 5$. The number of known clusters is $g = 3$ (1 = normal, 2 = hyper, 3 = hypo). We have to search among $N(215, 5) = 1.5826 \times 10^{148}$ partitions. We downloaded the data set from the URL http://mlearn.ics.uci.edu/databases/thyroid-disease (Hettich and Bay, 1999). The variables correspond to the following measurements.

1. T3-resin uptake test. (A percentage)
2. Total Serum thyroxin as measured by the isotopic displacement method.
3. Total serum triiodothyronine as measured by radioimmuno assay.
4. basal thyroid-stimulating hormone (TSH) as measured by radioimmuno assay.
5. Maximal absolute difference of TSH value after injection of 200 micro grams of thyrotropin-releasing hormone as compared to the basal value.

The GGA has been run on this data set using the following parameters.

- Population size $s = 40$,
- maximum number of iterations $N = 2000$,
- probability of crossover $p_c = 0.8$,
- probability of mutation $p_m = 0.01$,
- probability of inversion $p_i = 0.01$,
- elitist strategy,
- generational gap 1.

Four fitness functions have been used and results recorded for each one. The Calinski and Harabasz's variance ratio criterion (VRC) (Calinski and Harabasz, 1974) has been introduced already in Sect. 7.1.2.1. Then a version of the index suggested by Marriott (1982) has been used defined as

$$M = g^{-2} \det(T)/\det(W)$$

which is intended to be maximized. Two other indexes have been considered, the first one suggested by Banfield and Raftery (1993, p. 805) defined as

$$S^* = \sum_{k=1}^{g} n_k \log\left(S_k/n_k\right),$$

where (for $k = 1, \ldots, g$) $S_k = \text{trace}(A^{-1}\Omega_k)$, A is a known matrix and Ω_k is the diagonal matrix of the eigenvalues of the within-cluster scatter matrix W_k. Here we chose to set $A = \text{diag}(\alpha_1, \ldots, \alpha_p)$ where $\alpha_i = \lambda_i/\lambda_1$, $(\lambda_1, \ldots, \lambda_p)$ are the eigenvalues of W/n arranged in descending order and W is the pooled within-cluster scatter matrix. The second index has been considered the criterion given in Symons (1981, equation (12) p. 37). This index (let us call it $S(g, p)$) includes the term $\sum_{k=1}^{g} n_k \log\{\det(W_k/n_k)\}$ and further terms which take into account the data dimension p. These latter two criteria have to be minimized, so the fitness function has been set to $\exp(-S^*)$ and $\exp\{-S(g, p)\}$.

The behavior of the four fitness functions is displayed in Fig. 7.5. We may note the usual shape of an increasing step function with frequent large jumps at the first iterations and rare smaller jumps at later iterations. An exception is the S^* criterion that increases almost continuously almost until the last iteration. The difference resides in that S^* is a function of the eigenvalues while the other criteria are functions either of the trace or the determinant of the within-cluster scatter matrices.

The GGA estimate for the number of clusters is 3 regardless of the fitness function used. In Table 7.8 the partitions obtained by the GGA using each of the four fitness functions are evaluated by two external indexes of cluster validity, the mis-

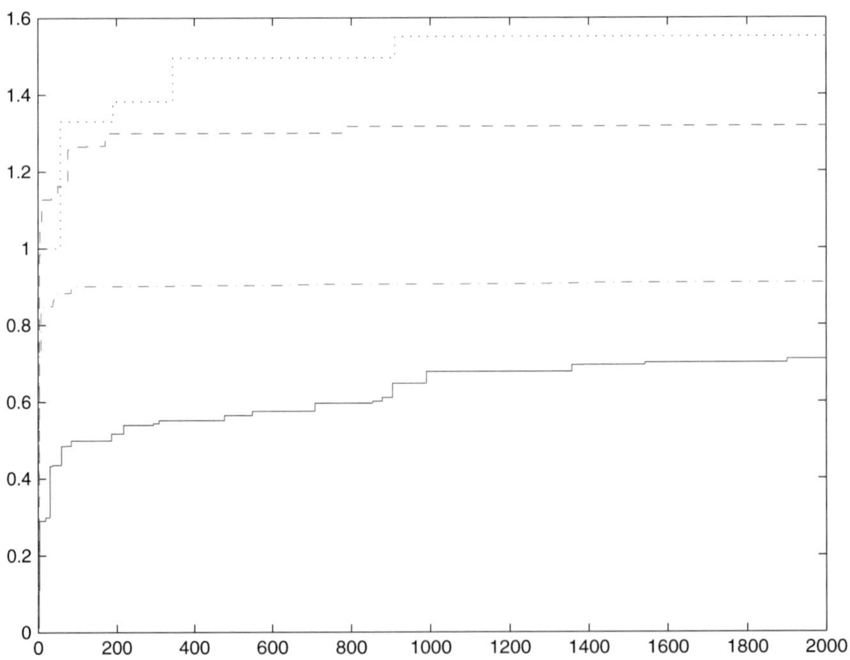

Fig. 7.5 Evolution of four fitness function used in the GGA algorithm applied to the Thyroid data. Symons index (*Solid line*), variance ratio criterion (*dashed line*), Marriott's criterion (*dotted line*) and Banfield and Raftery's S^* index (*dashed dotted line*) are displayed. Each of the GAs run 2000 iterations

Table 7.8 Results obtained from the GGA algorithm using 4 fitness function specifications evaluated by the misclassification rate and the corrected Rand index

Fitness function	VRC	M	S^*	$S(g, p)$
Misclass.rate (%)	18.60	22.79	23.72	4.19
Rand index	0.5791	0.3501	0.3966	0.8603

classification rate and the corrected Rand index. The indexes yield the same ranking but differences among the results become more or less apparent. The best result is obtained by using the fitness function based on the $S(g, p)$ criterion, with the corrected Rand index equal to 0.8603 and 9 cases misclassified out of 215 (4.19%). Then the VRC yields a rather satisfactory result while the remaining two criteria seem to have less discriminant power. According to the misclassification rate, the differences among the three fitness functions that give inferior results are not too much apparent because there are between 40 and 50 misclassified cases. The performance of the $S(g, p)$-based fitness function may be explained by following the discussion in Banfield and Raftery (1993). The clusters in the data set are ellipsoidal and differ for orientation, size and shape so that the criterion $S(g, p)$ may give the best performance because it does not impose constraints on clusters. The index S^* assumes that the clusters have the same shape, and the other two criteria, based on trace and determinant of the pooled within-cluster scatter matrix, assume the same size and shape.

7.2.5 Genetic Clustering of Large Data Sets

The clustering algorithm of Tseng and Yang (2001) is oriented to the cluster analysis of very large databases. The algorithm proceeds in two steps, the first one for preliminary aggregation of objects in "first level" clusters, called connected components, the second one to further aggregate the connected components obtained in the first step to yield the final objects partition. A suitable threshold $\bar{d}$ is computed from the data and objects are considered one at the time in arbitrary order. The first one constitutes the first connected component, the second one enters the same component if its distance is less than $\bar{d}$, otherwise it starts a new connected component, and so on. If an object may belong to two connected components or more, the one such that its first element has smallest distance is chosen. This first step reduces the number of objects from n to m, where it is hoped that $m \ll n$. In the second step a fitness function is defined and computed basing on the information obtained in the first step. Then a population of s binary string of length m is generated at random. A one-to-one mapping is defined between the characters of a binary string and the connected components. If the connected component corresponds to 1 then it is considered an "aggregation point" while any connected component that corresponds to "0" is aggregated to the nearest aggregation point. The binary string population is evolved by a GA that uses standard genetic operators for binary chromosomes. Usually a good partition is achieved corresponding to a large value of the fitness function.

7.3 Fuzzy Partition

Fuzzy partition (see, for instance, Hoppner et al., 1999) may be thought of as a generalization of hard partition in that, given n objects $\{x_1, \ldots, x_n\} = \mathcal{O} \subseteq \mathbb{R}^p$, membership of an object x_i to a cluster C_h, $h = 1, \ldots, c$, is not exclusive. Notice that we use the convention usual in fuzzy partition to denote c the number of clusters instead of g. Property (7.7) still has to hold while the validity of property (7.8) is no longer required. A certain amount of overlapping among subsets $\{C_1, \ldots, C_c\} \subset \mathcal{O}$ is allowed. The $n \times c$ fuzzy partition matrix U defines the degree of membership μ_{ik} of the object x_i in the group C_k provided that the following conditions are fulfilled

$$
\begin{aligned}
\mu_{ik} \in [0, 1], \quad 1 \le i \le n, &\quad 1 \le k \le c, \\
\sum_{k=1}^{c} \mu_{ik} = 1, &\quad 1 \le i \le n, \\
0 < \sum_{i=1}^{n} \mu_{ik} < n, &\quad 1 \le k \le c.
\end{aligned}
\tag{7.15}
$$

Knowledge of the matrix U allows a fuzzy partition to be uniquely identified. Notice that a hard partition could be defined in exactly the same way but the μ_{ik}'s would have to assume only the values 0 and 1.

7.3.1 *The Fuzzy c-Means Algorithm*

The most popular algorithm to obtain an optimal fuzzy partition according to a suitable criterion is the fuzzy c-means (FCM) algorithm (Bezdek, 1981). The FCM is an iterative method which yields the fuzzy partition that minimize the Dunn's criterion (Dunn, 1974), essentially the weighted within-group sum of squared errors with respect to the degrees of membership μ_{ik}'s and a set of p-dimensional cluster centers (centroids or in general medoids) $V = \{v_1, \ldots, v_c\}$. Given the data matrix (7.2) such objective function may be written

$$
J_q(U, V) = \sum_{k=1}^{c} \sum_{i=1}^{n} \mu_{ik}^{q} \|x_i - v_k\|_D^2, \tag{7.16}
$$

where q is a weighting exponent on each fuzzy membership and

$$
\|x_i - v_k\|_D^2 = (x_i - v_k)' D (x_i - v_k)
$$

is the squared Mahalanobis-type distance

$$
d(x_j, x_r) = \sqrt{\{(x_j - x_r)' D (x_j - x_r)\}}, \tag{7.17}
$$

where D is a p-dimensional positive definite square matrix. If, for instance, $D = I$, then (7.17) is the Euclidean distance between x_j and x_r. A Mahalanobis-like distance may be defined as well by taking $D = T^{-1}$, where T is now the variance-covariance matrix of X, that is (7.10) divided by n. Other objective functions may be built by replacing the difference norm in (7.16) by any distance measure (7.6) between the object x_i and the center v_k that we may denote $d(x_i, v_k)$. We have to choose a maximum number of iterations N and possibly a small positive real number ε that may serve to stop the iterations before N if appreciable improvement of the objective function is not likely to be obtained further. The skeleton of the FCM algorithm is as follows.

1. Assign proper values to the number of clusters c and to weighting exponent q, and initialize the fuzzy partition matrix U,
2. Calculate the p-dimensional cluster centers

$$v_k = \frac{1}{\sum_{i=1}^{n} \mu_{ik}^q} \sum_{i=1}^{n} \mu_{ik}^q x_i, \qquad k = 1, \ldots, c,$$

3. Update the fuzzy group membership weights

$$\mu_{ik}^* = \frac{1}{\sum_{j=1}^{c} \left(\|x_i - v_k\|_D^2 / \|x_i - v_j\|_D^2 \right)^{2/(q-1)}}, \qquad i = 1, \ldots, n, \qquad k = 1, \ldots, c,$$

4. If either the number of iterations exceeds N or $\|\mu_{ik} - \mu_{ik}^*\| < \varepsilon$ stop, otherwise set $\mu_{ik} = \mu_{ik}^*$ and go to step 2.

Note that if for object x_i we have $\|x_i - v_j\|_D^2 = 0$ for some $j \in [1, c]$ then in step 3 we have to set $\mu_{ik}^* = 0$ if $k \neq j$ and $\mu_{ij}^* = 1$.

It may be shown (see,e.g., Bezdek, 1981) that, given starting points μ_{ik}'s, the FCM algorithm always converges to some local minimum of the objective function (7.16). In general different choices of the initial degrees of membership yield different local minima.

Example 7.3.1.1 Wine data

These data are the results of a chemical analysis of wines grown in the same region in Italy but derived from three different cultivars. The analysis determined the quantities of 13 constituents found in each of the three types of wines. There are $n = 178$ observations in the data set. The number of possible partitions in $g = 3$ clusters is $N(178, 3) = 1.4107 \times 10^{84}$. The $p = 13$ variables are as follows.

1. Alcohol
2. Malic acid
3. Ash
4. Alcalinity of ash

5. Magnesium
6. Total phenols
7. Flavanoids
8. Nonflavanoid phenols
9. Proanthocyanins
10. Color intensity
11. Hue
12. OD280/OD315 of diluted wines
13. Proline

The known classification includes $g = 3$ clusters the first one with 59, the second one with 71 and the third one with 48 observations. The data have been downloaded from the URL http://archive.ics.uci.edu/ml (Asuncion and Newman, 2007). We run the fuzzy c-means algorithm described in Sect. 7.3.1. The Matlab toolbox FUZZCLUST (Abonyi et al., 2005) has been used for computation. We chose the Dunn's index as internal index of cluster validity and obtained the optimal partition corresponding to the value 0.1423 for this index. This solution may be considered a rather satisfactorily result. The misclassification rate is equal to 5.06% and the Rand and Jaccard external indexes of cluster validity equal 0.8498 and 0.8183 respectively. A principal component analysis provided the first two components displayed in Fig. 7.6. The three clusters obtained from the fuzzy c-means algorithm are well visualized with their centers.

7.3.2 Genetic Fuzzy Partition Algorithms

Genetic algorithms-based fuzzy clustering methods have been suggested to deal with two limitations of FCM, namely the number of clusters c has to be prespecified, and the initial values needed to start the algorithm may lead to a suboptimal solution (Maulik and Bandyopadhyay, 2003). Other applications of GAs have been proposed to solve special problems in the fuzzy partition framework, for instance discretization of continuous data in partially overlapping intervals (Choi and Moon, 2007).

The variable string length genetic algorithm (VGA) proposed by Maulik and Bandyopadhyay (2003) will be described that does not require prior knowledge of the number of clusters c. This latter is considered an additional parameter that is implicit in the objective function definition. Moreover, in the GAs framework, searching for the optimal solution is performed usually by maximizing an objective function which is positive real-valued (fitness function). A feasible choice is the Xie-Beni (XB) index (Xie and Beni, 1991) which is positive and, unlike the Dunn's index, depends on c. However, as the optimal solutions are to be found among the partitions that minimize XB, the fitness function will be defined $f = 1/XB$.

Let U and V denote as in Sect. 7.3.1 the fuzzy partition matrix with entries the degrees of membership μ_{ik}'s and the center coordinates matrix with entries the p-dimensional arrays v_k's respectively. Furthermore, let X be the $n \times p$ data

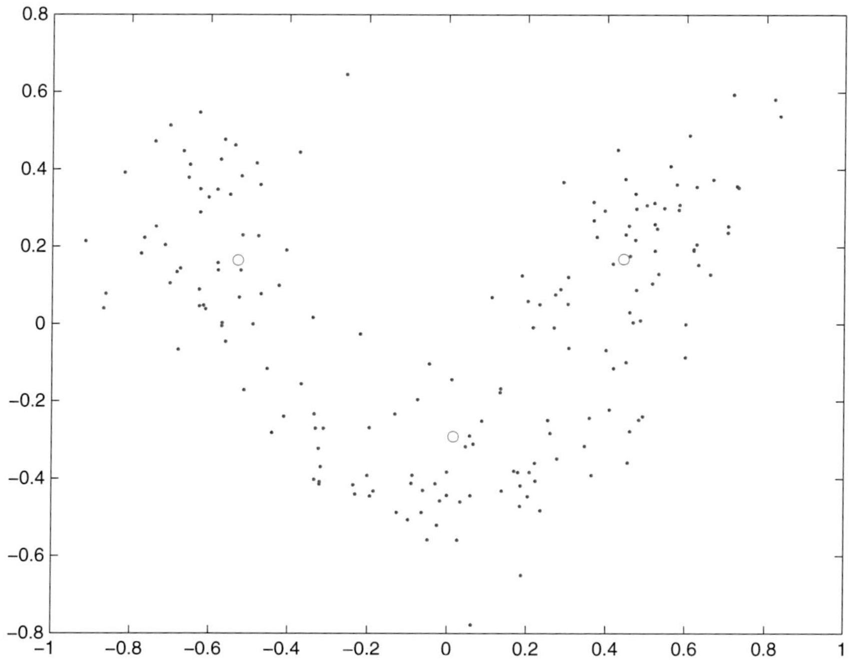

Fig. 7.6 Scatter diagram of the first two principal components of the wine data with the cluster centers (*circles*) computed by using the fuzzy *c*-means algorithm

matrix (7.2) defined in Sect. 7.1.1. The XB index is a function of the ratio of the total variation $\sigma(U, V; X)$ to the minimum separation $\text{sep}(U, V; X)$ of the clusters, where the dependence of both σ and sep on U, V and X is emphasized. Note that X is fixed while we are searching for optimal U and V parameters. Let

$$\sigma(U, V; X) = \sum_{k=1}^{c} \sum_{i=1}^{n} \mu_{ik}^2 \|x_i - v_k\|^2$$

and

$$\text{sep}(V) = \min_{k \neq j} \|v_k - v_j\|^2,$$

where $\|\cdot\|$ is now the Euclidean norm. The XB index may be written

$$\text{XB}(U, V; X) = \frac{\sigma(U, V; X)}{n\,\text{sep}(V)}, \tag{7.18}$$

and the fitness function is

$$f_{\mathrm{XB}}(U, V; X) = \frac{1}{\mathrm{XB}(U, V; X)}. \tag{7.19}$$

The set of the potential solutions has the cluster centers as elements. Let s denote the population size, and let the hth individual element be the chromosome $\xi^{(h)} = \left(v_1^{(h)}, \ldots, v_{c_h}^{(h)}\right)$. The chromosome has variable length as each chromosome may encode c_h centers, $h = 1, \ldots, s$. The genes are p-dimensional vectors each of which is a center representative of a cluster. A gene cannot be split into its coordinates though these latter are allowed to mutate according to a random mechanism that produces small changes with small probability. We assume that the constraint $2 \leq c_h \leq c_{\max}$ holds for each chromosome in each generation for some maximum pre-specified number of clusters $c_{\max}$.

Before the starting of the VGA we have to choose, as usual in GAs, a maximum number of iterations N and the crossover and mutation probability p_c and p_m respectively. Then the following steps are executed.

1. *Selection*. For $h = 1, \ldots, s$ the set of centers $\{v_1^{(h)}, \ldots, v_{c_h}^{(h)}\}$ are extracted from the chromosome $\xi^{(h)}$ and a set of weights μ_{ik}^* is computed by using equation in step 3 of the FCM algorithm in Sect. 7.3.1. Then (7.18) and (7.19) are computed and proportional selection is applied on the population according to the roulette wheel rule. Moreover, the elitist strategy is adopted to ensure that the fitness function of the best chromosome never decreases throughout generations.
2. *Crossover*. A special crossover is needed as the chromosomes have no fixed length. Moreover, the constraint on the number of clusters has to be fulfilled. Let $\xi^{(1)}$ and $\xi^{(2)}$ denote the parent chromosomes and let c_1 and c_2 be the respective number of clusters. Generate for the first chromosome a crossover point τ_1 uniformly randomly in the interval $[1, c_1]$. The crossover point τ_2 for the second chromosome is generated uniformly randomly in the interval $[\mathrm{LB}(\tau_2), \mathrm{UB}(\tau_2)]$. The genes in locations $\tau_1, \ldots, c_1$ of chromosome $\xi^{(1)}$ are replaced by the genes sequence $\tau_2, \ldots, c_2$ from chromosome $\xi^{(2)}$. Likewise, the genes in locations $\tau_2, \ldots, c_2$ of chromosome $\xi^{(2)}$ are replaced by the genes sequence $\tau_1, \ldots, c_1$ from chromosome $\xi^{(1)}$. So the two new chromosomes have $\tau_1 + c_2 - \tau_2$ and $\tau_2 + c_1 - \tau_1$ genes respectively. As the chromosome length is required to exceed 2 and to be less than $c_{\max}$ the lower and upper bounds $[\mathrm{LB}(\tau_2), \mathrm{UB}(\tau_2)]$ are constrained to the inequalities

$$\begin{aligned} \mathrm{LB}(\tau_2) &\geq \max\{2 - c_1 + \tau_1, \tau_1 + c_2 - c_{\max}\} \\ \mathrm{UB}(\tau_2) &\leq \min\{\tau_1 + c_2 - 2, c_{\max} - c_1 + \tau_1\}. \end{aligned}$$

3. *Mutation*. For each $h = 1, \ldots, s$ and each $j = 1, \ldots, c_h$, with probability p_m the value $v_j^{(h)}$ becomes $(1 \pm 2\delta)v_j^{(h)}$ if $v_j^{(h)} \neq 0$ and $\pm 2\delta$ if $v_j^{(h)} = 0$ where δ is a number generated from the uniform distribution in the interval $[0, 1]$. The $+$ or $-$ sign occurs with equal probability.

7.4 Multivariate Mixture Models Estimation by Evolutionary Computing

Multivariate mixture models constitute a convenient framework to make inference on grouped data (see McLachlan and Peel, 2000, for a comprehensive review). Assume that each row $(x_j)'$ (7.1) of the observed data X in (7.2), for $j = 1, \dots, n$, be a realization of a random variable distributed as a multivariate mixture density with g components $f_i(x_j)$, $i = 1, \dots, g$, defined by

$$f(x_j) = \sum_{i=1}^{g} \pi_i f_i(x_j), \tag{7.20}$$

where $0 \le \pi_i \le 1$, and $\sum_{i=1}^{g} \pi_i = 1$. The weights $\pi_1, \dots, \pi_g$ are the mixing proportions, while the $f_i(x_j)$ are the multivariate mixture component densities. The density function (7.20) is a g-component finite mixture density. We assume that g is some fixed positive integer, $g > 1$ and $g \ll n$. If $g = 1$ obviously (7.20) is still a density but not a mixture anymore. In order to check the existence of different models that generated the data a preliminary cluster analysis may be performed or the split and recombine (SAR) procedure introduced by Peña and Tiao (2003) may be used.

If the component densities are multivariate normal, we have

$$f_i(x_j|\mu_i, \Sigma_i) = (2\pi)^{-\frac{p}{2}} |\Sigma_i|^{-\frac{1}{2}} \exp\left\{-\frac{1}{2}(x_j - \mu_i)' \Sigma_i^{-1} (x_j - \mu_i)\right\}.$$

The likelihood function for given X reads

$$L(\theta|X) = \prod_{j=1}^{n} f(x_j), \tag{7.21}$$

where, under Gaussianity assumption, the parameter array θ includes the weights π_i's, the averages μ_i's and the variance-covariance matrices Σ_i's. According to the likelihood approach, estimating the multivariate mixture parameter vector is done by maximizing (7.21) with respect to θ. As the weights are constrained to be non-negative and sum to unity, and by the symmetry property of the variance-covariance matrices, the array θ has $g - 1 + gp + gp(p+1)/2$ essentially independent elements.

The likelihood approach for parameters estimation has been extensively studied and several methods are available. The favorite device is maybe the EM-algorithm, and its variants, as in general the maximization of (7.21) with these methods is easier than using other estimation techniques such as the quasi-Newton methods, for instance (McLachlan and Krishnan, 1997). Bayesian approaches used in conjunction with Markov chain Monte Carlo methods have been experienced as well (see, for instance Bensmail et al., 1997). Estimating the parameter vector θ is in general a difficult task, and it is worth the while to explore either alternative or complementary approaches. Some GAs-based procedures have been introduced by Baragona and Battaglia (2003). We shall describe in the next sections an estimation procedure that entirely relies on GAs and an hybrid algorithm that combines GAs and the EM-algorithm. Hybridization techniques are also suggested to deal with the case where the number of density mixtures is unknown.

7.4.1 Genetic Multivariate Mixture Model Estimates

Let n p-dimensional observations be available and form the array X. In order to fit a multivariate normal mixture model to the data, we define first the component indicator array Z with g rows and n columns. We may give Z one of the following definitions.

$$Z(i,j) = \{ \begin{matrix} 1 \text{ if the component of origin of } x_j \text{ in the mixture is } i \\ 0 \qquad\qquad\qquad \text{otherwise} \end{matrix} \tag{7.22}$$

where the constraints

$$\sum_{i=1}^{g} Z(i,j) = 1, \qquad j = 1, \ldots, n,$$

are assumed to hold, that is each observation originates from one and only one component.

$$Z(i,j) = \{ \begin{matrix} 1 \text{ if the component of origin of } x_j \text{ in the mixture is (possibly) } i \\ 0 \qquad\qquad\qquad \text{otherwise} \end{matrix} \tag{7.23}$$

where no constraints are imposed. So, some uncertainty is allowed whether which the component of origin of x_j may be.

$$Z(i,j) = \{ \begin{matrix} v \text{ if the component of origin of } x_j \text{ in the mixture is (possibly) } i \\ 0 \qquad\qquad\qquad \text{otherwise} \end{matrix} \tag{7.24}$$

where v is a nonnegative integer in a pre-specified interval $[0, q]$. The integer v may be regarded as a score assigned to the confidence that the observation x_j originates from the component i. Either of the three definitions (7.22), (7.23) or (7.24) may be employed in the GAs-based estimation procedure but they differ as to the requested amount of a priori knowledge on the objects grouping structure.

The probability that the component of origin of x_j in the mixture is i may be estimated

$$z(i,j) = \frac{Z(i,j)}{\sum_{i=1}^{g} Z(i,j)}, \qquad i = 1, \ldots, g, \quad j = 1, \ldots, n. \tag{7.25}$$

Then, the mixing proportions are computed

$$\pi_i = \frac{\sum_{j=1}^{n} z(i, j)}{n}, \qquad i = 1, \ldots, g. \tag{7.26}$$

Finally, the p-dimensional mean vectors μ_i and the variance-covariance $p \times p$ matrices may be computed

$$\mu_i = \sum_{j=1}^{n} \frac{z(i, j)}{\sum_{h=1}^{n} z(i, h)} x_j, \qquad i = 1, \ldots, g, \tag{7.27}$$

and

$$\Sigma_i = \sum_{j=1}^{n} \frac{z(i, j)}{\sum_{h=1}^{n} z(i, h)} (x_j - \mu_i)(x_j - \mu_i)', \qquad i = 1, \ldots, g. \tag{7.28}$$

The preceding equations (7.22) through (7.28) outline the procedure that we may embed into a genetic algorithm. Different encodings have to be adopted whether definition (7.22), or (7.23), or (7.24) is chosen. Binary encoding is well suited for the former two while the integer encoding has to be preferred for the latter. We have to notice, however, that any matrix Z yields a solution to the optimization problem because, given Z, it is straightforward to compute the parameter estimates by using equations (7.25), (7.26), (7.27) and (7.28). Moreover, the likelihood (7.21) is a positive valued function that has to be maximized and may be computed by substituting such estimates into its expression. So we are allowed to assume Z as a chromosome and (7.21) as the fitness function. Both for convenience and to adhere to the usual representation we may transform the matrix Z by stacking either its columns or its rows into a vector ζ that we may assume as a chromosome of length $\ell = gn$.

Let s be the population size and N the number of iterations. The gene placed in locus u which is included in the chromosome ζ of the kth element of the population in generation t may be denoted $\zeta_u(k, t)$, $k = 1, \ldots, s$, $t = 1, \ldots, N$. The term individual will be often used as synonym of element according to the word population which is used to denote the set of potential solutions at each iteration. A detailed explanation concerned with building the initial population and implementing the selection, crossover and mutation operators follows.

- *Initial population*. To start the genetic algorithm, s strings ζ have to be supplied. This may be done either at random or by exploiting the information contained in the data. If we want to choose the component indicator (7.22), then, for each column j of Z, a location between 1 and g has to be selected uniformly randomly and set equal to unity. All other entries in the column j are zero. In case (7.23), all entries in Z are filled with either 1 or 0 with equal probability. So, we may consider that the observation x_j originates from any component that shows unity in the corresponding jth column. In case (7.24), each entry in the column j of Z may be zero or greater than zero with equal probability. If greater than zero, then another integer random number v between 1 and q has to be generated. The integer v denotes the confidence that the component of origin of x_j in the mixture is i. This procedure for building the initial population is rather blind. Its advantage resides in that it assumes that we have no knowledge about the data structure, so that we do not impose any prior (maybe misleading) belief. On the other hand, convergence may be rather slow and time consuming and may require a large number of iterations. We may suggest an alternative procedure, which does not seem too much demanding, that takes into account the distance between observations. For each individual k, a binary string n bits long is generated, where g 1's are randomly placed, and the other characters are set equal to zero. The 1's indicate g observations which we consider merely aggregation centers. If, for instance, the rth location in the binary string is equal to 1, then compute the Mahalanobis-like distance $d(x_j, x_r)$ according to equation (7.17). Computation has to be repeated for each and every 1 in the binary string. If r^* is the index for which the smallest distance is computed, then the r^*th entry in column j of Z is set to unity, and other entries are set to zero. If we want possibly more than a single 1 in each column, as in (7.23), then the next index r in the ascending order of the distances may be taken as the location for another unity. The number of 1's in each column may be selected at random. In case (7.24), the integers v in each column may be given values inversely proportional to the distance (7.17) rounded to the nearest integer.

- *Selection.* The roulette wheel rule may be used, that is each individual chromosome in the current population is copied into a individual chromosome in the next generation with probability proportional to its fitness function value. The new generation entirely replaces the current population excepted possibly the single individual concerned with the application of the elitist strategy.
- *Crossover.* Let p_c be the pre-specified probability for a couple of individuals to undergo the crossover. So we may select at random $[sp_c/2]$ individual pairs in the current generation t. Simple crossover performs as follows. Let us randomly select the individuals k_1 and k_2, and let $\zeta(k_1, t)$ and $\zeta(k_2, t)$ be their chromosomes. Let c be an integer chosen uniformly randomly between 1 and $\ell - 1$. The integer c is called cutting point. The genes from locus $c + 1$ to ℓ are exchanged between the two chromosomes. The offsprings are the chromosomes of two new individuals that replace the old ones. In the present context, however, the simple crossover seems too disruptive because it does not take into account the structure of the matrix Z. In fact, the cutting point may split a column of the matrix Z, and a problem may arise in case (7.24). For instance, let $g = 3$ and let the cutting point divide the columns 111 of the first chromosome and 999 of the second one in such a way the offsprings 119 and 991 are generated. The probability for the observation to belong to the third component becomes large in the first chromosome and small in the second one in spite of the fact that the probabilities in each of the parent string are equal. We suggest to implement the crossover operator in two ways, either for observations or for components. If the former alternative is

chosen, then ζ has better be built by stacking the columns of Z. Let us choose uniformly randomly an integer c between 1 and $n-1$. The new individuals have to exchange their genes from locus $(g-1)c+1$ to $gn = \ell$. In practice, we consider the columns of Z as blocks g characters long which are not allowed to split. On the other hand, we may stack the rows of the matrix Z and consider any row separately. Note that each row i describes a component, that is it indicates which observations originate from the component i. Then, for each row, let us choose uniformly randomly an integer c between 1 and $g-1$. The new individuals have to exchange their genes from locus $(n-1)c+1$ to $ng = \ell$. This latter crossover procedure is more flexible, but it is not suitable in case (7.24) obviously because it does not ensure that the constraints required in this case will be fulfilled.

- *Mutation*. For binary chromosomes (7.22) and (7.23) each gene may change its value from 0 to 1 or vice versa with probability p_m. In case (7.24), if the value of the gene is greater than zero, then it may become zero with probability p_m. If the gene value is zero, then it may change with probability p_m. Its new value is chosen uniformly randomly between 1 and q.

Example 7.4.1.1 Mixture models for Iris Plants and Diabetes data (g known)

We illustrate the estimation of mixture models with the number of groups g known by using the method described in this Sect. 7.4.1 on the data sets Iris Plants and Diabetes. Let us call GA11 the version of the algorithm that uses the binary encoding (7.23) and GA21 the version that uses the integer encoding (7.24). For comparison we developed algorithms GA12 and GA13 that use the binary encoding (7.23) while the crossover is performed on observations and on components respectively and the initial population is formed by taking the distances into account. Two further versions, GA22 and GA23, use the integer encoding (7.24) with the same modifications as GA12 and GA13 respectively.

We run the six algorithms for each of the two sets by assuming the number of mixture components $g = 3$ and using the following GA parameters.

- Population size $s = 50$,
- Number of generations $N = 100000$,
- Crossover probability $p_c = 0.8$,
- Mutation probability $p_m = 0.005$.

The results given in Table 7.9 include the logarithm of the likelihood function computed from the best chromosome in the final population and the GA iteration where the last increase of the fitness function has been recorded. Comparison may be based on the log-likelihood because the number of parameters is always the same for all algorithms. Note that if the known partition is assumed then the logarithm of the likelihood is equal to -182.92 for the Iris data and -2329 for the Diabetes data so that we may consider that all algorithm perform rather satisfactorily. For the binary encoding the algorithm GA13 yields the largest log-likelihood for both data sets and in the smallest number of iterations. It has to be noticed, however, that for Diabetes data all algorithm end with the identical log-likelihood value. For the

Table 7.9 Results of GAs-based multivariate normal mixture models estimation on the Iris data and Diabetes data. The number of components is assumed known

	Iris data		Diabetes data	
Genetic algorithm version	Largest log-likelihood	Obtained at generation	Largest log-likelihood	Obtained at generation
GA11	−189.38	74406	−2304	52576
GA12	−180.25	95744	−2304	56437
GA13	−180.23	19721	−2304	43184
GA21	−297.85	93230	−2371	94824
GA22	−180.21	24566	−2304	97625
GA23	−180.20	99319	−2304	61407

integer encoding the algorithm GA23 again yields the best results but the number of iterations is considerably larger. However, the algorithm GA22 yields results slightly worse (Iris data) or identical (Diabetes data) and takes a number of iterations much less than GA23 for the Iris data.

7.4.2 Hybrid Genetic Algorithms and the EM Algorithm

The version of the genetic algorithm that we will describe in this section may be used to provide another local search algorithm, the EM algorithm, for instance, with suitable starting points. Similar procedures are often found in practical applications. For example, a model-based approach to clustering has been suggested by Banfield and Raftery (1993). Dasgupta and Raftery (1998) used a hierarchical clustering algorithm to find an initial proposal solution and assumed such a solution to initialize the EM algorithm to estimate the parameters of a mixture model. A similar device has been proposed by Brooks and Morgan (1995) for simulated annealing. Likewise, the genetic algorithm may be used conveniently to explore the solution space to locate the subsets that are likely to include the global maximum. Then, confining to these subsets only, some specific maximization algorithm may be used for refining the search to obtain the global maximum, or a close approximation at least. The genetic algorithm to be used within this hybrid approach may be better developed along the guidelines provided in Chatterjee et al. (1996); Chatterjee and Laudato (1997). Their procedure addresses the maximization of the likelihood function by direct encoding of the full parameter vector into a chromosome. The floating-point encoding may be used, that is each gene is a real number. If we want to maintain the binary encoding instead, then a one-to-one correspondence between the real parameter θ and the binary string ξ may be established according to the formula

$$\theta = a + \xi(b - a)/(2^{\ell} - 1), \tag{7.29}$$

where θ belongs to the interval (a, b) and ℓ is the pre-specified length of the binary string ξ. For calculations ξ in (7.29) is assumed the corresponding non negative integer.

Under Gaussianity assumption we have to estimate the parameter vector θ of the multivariate mixture model (7.21) which contains $h = g - 1 + gp + gp(p+1)/2$ entries, that is h distinct scalar parameters. These parameters are represented by a sequence of either h real numbers or h binary strings of length ℓ each. The fitness function is assumed equal to the likelihood function (7.21) as before. The GA may be implemented by specifying the number of generations N and the population size s and defining each and every chromosome in the initial population (often we shall refer to a chromosome as an individual) and the genetic operators selection, crossover and mutation.

- *Initial population.* The initial population is randomly generated to include s chromosomes each of which is a sequence of parameters as follows. For the mixing proportions, g values are generated at random and re-scaled to sum to unity. The effective number of parameters is $g - 1$. To generate the mean vector μ_i, $i = 1, \ldots, g$, for each of the p variable the interval (a, b) is taken with a equal to the minimum and b equal to the maximum computed on all observations. The same has been done for the variances, for each variable in each component. Let $\sigma_{i,j}^2$ denote the variance of the jth variable in the ith component. Its value is determined by choosing a string ξ ℓ bits long uniformly randomly, and using (7.29) with a equal to zero and b equal to a fraction of the variance computed for that variable by using all observations. The off-diagonal entry of the matrix Σ_i in row k and column j, $k > j$, are randomly generated, according to (7.29), in the interval $(-\sigma_{i,k}\sigma_{i,j}, \sigma_{i,k}\sigma_{i,j})$.
- *Selection.* (Tournament selection) The fitness evaluation is performed for each chromosome in the current population by using the encoded solution as the starting point to initialize the EM algorithm. This latter yields the chromosome fitness function. Then the chromosomes are paired, and, in each couple, the one which possesses the larger fitness function is copied into the other with probability p_s. This probability is the selection pressure, with obvious meaning, and has to be pre-specified.
- *Crossover.* The probability p_c is pre-specified, and $sp_c/2$ pairs are randomly chosen. For each pair, a cutting point c, say, is randomly chosen in the interval $(1, \ell - 1)$. The bits from $c + 1$ to ℓ of the first chromosome in the couple replace the corresponding ones in the second chromosome, and vice versa. Even in case of binary encoding the real numbers are not to be split.
- *Mutation.* Mutation may occur with pre-specified probability p_m per bit. The bit changes from 1 to 0 or vice versa. If floating-point encoding is used, then each gene ν becomes either $\nu \pm 2\delta\nu$ if $\nu \neq 0$ or $\pm 2\delta$ if $\nu = 0$. δ is a number generated from the uniform distribution in [0, 1] and the + or − sign occurs with equal probability.

The steps of the genetic algorithm described above are much alike that of the simple genetic algorithm. Nonetheless, there are reasons to prefer the tournament selection instead of the roulette wheel rule for selection because the former implements the elitist strategy at no additional computation cost. This is important because the hybrid algorithm needs fast execution of the genetic algorithm to counterbalance the computing time needed by the local optimization algorithm to perform its supplementary search. The drawback, however, consists in that in tournament selection a smaller number of copies of the fittest individuals are expected to pass to the next generations. This circumstance may slow the GAs convergence but in hybrid GAs the co-operating algorithm improves the convergence rate considerably so that this effect is less serious.

7.4.3 Multivariate Mixture Model Estimates with Unknown Number of Mixtures

The GAs-based procedure in Sect. 7.4.1 and the hybrid algorithm described in Sect. 7.4.2 could be extended to the case of unknown number of clusters provided that the fitness function depends on the number of mixtures g. The likelihood function (7.21) is not suited for the purpose of estimating both the number of mixtures and the mixture model parameters as g is assumed as a fixed parameter. A suitable objective function may be obtained by using the asymptotic information criterion (AIC) (Akaike, 1974) or the Schwarz's information criterion (SIC) (Schwarz, 1978). A comparison of the two criteria is discussed in Koehler and Murphree (1988). Estimates of the number of clusters g and the mixture model parameter vector θ may be obtained by minimizing either AIC or SIC. We have

$$\begin{aligned} \text{AIC} &= -2\log L(\theta, g|X) + 2h, \\ \text{SIC} &= -2\log L(\theta, g|X) + \log(n)h, \end{aligned} \tag{7.30}$$

where h denote the total number of parameters, that is $h = (g-1) + gp + gp(p+1)/2 + 1$, and n is the number of observations. A transform of (7.30) has to be applied to obtain the fitness function. For instance, the transform

$$f(g, \theta) = \exp(-\text{AIC}/c) \tag{7.31}$$

provides us with a real positive objective function to be maximized. The positive real constant c may be included to scale the function values and avoid the possible occurrence of overflows during the calculations.

Genetic algorithms for cluster analysis with unknown number of groups have been introduced in Sects. 7.2.3 (the GCUK algorithm) and 7.2.4 (the GGA algorithm). These GAs aim at estimating simultaneously the number of groups and the group membership. Usually, such algorithms seek for a partition of the observations into a variable number g of groups, and we are allowed to apply genetic algorithms to estimate the parameter vector of the multivariate mixture model when the number of components g is unknown. It suffices to include in the chromosome ζ a sub-string which encodes possible values for the number of clusters by either binary or integer code. Equation (7.31) provides the genetic algorithm with an appropriate fitness function. The problem, however, is rather difficult to handle and we expect to obtain only an approximate solution unless the number of generations N is very large. An alternative is to resort to the hybrid algorithm introduced in Sect. 7.4.2. The performance of the algorithm could be improved further by exploiting not only the individual with the largest fitness function but a subset of the population. For example, from the first 10 best individuals in the final population we may decode 10 estimated parameter vectors to be used as initial values to start some steps of the EM algorithm. This procedure is likely to yield more accurate solutions than using either the genetic algorithm or the EM algorithm alone.

Example 7.4.1.1 Mixture models for Iris Plants and Diabetes data (g unknown)

We consider the Iris plants and Diabetes data sets for checking the capability of hybrid GAs at estimating mixture models if the number of components is unknown. In Table 7.10 the performances of GCUK and GGA when the number of components g is unknown are displayed. The SIC criterion (7.30) has been chosen as objective function rather than the AIC criterion because this latter leads to over-estimate the number of components for the two data sets. The GAs yield a solution that maximizes the fitness function whilst we found that not always the number of components and the starting points provided by such best solution allow the EM algorithm to attain the maximum of the objective function. In some cases the second best GAs solution provided the EM algorithm with starting values that produced a superior performance. For the Iris data, the GGA performs better than the GCUK, which in some instances tends to explore solutions with the wrong number of components. In all cases the best solution provided by the GAs corresponds to the best solution provided by the EM algorithm. For the Diabetes data, the two GAs performs nearly the same. The best solution provided by the GCUK algorithm, if used to initialize the EM algorithm, allows this latter to yield the overall optimal solution. On the contrary, the second best solution from the GGA algorithm is able to provide the EM algorithm with initial values such that the overall optimal solution is attained.

Table 7.10 Mixture models estimation for the Iris and the Diabetes data. The number of components g is unknown. The SIC criterion is assumed as the objective function to be minimized. The GAs, either GCUK or GGA, find proposal g values in the interval $2 \leq g \leq 30$ and provide the EM algorithm with starting points

	Iris data		Diabetes data	
Algorithm	# groups	SIC	# groups	SIC
GCUK (best)	2	600	3	4790
+EM		574		4774
GCUK (2nd best)	3	643	3	4815
+EM		585		4751
GGA (best)	4	564	3	4782
+EM		521		4774
GGA (2nd best)	3	513	3	4809
+EM		506		4751

7.5 Genetic Algorithms in Classification and Regression Trees Models

Classification and regression tree (CART) models have been introduced by Breiman et al. (1984) as a method for predicting continuous dependent variables and categorical predictor variables. The former task refers to the regression framework while the latter regards classification. A Bayesian approach for finding CART models has been suggested by Chipman et al. (1998). The CART method aims at building a binary decision tree by splitting the data set according to the variables that lead to minimization of a heterogeneity criterion. Algorithms that implement the CART method typically generate a sequence of trees, each of which is an extension of the previous tree. To avoid over-fitting due to the presence of large trees a pruning process is adopted for grouping nodes that have been split in previous steps. Such algorithms are expected to produce valuable results with low computational cost if a single variable may explain most of the heterogeneity in the data set. Many variables and large data sets may require instead a heavy computational burden specially if a single variable cannot be found which determines the heterogeneity in the data.

Genetic algorithms have been suggested to deal with the issues related with time consuming computations (Mola and Miele, 2006). Let X be the $n \times p$ data matrix where n observations taken on p variables are stored row-wise and let k denote the number of values for each variable. Then it may be checked easily that the number of possible splits is $2^{k-1} - 1$, a large number even for moderate k. Another problem stems from the fact that past splitting may need revision in the view of an attempt to attain the global optimality of the solution.

We shall summarize the GAs-based procedure for finding the best split for each node of the tree at a given step. Let s be the population size and define s binary chromosomes of length $\ell = kp$. Each chromosome is composed of p fragments of length k and a GA has to be used to locate the point where the variable values interval has to be split according to an optimality criterion. This latter may be assumed in straightforward manner the impurity decrease proposed by Breiman et al. (1984). The genetic operators may be assumed as follows.

- *Selection*. Roulette wheel rule with elitist strategy,
- *Crossover*. Single cutting point crossover,
- *Mutation*. Any bit may flip with pre-specified probability.

This algorithm is to be used as an auxiliary algorithm that operates within a main algorithm that drives the whole procedure for building the sequence of trees.

7.6 Clusters of Time Series and Directional Data

Grouping a set of time series in smaller subsets may provide us with interesting information about the time series structure. Wide application fields and close connection to data mining problems and techniques contributed to the increasing interest on this subject matter. Methods for clustering time series have been developed based on many different time series properties and on several clustering algorithms. Comprehensive accounts may be found in Keogh and Kasetty (2003) and Liao (2005). Wang et al. (2005) made an attempt to select all time series characteristics that are believed to be really important for a reliable and accurate clustering procedure. Meta-heuristic methods for clustering time series have been suggested by Baragona (2001). The time series may be taken to belong to the same subset (cluster) either if they follow similar models, or if they are strongly correlated in some sense. Several measures of similarity (or dissimilarity) have been proposed. For grouping according to similarity in the model, the comparison between model parameters is the most obvious basis for a suitable procedure. If measures of correlation are to be taken into account, then the cross correlation coefficients, possibly computed from the time series model residuals after pre-whitening (see Box et al., 1994) are the most useful tool. It is often useful grouping time series according to time delay or phase difference to check, for instance, if time series are in-phase or out-of-phase with respect to one or more reference series. In this latter case clustering directional data methods have to be considered (Lund, 1999).

7.6.1 GAs-Based Methods for Clustering Time Series Data

Let n time series be available for clustering purpose and let p denote the number of features of interest. Feature extraction may be performed to provide us with the $n \times p$ matrix X where there is a row-wise correspondence to the time series data set. The columns are in correspondence with the extracted features. Then any of the techniques described in Sect. 7.2 may be of use for genetic cluster analysis. For instance, let the model structure similarity be of interest as a criterion for grouping the time series data into clusters. Then for any pair of time series $\{x_{it}, x_{jt}\}$ in a given data set ($t = 1, \ldots, T$) we consider the squared autoregressive distance

$$\hat{d}_{ij}^2 = \sum_{k=1}^{m} \left(\hat{\pi}_{ik} - \hat{\pi}_{jk}\right)^2,$$

where $\{\hat{\pi}_{ik}, \hat{\pi}_{jk}\}$ denote the least squares estimates of the parameters of the autoregressive models of order m (Piccolo, 1990). The model order m has to be pre-specified large enough to take the model dependence structure into account properly.

Finding a partition of a set of time series according to their cross correlations computed after pre-whitening requires a different approach. Such a partition may be useful if we want each cluster to group together time series that may be joint modeled, or share properties of interest, for example correlation with some composite indicator. In this context, we shall define a cluster as a set (group) of time series that satisfy the following condition (Zani, 1983). Given a set of k stationary time series $\{x_1, \ldots, x_k\}$, where $x_i = \left(x_{i,1}, \ldots, x_{i,T}\right)$, $i = 1, \ldots, k$, a subset C which includes k' series ($k' < k$) is said to form a group if, for each of the $k'(k'-1)/2$ cross-correlations $\rho_{i,j}(\tau)$, we have

$$|\rho_{i,j}(\tau)| > c(\alpha) \tag{7.32}$$

for at least a lag τ between $-m$ and m, and $i, j \in C, i \neq j$. A positive integer m has to be pre-specified which denotes the maximum lag. The cross-correlations $\rho_{i,j}(\tau)$ have to be computed from the pre-whitened time series (see, for instance, Brockwell and Davis, 1996, p. 232). If all time series have T as a common number of observations, then choosing, for instance, the significance level $\alpha = 0.05$ gives the figure $c(\alpha) = 1.96/\sqrt{T}$ in (7.32). The previously stated definition does not exclude that a time series may belong to more than a single group. Then there are possibly several allowable partitions to consider, and their number may be very large. This circumstance suggests that the quick partition clustering procedure described in Sect. 7.2.2 could be used. The only features to account for are the definition of a distance and the choice of a suitable fitness function. For any pair of time series (x_i, x_j) let us define the distance $d_{i,j}$ as follows (Bohte et al., 1980)

$$d_{i,j} = \sqrt{\{1 - \rho_{i,j}^2(0)\}/\sum_{\tau=1}^{m} \rho_{i,j}^2(\tau)}. \tag{7.33}$$

We may adopt as objective function to minimize for a good clustering the k-min cluster criterion (Sahni and Gonzalez, 1976)

$$f(C_1, C_2, \ldots, C_g) = \sum_{\omega=1}^{g} \sum_{i,j \in C_\omega, i \neq j} d_{i,j}. \tag{7.34}$$

In this case, the number of clusters g must be supplied for, otherwise, any algorithm which uses (7.34) as objective function is likely to assign each time series a separate cluster, by letting $g = k$ at the end. On the other hand, if g is specified as the maximum allowable number of clusters, then the solution will display exactly g clusters. In order to let the procedure itself determine the number of clusters g, the following objective function may be employed to be maximized

$$f^{+}(C_1, C_2, \ldots, C_g; g) = \sum_{\omega=1}^{g} \sum_{i,j \in C_\omega, i \neq j} d_{i,j}^{+}, \tag{7.35}$$

where $d_{i,j}^{+} = \exp(-d_{i,j})$ and g is assumed unknown. When using (7.35) each cluster has to be a group, according to (7.32), for, otherwise, any algorithm, unless prematurely ended, will put together all time series into a single cluster.

Example 7.3.1.1 The Seven-country data set

Let us consider the seven-country data set referenced in Stock and Watson (2004). The data consist in several quarterly macroeconomic time series from 1969 to 1999 and have been used to compute combination forecasts of output growth. We use here only a part of this data set which covers France, Germany and Italy and only the time series marked 'a' in table Ib in Stock and Watson (2004). The largest time span for which as many as possible time series data are available ranges from the second quarter of 1960 to the fourth quarter of 1999. We transformed the data as suggested in Stock and Watson (2004) and due to this transforms the first data are lost. The remaining data set that we shall examine has starting and ending times the third quarter of 1960 (III/60) and the fourth of 1999 (IV/1999) respectively. As a result the time series in the data set that we shall consider here are $n = 27$ and have $T = 254$ observations each. In Table 7.11 for each time series a label and a short explanation are given, the applied transforms are specified and the countries for which data are available are displayed.

Each time series may be identified by the macroeconomic variable and country. For instance, RBNDL(G) will identify the Germany interest rate of long-term government bonds. There is no known classification for the time series in this data set.

We performed the cluster of this set of time series by using three different methods based on GAs. The first one is the method based on the cross-correlations described in detail in this Sect. 7.6.1. The second one consists in fitting an autoregressive (AR) model of order p to each transformed series and then using the autoregressive coefficients as the features set for each time series (the π-weights). The cluster of time series is performed by clustering the $n \times p$ features data set X. The third method is similar to the second one as for each time series a set of features is extracted on which the clustering procedure is performed. The time delays computed for each time series with respect to a time series in the set considered as a reference series may be used as extracted features (details may be found in Baragona and Carlucci (1997)).

Table 7.11 The quarterly macroeconomic time series labels and preliminary transformations and countries for which data are available (France = F, Germany = G and Italy = I)

Label	Description	Transform	Countries		
CPI	Consumer price index	$\Delta^2 \ln$	F	G	I
IP	Index of industrial production	$\Delta \ln$	F	G	I
PGDP	Gross domestic product deflator	$\Delta^2 \ln$		G	I
RBNDL	Interest rate of long-term government bonds	Δ	F	G	I
RBNDM	Interest rate of medium-term government bonds	Δ			I
RCOMMOD	Real commodity price index	$\Delta \ln$	F	G	I
RGDP	Real gross domestic product	$\Delta \ln$		G	I
ROIL	Real oil prices	$\Delta \ln$	F	G	I
RGOLD	Real gold prices	$\Delta \ln$	F	G	I
RSTOCK	Real stock price index	$\Delta \ln$	F	G	I
UNEMP	Unemployment rate	Δ			I

For all methods the GA parameters have been chosen as follows.

- Population size $s = 50$
- Maximum number of GA iterations $N = 1000$
- Crossover probability $p_c = 0.8$
- Mutation probability $p_m = 0.1$.

The AR order has been $p = 9$ and the correlations have been computed at lags $0, 1, \ldots, 36$ (cross-correlations include negative lags as well).

Cross-correlation-based method. In this case we need a threshold to be pre-specified according to (7.32). As $T = 154$ the threshold to be compared with each cross-correlation absolute value may be computed equal to $c(0.05) = 0.1579$, namely a pair of time series may join the same cluster only if their cross-correlation absolute value exceeds this threshold. The algorithm attains the largest fitness function at iteration 204. $g = 7$ clusters are found. The group membership is displayed in Table 7.12. We may note that the time series form clusters according to the macroeconomic variables rather than countries. This circumstance may suggest that since 1960 the economies of France, Germany and Italy have been interdependent each other. For instance, the consumer price indexes form a single cluster, namely this index is contemporaneously correlated (zero lag) across the three countries. Cluster 2 includes the interest rate of long-term (and in addition medium-term for Italy) government bonds and the real oil prices for the three countries. So these indexes are not only correlated across countries but there is an appreciable correlation between the two macroeconomic variables with a lag of some quarters, the real oil prices leading the interest rate of government bonds. Cluster 3 includes the index of industrial production and the real gross domestic product with largest cross-correlations at lags 0 and 1. This correlation is rather natural and has been detected for the three countries together. The remaining large cluster is cluster 6 that includes the real gold prices and the real stock price indexes whilst this latter variable for France is included in cluster 2. The real gold price lags the real stock price index for about 1 year. The remaining three clusters are small clusters including two time series each.

Table 7.12 Group membership for clusters found by the cross-correlation-based method

Cluster	# Time series	Time series included in the cluster
1	3	RCOMMOD(F), RCOMMOD(G), RCOMMOD(I)
2	8	RBNDL(F), RBNDL(G),RBNDL(I), RBNDM(I), ROIL(F), ROIL(G), ROIL(I), RSTOCK(F)
3	5	IP(F), IP(G), IP(I), RGDP(G), RGDP(I)
4	2	CPI(G), UNEMP(I)
5	2	CPI(F), CPI(I)
6	5	RGOLD(F), RGOLD(G), RGOLD(I) RSTOCK(G), RSTOCK(I)
7	2	PGDP(G), PGDP(I)

Table 7.13 Group membership for clusters found by the π-weights-based method

Cluster	# Time series	Time series included in the cluster
1	8	CPI(G), IP(G), PGDP(G), RGDP(G), RSTOCK(G) CPI(I), PGDP(I), RGDP(I)
2	12	CPI(F), IP(F), RBNDL(F), RSTOCK(F), RBNDL(G), RGOLD(G), IP(I), RBNDL(I), RBNDM(I), RCOMMOD(I), ROIL(I), RSTOCK(I)
3	7	RCOMMOD(F), ROIL(F), RGOLD(F), RCOMMOD(G), ROIL(G), RGOLD(I), UNEMP(I)

π-weights-based method. The clustering performed using the autoregressive coefficients as features representing the time series in the data set yields an optimal partition in $g = 3$ clusters. The time series in the same cluster are supposed to share the behavior and the underlying model structure and are not necessarily highly correlated. In this framework the country seems to have some importance though some time series that correspond to the same macroeconomic variable are included in the same cluster for all countries. The group membership is displayed in Table 7.13. For instance cluster 1 is chiefly composed of time series concerned with Germany. On the other hand, the interest rate of log-term and medium-term government bonds time series are included in the same cluster for all countries in this partition too. Only the real oil price in Italy is included in this cluster, whilst this same macroeconomic variable for France and Germany has a different behavior through time and both are included in the third cluster. The gross domestic product deflator and the real gross domestic product for Germany and Italy are included in the same cluster as for the cross-correlation-based method, but note that the gross domestic product deflator for France is not available.

Time delay-based method. According to this method the features extracted are the time delays of each time series with respect to a reference series. The time delay is a measure in time units (quarters in the present context) of a leading or lagging relationship between two time series. The cross-spectrum is the statistics that has to be estimated to compute the phase and the time delay. If time series x_j leads x_i by 4 time units we may expect for instance that an increase of x_j at time t will be followed by an increase (or decrease, in case of inverse relationship) of x_i at time $t + 4$. The relationship is approximate because we may compute a time delay at each frequency in the interval $(0, \pi)$ and we cannot expect in general that the same time delay will be computed at each frequency. If we assume m the maximum lag, then we may compute the time delay at the discrete set of angular frequencies $\{\pi/m, 2\pi/m, \ldots, (m-1)\pi/m\}$ (unit of radians). A frequency may be better understood if it is translated to the corresponding period. This latter is easier to interpret because it is expressed in time units. The relationship is $P = 2\pi/\omega$, where P is the period in time units and ω the frequency in radians. We may consider some frequencies of special interest only. For this time series data set we assumed $m = 36$ and considered the frequencies $2\pi/36$, $6\pi/36$ and $18\pi/36$, i.e. periods 36, 12 and 4 quarters. We chose these frequencies because the periods are 9 years,

Table 7.14 Group membership for clusters found by the time delay-based method

Cluster	# Time series	Time series included in the cluster
1	13	CPI(F), RSTOCK(F), CPI(G), PGDP(G), RBNDL(G), RGDP(G), RSTOCK(G), IP(I), PGDP(I), RBNDL(I), RCOMMOD(I), RGDP(I), UNEMP(I)
2	7	IP(F), RBNDL(F), RCOMMOD(F), RGOLD(F), RGOLD(G), CPI(I), RGOLD(I)
3	7	ROIL(F), IP(G), RCOMMOD(G), ROIL(G), RBNDM(I), ROIL(I), RSTOCK(I)

3 years and 1 year, to be assumed as long term, medium term and short term. The clustering algorithm has been applied to a data set of $n = 27$ cases (time series) and $p = 3$ variables. The reference series has been computed the interest rate of long-term government bonds for Germany. We obtained the partition in $g = 3$ clusters displayed in Table 7.14. In this case a leading time series may be used to predict the time series in the same cluster or a set of leading time series may be assumed as the basis to define a leading composite index. The cluster 1 includes the reference series and it is supposed to include the time series that leads or lags the reference series within a short time. In cluster 1 the interest rate of long-term government bonds are included for Germany and Italy only, and so the gross domestic product deflator and the real gross domestic product for Germany and Italy. Only two time series for France are present, the consumer price index and the real stock price index, and both are present for Germany too. Cluster 2 includes the real gold prices for all three countries which is found to lead for 7 quarters the reference series at the lowest frequency whilst it is lagging at higher frequencies. In cluster 3 there are the real oil prices for the three countries. In this case too this variable leads at low frequencies while lags at high frequencies the reference series.

In Fig. 7.7 the interest rate of long-term government bonds for the three countries (plus the interest rate of medium-term government bonds for Italy), the consumer price index and the index of industrial production are plotted. The plot shows that the government bonds are strictly related though some lead and lag relationships may occur. The other time series have been found in different clusters using the three methods. The consumer price index shows a peculiar behavior with marked oscillations in the eighties for Italy and in the nineties for France. The index of industrial production for Italy shows marked oscillation at the beginning and at the end of the seventies. This may suggest an explanation for the reason why these time series have been included almost always in different clusters.

7.6.2 GAs-Based Methods for Clustering Directional Data

Let $\{\theta_1, \theta_2, \ldots, \theta_n\}$ be a set of angular measurements in $[0, 2\pi)$, and g the number of clusters. Such directional (or circular) data may be partitioned so that the objective function (Lund, 1999)

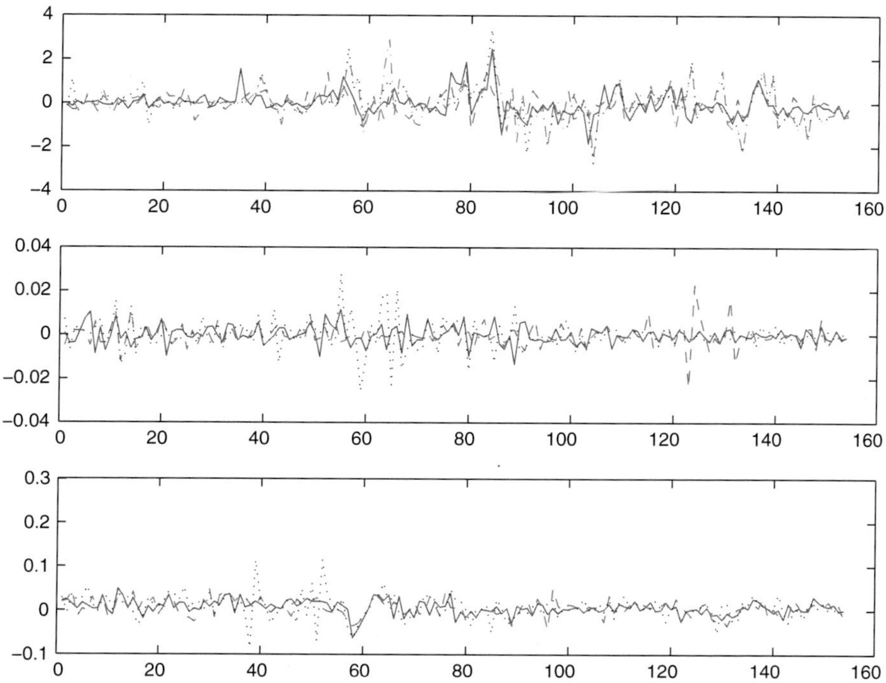

Fig. 7.7 Interest rate of long-term government bonds (*top panel*), consumer price index (*middle panel*) and index of industrial production (*bottom panel*) for France (*solid line*), Germany (*dashed line*) and Italy (*dotted line, dash dotted* for the interest rate of long-term government bonds)

$$S(g) = \sum_{j=1}^{g} (\bar{r}_j - p_j) \tag{7.36}$$

is maximized, where

$$\bar{r}_j = \frac{\sqrt{S_j^2 + C_j^2}}{|J|}, \; S_j = \sum_{i \in J} \sin\theta_i, \; C_j = \sum_{i \in J} \cos\theta_i .$$

$\bar{r}_j \in [0, 1]$ is the mean resultant length of cluster j and decreases as soon as the dispersion of the angular measurements increases. J denotes the set of all indexes of the objects that belong to the cluster j. The p_j's are penalties that have to be introduced as the sum of the $\bar{r}_j$'s increases with g. Clusters of the θ_j's are defined by placing on the unit circle a set of g points that separate the adjacent clusters. Let $m_1, m_2, \ldots m_g$, $0 < m_j < 2\pi$, denote such cut-points. The penalties p_j's are computed

$$p_j = \frac{\sin(\|m_j, m_{j+1}\|/2)}{\|m_j, m_{j+1}\|/2},$$

where $\|m_j, m_{j+1}\| = m_{j+1} - m_j (\text{mod } 2\pi)$ is the amplitude, measured in radians, of the jth cluster. By definition, $m_{g+1} = m_1$.

We shall summarize the GAs-based procedure outlined in Baragona (2003a). Two distinctive features are needed to deal with directional data.

- The cut-points are searched for instead of the cluster centers,
- The statistic (7.36) replaces the Euclidean metric-based fitness function.

The GA-clustering genetic algorithm for directional data performs as follows. Let s denote the population size, p_c and p_m the crossover and mutation probabilities respectively, N the number of iterations and $g_{\max}$ the maximum number of clusters. Let g be a fixed positive integer in the interval $[1, g_{\max}]$. For $i = 1, \ldots, s$, g cut-points are selected in $[0, 2\pi)$. The first cut-point is selected uniformly randomly, while the remaining $g - 1$ are taken equispaced on the unit circle. The s sets of cut-points form the initial population. In each of N iterations the genetic operators selection, crossover and mutation are defined as follows.

- *Selection*. The roulette wheel rule is used for selection with complete replacement of the past population and the correction given by the elitist strategy.
- *Crossover*. The single point crossover is implemented. $\lfloor s/2 \rfloor$ pairs of cut-point sets are formed at random. A pair undergoes the crossover with probability p_c. A positive integer ℓ is generated from the uniform distribution on the interval $[1, g-1]$. The cut-points from $\ell + 1$ to g of the first set replace the corresponding cut-points of the second set and vice versa to yield two new cut-point sets.
- *Mutation*. Any cut-point v in any set is allowed to mutate with probability p_m. A value $v \neq 0$ changes to $v \pm 2\delta v$ while $v = 0$ becomes $\pm 2\delta$. The "+" or "−" sign occurs with equal probability and the real number δ is a fixed pre-specified positive constant which is to be chosen in [0, 1].

This procedure is similar to the procedures described in Sect. 7.2.3. The optimum number of clusters is chosen by replicating the procedure for $g = 1, \ldots, g_{\max}$ and retaining the solution which yields the largest fitness function.

Example 7.6.2.1 Phase-based cluster of the Seven-country data

The procedure described in this Sect. 7.6.2 has been applied to the Seven-country data set. The phase spectrum has been computed for the frequency $2\pi/36$ that corresponds to 9 years. The phase is in radians in the interval $(-\pi, \pi)$ and is an example of directional data. The GA has been used with the following parameters.

- Population size 30
- Maximum number of iterations 1000
- Chromosome length 360
- Probability of crossover 0.08
- Probability of mutation 0.001
- Elitist strategy
- Generational gap 1

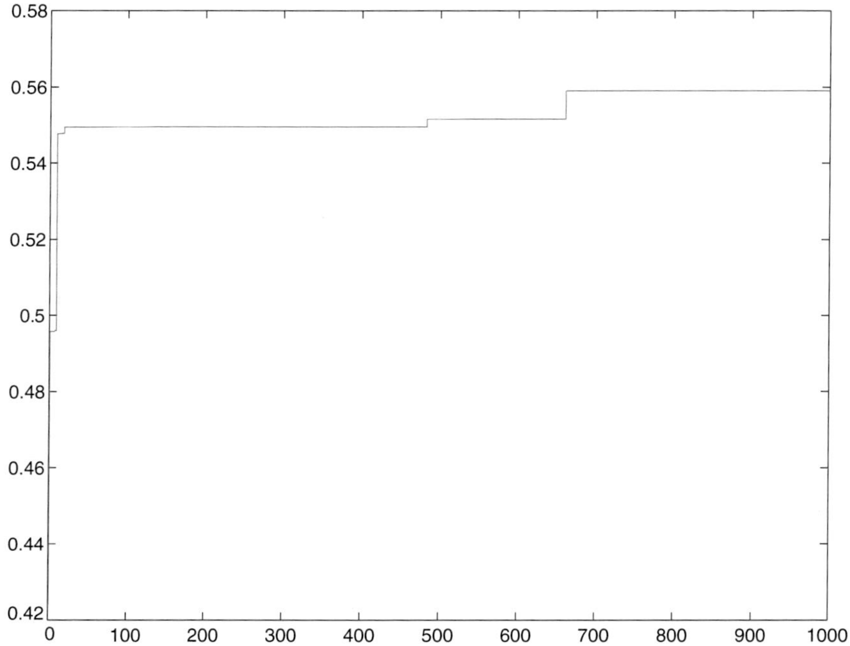

Fig. 7.8 Fitness function for the directional data clustering against the number of iterations

The fitness function values at each iteration are plotted in Fig. 7.8. The usual behavior is displayed, i.e. a steep increase in the first iterations and some improvements in late iterations. The largest fitness function value is attained at iteration 661. The initial value is 0.4240 the largest one 0.5590. The results concerned with the final partition are displayed in Table 7.15. The algorithm finds 4 clusters but two include a time series each while the other time series are included in the remaining two clusters. The largest cluster ranges from 308 to 179° counterclockwise and includes the reference series "interest rate of long-term government bonds" for Germany. The time series included in each of the four clusters are listed in Table 7.16. Most time series are in the same cluster with the reference series. The industrial production index and the real gross domestic product are in-phase for all countries and form the other relevant cluster. The real stock price index is the only variable such

Table 7.15 Cluster structure of the final partition found by the GAs-based algorithm on the phase spectrum computed for the Seven-country data set

Cluster	# Time series	Midpoints (degrees)	Average phase (radians)	Mean resultant (length)	Penalty
1	1	(179, 181)	−3.1343	1.0000	0.9999
2	7	(181, 306)	−1.5282	0.9529	0.8132
3	1	(306, 308)	−.9285	1.0000	0.9999
4	18	(308, 360) +(0, 179)	0.5257	0.8669	0.4477

Table 7.16 Group membership for clusters found by the phase-based method

Cluster	# Time series	Time series included in the cluster
1	1	RSTOCK(G)
2	7	IP(F), IP(G), IP(I), RGDP(G), RGDP(I), RSTOCK(F), UNEMP(I)
3	1	RSTOCK(I)
4	18	CPI(F), CPI(I), CPI(G), PGDP(G), PGDP(I), RBNDL(F), RBNDL(G), RBNDL(I), RBNDM(I), RCOMMOD(F), RCOMMOD(G), RCOMMOD(I), ROIL(F), ROIL(G), ROIL(I), RGOLD(F), RGOLD(G), RGOLD(I)

that the corresponding time series are not in-phase across the three countries. The real stock price index for France is in the same cluster with the industrial production index and the real gross domestic product of the three countries while the real stock price index for Germany and Italy each forms a separate cluster.

7.7 Multiobjective Genetic Clustering

We have considered in general clusters of objects as the result of some optimization algorithm. Several indexes of internal cluster validity are available to provide the algorithm with a convenient objective function. Though sometimes the results do not depend on the particular criterion, more often different criteria lead to different partitions. As a matter of fact, any criterion produces an optimal partition according to some special cluster property, for instance compactness, connectedness or spatial separation. The multiobjective clustering encompasses the limitation inherent to the single objective optimization algorithms by using many optimality criteria simultaneously. The GAs are so often used as the underlying search technique in multiobjective clustering chiefly because in a single iteration a population of partitions is considered instead of a single one. This circumstance allows the concept of Pareto optimality to be fully exploited in a multiobjective clustering algorithm design. Deb (2001), Coello Coello et al. (2002) and Handl and Knowles (2007) developed multiobjective clustering methods while utilizing the search capability of GAs. A new model of multiobjective simulated annealing algorithm called AMOSA (Bandyopadhyay et al., 2008) has been developed as well. Also fuzzy clusters have been considered in the multiobjective optimization framework (Deb, 2001). An algorithm that performs the multiobjective genetic fuzzy clustering for a special application may be found in Bandyopadhyay et al. (2007).

7.7.1 *Pareto Optimality*

The multiobjective optimization problem in a clustering context consists in finding a partition $C = \{C_1, \ldots, C_g\}$ that simultaneously optimizes the m objective functions

$$\{f_1(C), f_2(C), \ldots, f_m(C)\}.$$

Constraints may be possibly imposed on the partitions set which define the feasible region F which contains all the admissible solutions. Any solution outside this region is inadmissible since it violates one or more constraints. C denotes an optimal solution in F. In this framework a convenient definition of optimality is difficult to be delivered since it happens seldom that a unique partition C represents the optimum solution to all the m objective functions.

Most multiobjective optimization techniques use the concepts of dominance relation and Pareto optimality. Let all objective functions have to be maximized. Then a solution $C^{(i)}$ is said to dominate $C^{(j)}$ if

$$\forall k \in \{1, 2, \ldots, m\} \quad f_k(C^{(i)}) \geq f_k(C^{(j)})$$

and

$$\exists k \in \{1, 2, \ldots, m\} \quad \text{such that } f_k(C^{(i)}) > f_k(C^{(j)}).$$

Among a set of solutions P, the non-dominated set of solutions P' are those that are not dominated by any member of the set P. A solution C is said to be non-dominated in P if there exist no solution C^* which dominates C. The non-dominated set of the entire search space F is the globally Pareto optimal set. The globally Pareto optimal set is often simply referred to as the Pareto optimal set. The image of the globally Pareto optimal set in the objective space is known as the Pareto front.

7.7.2 Multiobjective Genetic Clustering Outline

We present a genetic algorithm that produces a partition optimal with respect to m objective functions. For example we may assume the DB index and the VRC criterion as two objective functions to be optimized simultaneously. The algorithm encodes the partitions in the chromosome ξ as cluster centers. The different steps of the algorithm are as follows.

1. The population P at each generation is split into a set of non-dominated solutions P' and a set of dominated solutions P''. The former (P') are set apart and are evaluated for entering the new generation as in the ordinary elitist strategy.
2. At the end of the iterative procedure the best solution is searched for only within the current set P'.
3. The assignment of objects to clusters is done by taking the m criteria into account simultaneously. A 'voting' mechanism may be adopted that assigns an item to the cluster to which it is assigned by the majority of the criteria. As an alternative, an 'amount of dominance' may be defined by assuming an overall fitness as the sum of the fitnesses computed for each objective. In this latter case the m fitness functions are conveniently normalized in such a way that this comparison is meaningful.

The algorithm replicates these steps for a pre-specified number N of iterations.

7.7.2.1 String Representation and Population Initialization

We assume that the number of clusters is known *a priori* and is equal to g. Each chromosome ξ in the population represents a collection of the centers to which the objects are to be aggregated to form each cluster.

Let s denote the population size and assume that p measurements are available for each object. We use the real encoding, so a chromosome ξ_j, $j \in \{1, 2, \ldots, s\}$, is a row vector of length $\ell = p \times g$. The first g entries are the coordinates of the first center, the entries from $g+1$ to $2g$ are the coordinates of the second center and so on. Then m initial populations are generated at random, one for each criterion. Consider the criterion i , $i \in \{1, 2, \ldots, m\}$. Within each population the fitness function is evaluated so that the values $\{f_{i,j}\}$, $i \in \{1, 2, \ldots, m\}$ and $j \in \{1, 2, \ldots, s\}$, may be computed.

7.7.2.2 Genetic Operators

The genetic operators may be described as follows.

1. *Selection*. According to the fitness function values the set of non-dominated solutions P' is set apart while the roulette wheel selection is performed as usual within the whole population P. If a generational gap G $(0 < G < 1)$ is assumed, $G \times s$ chromosomes are replaced in P by the selected solutions, otherwise P is entirely replaced by the selected chromosomes.
2. *Pareto optimality elitist strategy*. The new set P is augmented with the set P' of non-dominated solutions found in the past generation and non-dominated solutions are selected within the set $P \cup P'$. If the selected solutions exceed s, then the best s form the next generation, otherwise non-dominated solutions are added to yield all s chromosomes needed for complete replacement.
3. *Crossover*. The single point crossover may be used with a pre-specified crossover probability p_c. The cutting point t is selected in the interval $[1, \ell - 1]$ in such a way that the exchange regards only complete sets of center coordinates. In practice a uniform random number u is chosen in $[1, g - 1]$ and the cutting point is $t = u \times p$. The genes from $t + 1$ to ℓ of the first chromosome are replaced by the corresponding genes of the second one, and vice versa.
4. *Mutation*. Any gene may mutate with pre-specified probability p_m. The floating point mutation has to be used. A uniform random number δ is generated. Let v denote the value of a gene. After mutation the gene value becomes $v = v \pm 2\delta v$ if $v \neq 0$ and $v = v \pm 2\delta$ if $v = 0$. The positive or negative sign occurs with equal probability.

The assignment of objects to clusters is finally done along the guidelines previously outlined. Note that though the number of clusters g is pre-specified, the assignment process may leave some cluster empty. In this case the overall solution includes less than g clusters.

References

Abonyi J, Balasko B, Feil B (2005) Fuzzy clustering and data analysis toolbox. http://www.fmt.vein.hu/softcomp/fclusttoolbox. Accessed 21 Nov 2010

Akaike H (1974) A new look at the statistical identification model. IEEE Trans Autom Control 19:716–723

Akaike H (1977) An entropy maximisation principle. In: Krishnaiah PR (ed) Proceedings of the symposium on applied statistics. North-Holland, Amsterdam, pp 27–41

Alander JT (1992) On optimal population size of genetic algorithms. In: Proceedings of the CompEuro92. IEEE Computer Society Press, Washington, pp 65–70

Andrews DF, Pregibon D (1978) Finding the outliers that matter. J R Stat Soc B 40:85–93

Apolloni B, Bassis S, Marinaro M (2009) New directions in neural networks. IOS Press, The Netherlands

Asuncion A, Newman D (2007) UCI machine learning repository. http://archive.ics.uci.edu/ml. Accessed 21 Nov 2010

Atkinson A, Donev A, Tobias R (2007) Optimum experimental designs, with SAS. Oxford University Press, Oxford

Atkinson AC, Riani M (2000) Robust diagnostic regression analysis. Springer, New York, NY

Atkinson AC, Riani M (2002) Forward search added-variable t-tests and the effect of masked outliers in model selection. Biometrika 89:939–946

Aytug H, Koehler GJ (2000) New stopping criterion for genetic algorithms. Eur J Oper Res 126:662–674

Back T (1996) Evolutionary algorithms in theory and practice. Oxford University Press, Oxford

Bailey R (2008) Design of comparative experiments. Cambridge University Press, Cambridge

Balcombe K (2005) Model selection using information criteria and genetic algorithms. Comput Econ 25:207–228

Baldi Antognini A, Giovagnoli A, Romano D, Zagoraiou M (2009) Computer simulations for the optimization of technological processes. In: Erto P (ed) Statistics for innovation. Springer, Milan, pp 65–88

Bandyopadhyay S, Maulik U (2002) Genetic clustering for automatic evolution of clusters and application to image classification. Pattern Recognit 35:1197–1208

Bandyopadhyay S, Maulik U, Mukhopadhyay A (2007) Multiobjective genetic clustering for pixel classification in remote sensing imagery. IEEE Trans Geosci Remote Sens 45:1506–1511

Bandyopadhyay S, Saha S, Maulik U, Deb K (2008) A simulated annealing based multi-objective optimization algorithm: AMOSA. IEEE Trans Evol Comput 12:269–283

Banfield JD, Raftery A (1993) Model-based gaussian and non-gaussian clustering. Biometrics 49:803–821

Baragona R (2001) A simulation study on clustering time series with metaheuristic methods. Quad Stat 3:1–26

Baragona R (2003a) Further results on Lund's statistic for identifying cluster in a circular data set with application to time series. Commun Stat Simul Comput 32:943–952

DOI 10.1007/978-3-642-16218-3,

Baragona R (2003b) General local search methods in time series, contributed paper at the international workshop on computational management science, economics, finance and engineering, Limassol, Cyprus

Baragona R, Battaglia F (1995) Linear interpolators and the inverse correlation function of non stationary time series. J Time Ser Anal 16:531–538

Baragona R, Battaglia F (2003) Multivariate mixture models estimation: a genetic algorithm approach. In: Schader M, Gaul W, Vichi M (eds) Between data science and applied data analysis. Springer, Berlin, pp 133–142

Baragona R, Battaglia F (2007) Outliers detection in multivariate time series by independent component analysis. Neural Comput 19:1962–1984

Baragona R, Battaglia F, Calzini C (2001a) Genetic algorithms for the identification of additive and innovation outliers in time series. Comput Stat Data Anal 37:1–12

Baragona R, Battaglia F, Cucina D (2002) A note on estimating autoregressive exponential models. Quad Stat 4:71–88

Baragona R, Battaglia F, Cucina D (2004a) Estimating threshold subset autoregressive moving-average models by genetic algorithms. Metron 62:39–61

Baragona R, Battaglia F, Cucina D (2004b) Fitting piecewise linear threshold autoregressive models by means of genetic algorithms. Comput Stat Data Anal 47:277–295

Baragona R, Calzini C, Battaglia F (2001b) Genetic algorithms and clustering: an application to Fisher's iris data. In: Borra S, Rocci R, Vichi M, Schader M (eds) Advances in classification and data analysis. Springer, Heidelberg, pp 109–118

Baragona R, Carlucci F (1997) An optimality criterion for aggregating a set of time series in a composite index. J Time Ser Anal 18:1–9

Baragona R, Cucina D (2008) Double threshold autoregressive conditionally heteroscedastic model building by genetic algorithms. J Stat Comput Simul 78:541–558

Barnett V, Lewis T (1994) Outliers in statistical data, 3rd edn. Wiley, Chichester

Battaglia F (1984) Inverse covariances of a multivariate time series. Metron 42:117–129

Battaglia F (1988a) Bilateral autoregressive models for data validation in time series. Metron 46:275–286, invited lecture given at the 17th Conference on stochastic processes and their applications held in Rome, June 27th–July 1st, 1988

Battaglia F (1988b) On the estimation of the inverse correlation function. J Time Ser Anal 9:1–10

Battaglia F (2001) Genetic algorithms, pseudo-random numbers generators, and markov chain monte carlo methods. Metron 59(1–2):131–155

Battaglia F (2005) Outliers in functional autoregressive time series. Stat Probab Lett 72:323–332

Battaglia F (2006) Bias correction for outlier estimation in time series. J Stat Plan Inference 136:3904–3930

Battaglia F, Baragona R (1992) Linear interpolators and the outlier problem in time series. Metron 50:79–97

Battaglia F, Orfei L (2005) Outlier detection and estimation in non linear time series. J Time Ser Anal 26:107–121

Bedau M, Buchanan A, Gazzola G, Hanczyc M, McCaskill J, Poli I, Packard N (2005) Evolutionary design of a ddpd model of ligation. In: Proceedings of the 7th international conference on artificial evolution EA'05 (Lecture notes in computer science), Lille, France, vol 3871, pp 201–212

Bell AJ, Sejnowski TJ (1995) An information – maximization approach to blind separation and blind deconvolution. Neural Comput 7:1129–1159

Bensmail H, Celeux G, Raftery AE, Robert C (1997) Inference in model-based cluster analysis. Stat Comput 7:1–10

Berkhin P (2002) Survey of clustering data mining techniques. Technical report, Accrue Software, San Jose, CA. http://www.cs.iastate.edu/~honavar/clustering-survey.pdf. Accessed 21 Nov 2010

Beyer HG, Schwefel H (2002) Evolution strategies, a comprehensive introduction. Natural Comput 1:3–52

Bezdek JC (1981) Pattern recognition with Fuzzy objective function algorithms. Plenum, New York, NY

Bezdek JC, Pal NR (1998) Some new indexes of cluster validity. IEEE Trans Syst, Man Cybern B: Cybern 28:301–315

Bhansali RJ (1990) On a relationship between the inverse of a stationary covariance matrix and the linear interpolator. J Appl Probab 27:156–170

Blum C, Roli A (2003) Metaheuristics in combinatorial optimization: overview and conceptual comparison. ACM Comput Surv 35(3):268–308

Bohte Z, Cepar D, Košmelj K (1980) Clustering of time series. In: COMPSTAT 1980. Physica-Verlag, Heidelberg, Germany, pp 587–593

Boley D (1998) Principal direction divisive partitioning. Data Min Knowl Discov 2:325–344

Borgelt C, Kruse R (2002) Graphical models: methods for data analysis and mining. Wiley, New York, NY

Borrotti M, De Lucrezia D, Minervini G (2009) Evolutionary experimental design for synthetic protein. Working paper 24, European centre for living technology, Venice, Italy, 2nd workshop of the ERCIM working group on computing & statistics, Limassol, Cyprus

Box GEP (1957) Evolutionary operation: a method for increasing industrial productivity. Appl Stat 6:81–101

Box GEP, Jenkins GM (1976) Time series analysis: forecasting and control, 2nd edn. Holden-Day, San Francisco, CA

Box GEP, Jenkins GM, Reinsel GC (1994) Time series analysis: forecasting and control, 3rd edn. Prentice Hall, Englewood Cliffs, NJ

Bozdogan H (1988) Icomp: a new model-selection criterion. In: Bock HH (ed) Classification and related methods of data analysis. Elsevier (North Holland), Amsterdam, pp 599–608

Bozdogan H, Bearse P (2003) Information complexity criteria for detecting influential observations in dynamic multivariate linear models using the genetic algorithm. J Stat Plan Inference 114:31–44

Bradley AP (1997) The use of the area under the ROC curve in the evaluation of machine learning algorithms. Pattern Recognit 30:1145–1159

Breiman L, Friedman J, Olshen R, Stone C (1984) Classification and regression trees. Wadsworth, Belmont, CA

Bremer RH, Langevin GJ (1993) The genetic algorithm for identifying the structure of a mixed model. In: ASA proceedings of the statistical computing section. American Statistical Association, Alexandria, pp 80–85

Brockwell PJ, Davis RA (1996) Introduction to time series and forecasting. Springer, New York, NY

Brooks SP, Morgan BJT (1995) Optimization using simulated annealing. Statistician 44:241–257

Bruce AG, Martin RD (1989) Leave-k-out diagnostics for time series (with discussion). J R Stat Soc B 51:363–424

Cai Z, Fan J, Yao Q (2000) Functional-coefficient regression models for nonlinear time series. J Am Stat Assoc 95:941–956

Calinski T, Harabasz J (1974) A dendrite method for cluster analysis. Commun Stat 3:1–27

Cardoso JF, Souloumiac A (1993) Blind beamforming for non Gaussian signals. IEE Proc F 140:362–370

Cawse J (2003) Experimental design for combinatorial and high throughput material developments. Springer, New York, NY

Chang I, Tiao GC, Chen C (1988) Estimation of time series parameters in the presence of outliers. Technometrics 30:193–204

Chan WS, Wei W (1992) A comparison of some estimators of time series autocorrelations. Comput Stat Data Anal 14:149–163

Chatterjee S, Laudato M (1997) Genetic algorithms in statistics: procedures and applications. Commun Stat Theory Methods 26(4):1617–1630

Chatterjee S, Laudato M, Lynch LA (1996) Genetic algorithms and their statistical applications: an introduction. Comput Stat Data Anal 22:633–651

Chen C (1997) Detection of additive outliers in bilinear time series. Comput Stat Data Anal 24:283–294

Chen C, Liu LM (1993) Joint estimation of model parameters and outlier effects in time series. J Am Stat Assoc 88:284–297

Chen CWS, Cherng TH, Wu B (2001) On the selection of subset bilinear time series models: a genetic algorithm approach. Comput Stat 16:505–517

Chen R, Tsay RS (1993) Functional-coefficient autoregressive models. J Am Stat Assoc 88: 298–308

Chiodi M (1986) Procedures for generating pseudo-random numbers from a normal distribution of order p ($p > 1$). Stat Appl 1:7–26

Chiogna M, Gaetan C, Masarotto G (2008) Automatic identification of seasonal transfer function models by means of iterative stepwise and genetic algorithms. J Time Ser Anal 29:37–50

Chipman HA, George EI, McCulloch RE (1998) Bayesian cart model search. J Am Stat Assoc Theory Methods 93:935–948

Choi KS, Moon BR (2007) Feature selection in genetic fuzzy discretization for the pattern classification problem. IEICE Trans Inf Syst E90-D:1047–1054

Choy K (2001) Outlier detection for stationary time series. J Stat Plan Inference 99:111–127

Cleveland WS (1972) The inverse autocorrelations of a time series and their applications. Technometrics 14:277–298

Coello Coello CA, Van Veldhuizen DA, Lamont GB (2002) Evolutionary Algorithms for solving multi-objective problems. Kluwer, Norwell, MA

Cook RD, Weisberg S (1982) Residuals and influence in regression. Chapman and Hall, London

Cornell J (2002) Experiments with mixtures: designs, models, and the analysis of mixture data. Wiley, New York, NY

Cowell R, Dawid A, Lauritzen S, Spiegelhalter D (1999) Probabilistic networks and expert systems. Springer, New York, NY

Cox D (1953) Planning of experiments. Wiley, New York, NY

Cox D, Reid N (2000) The theory of the design of experiments. Chapman & Hall, London

Crawford KD, Wainwright RL (1995) Applying genetic algorithms to outlier detection. In: Eshelman LJ (ed) Proceedings of the 6th international conference on genetic algorithms. Morgan Kaufmann, San Mateo, CA, pp 546–550

Crawford KD, Wainwright RL, Vasicek DJ (1995) Detecting multiple outliers in regression data using genetic algorithms. In: Proceedings of the 1995 ACM/SIGAPP symposium on applied computing. 26–28 Feb 1995, ACM Press, Nashville, TN, pp 351–356

Darwiche A (2009) Modeling and reasoning with Bayesian networks. Cambridge University Press, Cambridge

Dasgupta A, Raftery AE (1998) Detecting features in spatial point processes with clutter via model-based clsutering. J Am Stat Assoc 93:294–302

Davies DL, Bouldin DW (1979) A cluster separation measure. IEEE Trans Pattern Anal Mach Intell 1:224–227

Davis L (1985) Applying adaptive algorithms to epistatic domains. In: Proceedings of the 9-th international joint conference on artificial intelligence, Morgan Kaufman San Francisco, pp 162–164

Davis LD (1991) Handbook of genetic algorithms. Van Nostrand, New York, NY

Davis R, Lee T, Rodriguez-Yam G (2006) Structural break estimation for nonstationary time series models. J Am Stat Assoc 101:223–239

Davis R, Lee T, Rodriguez-Yam G (2008) Break detection for a class of nonlinear time series models. J Time Ser Anal 29:834–867

Davis TE, Principe JC (1993) A markov chain framework for the simple genetic algorithm. Evol Comput 1(3):269–288

De Jong K (2006) Evolutionary computation. The MIT Press, Cambridge

De Jong KA (1975) An analysis of the behavior of a class of genetic adaptive systems. PH.D. thesis, Department of Computer and Communication Sciences, University of Michigan, Ann Arbor, MI

De Jong KA (1993) Genetic algorithms are not function optimizers. In: Whitley D (ed) Foundations of genetic algorithms 2. Morgan Kaufman, San Mateo, CA, pp 1–18

De March D, Forlin M, Slanzi D, Poli I (2009a) An evolutionary predictive approach to design high dimensional experiments. In: Serra R, Poli I, Villani M (eds) Artificial life and evolutionary computation: proceedings of WIVACE 2008. World Scientific Publishing Company, Singapore, pp 81–88

De March D, Slanzi D, Poli I (2009b) Evolutionary algorithms for complex experimental designs. In: Ermakov S, Melas V, Pepelyshev A (eds) Simulation, St. Petersburg VVM com., St. Petersburg, Russia, pp 547–552

Dean A, Voss D (1999) Design and analysis of experiments. Springer, New York, NY

Deb K (2001) Multi-objective optimization using evolutionary algorithms. Wiley, New York, NY

Delgado A, Prat A (1997) Modeling time series using a hybrid system: neural networks and genetic algorithm. In: Bellacicco A, Lauro NC (eds) Reti neurali e statistica. Franco Angeli, Milan, pp 77–88

Demsar J, Zupan B, Leban G (2004) Orange: from experimental machine learning to interactive data mining, white paper. www.ailab.si/orange. Accessed 21 Nov 2010

Donoho D, Johnston I (1994) Ideal spatial adaptation by wavelet shrinkage. Biometrika 81: 425–455

Dorigo M (1992) Optimization, learning and natural algorithms. Ph.D. thesis, Politecnico di Milano, Italy

Dorigo M, Gambardella M (1997) Ant colony system: a cooperative learning approach to the traveling salesman problem. IEEE Trans Evol Compu 1(1):53–66

Dorigo M, Stützle T (2004) Ant colony optimization. MIT Press, Cambridge

Drugan M, Thierens D (2004) Evolutionary markov chain monte carlo. In: Liardet P (ed) Proceedings of the 6th International Conference on Artificial evolution - EA 2003. Springer, Berlin, pp 63–76

Dunn JC (1974) Well separated clusters and optimal fuzzy-partitions. J Cybern 4:95–104

Edwards W, Cavalli-Sforza L (1965) A method of cluster analysis. Biometrics 21:362–375

Falkenauer E (1998) Genetic algorithms and grouping problems. Wiley, Chichester

Fan J, Li R (2006) Statistical challenges with high dimensionality: feature selection in knowledge discovery. In: Proceedings of the international congress of mathematicians, Madrid, Spain

Fan K, Lin D, Winker P, Zhang Y (2000) Uniform design: theory and application. Technometrics 42(3):237–248

Ferligoj A, Batagelj V (1992) Direct multicriteria clustering algorithms. J Classification 9:43–61

Fisher R (1935) The design of experiments. Oliver & Boyd, Edinburgh

Fitzenberger B, Winker P (1998) Threshold accepting to improve the computation of censored quantile regression. In: Paynem R, Green P (eds) COMPSTAT, proceedings in computational statistics. Physica-Verlag, Heidelberg, pp 311–316

Fogel DB (1998) Evolutionary computation: toward a new philosophy of machine intelligence. IEEE Press, New York, NY

Fogel LJ, Owens AJ, Walsh MJ (1966) Artificial intelligence through simulated evolution. Wiley, New York, NY

Forlin M (2009) A model-based evolutionary approach to high dimensional experimentation. In: Mola F, Conversano C, Vinzi V, Fisher N (eds) European regional meeting of the international society for business and industrial statistics - EURISBIS'09, Cagliari, Italy, TAPILA editore, pp 120–121

Forlin M, De March D, Poli I (2007) The model-based genetic algorithms for designing mixture experiments. Working paper 18, European centre for living technology, Venice

Forlin M, Poli I, De March D, Packard N, Gazzola G, Serra R (2008) Evolutionary experiments for self-assembling amphiphilic systems. Chemom Intell Lab Syst 90(2):153–160

Fox AJ (1972) Outliers in time series. J R Stat Soc B 43:350–363
Friedman HP, Rubin J (1967) On some invariant criteria for grouping data. J Am Stat Assoc 62:1159–1178
Friedman J (1987) Exploratory projection pursuit. J Am Stat Assoc 82:249–266
Gaetan C (2000) Subset arma model identification using genetic algorithms. J Time Ser Anal 21:559–570
Galeano P, Peña D, Tsay RS (2006) Outlier detection in multivariate time series by projection pursuit. J Am Stat Assoc 101:654–669
Gao Y (2003) Population size and sampling complexity in genetic algorithms. GECCO 2003 Workshop on Learning, Adaptation, and Approximation in Evolutionary Computation, 2003, Springer, Berlin Heidelberg, pp 178–181
Geyer CJ (1991) Markov chain monte carlo maximum likelihood. In: Keramidas EM (ed) Computing science and statistics, Proceedings of the 23rd Symposium on the interface, interface foundation, Fairfax Station, VA, pp 156–163
Ghaddar DK, Tong H (1981) Data transformation and self-exciting threshold autoregression. Appl Stat 30:238–248
Gilks WR, Richardson R, Spiegelhalter DJ (1996) Markov chain monte carlo in practice. Chapman and Hall/CRC, London
Glendinning RH (2000) Estimating the inverse autocorrelation function from outlier contaminated data. Comput Stat 15:541–565
Goldberg DE (1989a) Genetic algorithms in search, optimization and machine learning. Addison-Wesley, Reading, MA
Goldberg DE (1989b) Genetic algorithms in search, optimization and machine learning. Addison-Wesley, Reading, MA
Goldberg DE (1989c) Sizing populations for serial and parallel genetic algorithms. In: Schafer JD (ed) Proceedings of the 3rd conference on genetic algorithms. Morgan Kaufmann, San Mateo, CA
Goldberg DE, Deb KE, Clark JH (1992) Genetic algorithms, noise and the sizing of populations. Complex Syst 6:333–362
Goldberg DE, Lingle R (1985) Alleles, loci and the travelling salesman problem. In: Grefenstette JJ (ed) Proceedings of an international conference on genetic algorithms and their applications. Lawrence Erlbaum Associates, Hillsdale, NJ, pp 154–159
Gordon AD (1981) Classification. Chapman and Hall, London
Gorriz JM, Puntonet CG, Gomez AM, Pernia O (2005) Guided GA-ICA algorithms. In: Wang J, Liao X, Yi Z (eds) ISNN 2005, LNCS 3496. Springer, Berlin Heidelberg, pp 943–948
Goswami G, Liu JS (2007) On learning strategies for evolutionary monte carlo. Stat Comput 17:23–38
Gounder MK, Shitan M, Imon R (2007) Detection of outliers in non-linear time series: A review. In: Festschrift in honor of distinguished professor Mir Masoom Ali on the occasion of his retirement. 18–19, May 2007, Ball State University, Muncie, IN, USA, pp 213–224
Gower JC, Ross GJS (1969) Minimum spanning trees and single linkage cluster analysis. Appl Stat 18:54–64
Granger C, Andresen A (1978) Introduction to bilinear time series models. Vandenbroek and Ruprecht, Göttingen
Greenshtein E (2006) Best subset selection, persistence in high-dimensional statistical learning and optimization under l_1 constraint. Ann Stat 34(5):2367–2386
Greenshtein E, Ritov Y (2004) Persistency in high dimensional linear predictor-selection and the virtue of over-parametrization. Bernoulli 10:971–988
Grefenstette JJ (1986) Optimization of control parameters for genetic algorithms. IEEE Trans Syst Man Cybern 16(1):122–128
Grenander U, Rosenblatt M (1957) Statistical analysis of stationary time series. Wiley, New York, NY

Guo Q, Wu W, Massart DL, Boucon C, de Jong S (2002) Feature selection in principal component analysis of analytical data. Chemom Intell Lab Syst 61:123–132

Haggan V, Ozaki T (1981) Modelling nonlinear random vibrations using an amplitude-dependent autoregressive time series model. Biometrika 68:189–196

Handl J, Knowles J (2007) An evolutionary approach to multiobjective clustering. IEEE Trans Evol Comput 11:56–76

Hannan EJ, Rissanen J (1982) Recursive estimation of mixed autoregressive moving average order. Biometrika 69:81–94

Hartigan J (1975) Clustering algorithms. Wiley, New York, NY

Hartigan J, Wong M (1979) Algorithm as136: a k-means clustering algorithm. Appl Stat 28: 100–108

Heckerman D, Geiger D, Chickering D (1995) Learning bayesian networks: the combinations of knowledge and statistical data. Mach Learn 20:197–243

Heredia-Langner A, Carlyle W, Montgomery D, Borror C, Runger G (2003) Genetic algorithms for the construction of d-optimal designs. J Qual Technol 35(1):28–46

Hettich S, Bay SD (1999) The UCI KDD archive. http://kdd.ics.uci.edu. Accessed 25 Jul 2009

Holland JH (1975) Adaptation in natural and artificial systems. University of Michigan Press, Ann Arbor, MI

Holmes CC, Mallick BK (1998) Parallel markov chain monte carlo sampling. mimeo, Department of Mathematics, Imperial College, London

Hoppner F, Klawonn F, Kruse R, Runkler T (1999) Fuzzy cluster analysis: methods for classification, data analysis and image recognition. Wiley, Chichester

Hornik K (1993) Some new results on neural network approximation. Neural Netw 6:1069–1072

Hornik K, Leisch F (2001) Neural networks models. In: Peña D, Tiao GC, Tsay RS (eds) A course in time series analysis. Wiley, Hoboken, New Jersey, NJ, pp 348–362

Hosmer D, Lemeshow S (1989) Applied logistic regression. Wiley, New York, NY

Huber PJ (1981) Robust statistics. Wiley, New York, NY

Huber PJ (1985) Projection pursuit. Ann Stat 13:435–475

Hubert L, Arabie P (1985) Comparing partitions. J Classif 2:193–218

Hyvärinen A, Karhunen J, Oja E (2001) Independent component analysis. Wiley, New York, NY

Hyvarinen A, Oja E (2000) Independent component analysis: algorithms and applications. Neural Netw 13:411–430

ISTAT (2008) Italian statistical yearbook. Rome, Italy

Jaccard P (1901) Distribution de la florine alpine dans la bassin de dranses et dans quelques regiones voisines. Bull Soc Vaud Sci Nat 37:241–272

Jensen F (2001) Bayesian networks and decision graphs. Springer, New York, NY

Jones DR, Beltramo MA (1991) Solving partitioning problems with genetic algorithms. In: Belew RK, Booker LB (eds) Proceedings of the 4th international conference on genetic algorithms. Morgan Kaufmann, San Mateo, CA, pp 442–449

Kapetanios G (2007) Variable selection in regression models using nonstandard optimisation of information criteria. Comput Stat Data Anal 52:4–15

Kargupta H, Deb K, Goldberg DE (1992) Ordering genetic algorithms and deception. In: Männer R, Manderick B (eds) Parallel problem solving from nature, vol 2. Elsevier, Amsterdam, pp 47–56

Kaufman L, Rousseeuw PJ (2005) Finding groups in data. Wiley, Hoboken, NJ

Kemsley EK (1998) A genetic algorithm approach to the calculation of canonical variates. Trends Anal Chem 17:24–34

Kemsley EK (2001) A hybrid classification method: discrete canonical variate analysis using a genetic algorithm. Chemom Intell Lab Syst 55:39–55

Kennedy J, Eberhart R (1995) Particle swarm optimization. In: Proceedings of the IEEE Conference on neural networks, Piscataway, NJ, pp 1942–48

Kennedy J, Eberhart R (2001) Swarm intelligence. Morgan Kaufmann, San Mateo, CA

Keogh E, Kasetty S (2003) On the need for time series data mining benchmarks: a survey and empirical demonstration. Data Min Knowl Discov 7:349–371

Kim Hj, Shin Ks (2007) A hybrid approach based on neural networks and genetic algorithms for detecting temporal patterns in stock markets. Appl Soft Comput 7:569–576
Koehler AB, Murphree ES (1988) A comparison of the Akaike and Schwarz criteria for selecting model order. Appl Stat 37:187–195
Kohn R, Ansley CF (1983) Fixed interval estimation in state space models when some of the data are missing or aggregated. Biometrika 70:683–688
Koza JR (1992) Genetic programming: on the programming of computers by means of natural selection. MIT Press, Cambridge
Lance GN, Williams WT (1967) A general theory of classificatory sorting strategies: I. hierarchical systems. Comput J 9:373–380
Larrañaga P, Lozano JA (2002) Estimation of distribution algorithms: a new tool for evolutionary optimization. Kluwer, Boston, MA
Lauritzen SL (1996) Graphical models. Oxford University Press, Oxford
Lazic Z (2004) Design of experiments in chemical engineering. Wiley-VCH, Weinheim, Germany
Li CW, Li WK (1996) On a double-threshold autoregressive heteroscedastic time series model. J Appl Econ 11:253–274
Liang F, Wong WH (2000) Evolutionary monte carlo: applications to c_p model sampling and change point problem. Stat Sinica 10(2):317–342
Liang F, Wong WH (2001) Real-parameter evolutionary monte carlo with applications to bayesian mixture models. J Am Stat Assoc 96(454):653–666
Liao TW (2005) Clustering of time series data – a survey. Pattern Recognit 38:1857–1874
Liu GL (1968) Introduction to combinatorial mathemathics. McGraw Hill, New York
Liu LM, Hudak T (1992) Forecasting and time series analysis using the sca statistical system. Technical report, Scientific Computing Associates, DeKalb, IL
Lozano JA, Larrañaga P, Inza I, Bengoetxea G (2006) Towards a new evolutionary computation: advances in estimation of distribution algorithms. Springer, Berlin
Lund U (1999) Cluster analysis for directional data. Commun Stat Simul Comput 28(4):1001–1009
Man KF, Tang KS, Kwong S (1999) Genetic algorithms: concepts and designs. Springer, London
Mandic D, Chambers J (2001) Recurrent neural networks for prediction: architectures, learning algorithms and stability. Wiley, New York, NY
Maravall A, Peña D (1989) Missing observations, additive outliers and inverse autocorrelation function. Technical Report 89/384, European University Institute, Florence
Marinari E, Parisi G (1992) Simulated tempering: a new monte carlo scheme. Europhys Lett 19:451–458
Marriott FHC (1982) Optimization methods of cluster analysis. Biometrics 69:417–422
Maulik U, Bandyopadhyay S (2003) Fuzzy partitioning using real coded variable length genetic algorithm for pixel classification. IEEE Trans Geosci Remote Sens 41:1075–1081
McCullagh P, Nelder JA (1989) Generalized linear models, 2nd edn. Chapman and Hall, London
McCulloch WS, Pitts W (1943) A logical calculus of the ideas immanent in nervous activity. Bull Math Biophys 5:115–133
McLachlan G, Krishnan T (1997) The EM algorithm and extensions. Wiley, New York
McLachlan G, Peel D (2000) Finite mixture models. Wiley, New York
Meinshausen N, Bühlmann P (2006) High-dimensional graphs and variable selection with the Lasso. Ann Stat 34(3):1436–1462
Michalewicz Z (1996a) Genetic algorithms + data structures = evolution programs. Springer, Berlin
Michalewicz Z (1996b) Genetic algorithms + data structures = evolution programs, 3rd edn. Springer, Berlin
Miller AJ (1990) Subset selection in regression. Chapman and Hall, London
Milligan GW, Cooper MC (1986) A study of the comparability of external criteria for hierachical cluster analysis. Multivar Behav Res 21:441–458
Minerva T, Paterlini S (2002) Evolutionary approaches for statistical modelling. In: Fogel DB, El-Sharkam MA, Yao G, Greenwood H, Iba P, Marrow P, Shakleton M (eds) Evolutionary

computation 2002. Proceedings of the 2002 congress on evolutionary computation. IEEE Press, Piscataway, NJ, vol 2, pp 2023–2028

Minerva T, Poli I (2001a) Building arma models with genetic algorithms. In: Boers EJW, et al (eds) EvoWorkshop 2001, LNCS 2037. Springer, Berlin, pp 335–342

Minerva T, Poli I (2001b) A neural net model to predict high tides in Venice. In: Borra S, Rocci R, Vichi M, Shader M (eds) Advances in data analysis and classification. Springer, Berlin, pp 367–374

Minervini G, Evangelista G, Villanova L, Slanzi D, De Lucrezia D, Poli I, Luisi P, Polticelli F (2009) Massive non natural proteins structure prediction using grid technologies. BMC Bioinformatics 10(6):S22

Mitchell M (1996) An Introduction to genetic algorithms. The MIT Press, Cambridge, MA

Mola F, Miele R (2006) Evolutionary algorithms for classification and regression trees. In: Zani S, Cerioli A, Riani M, Vichi M (eds) Data analysis, classification and the forward search. Springer, Heidelberg, pp 255–262

Montgomery D (2009) Design and analysis of experiments. Wiley, New York, NY

Mühlenbein H, Schlierkamp-Voosen D (1993) Predictive models for the breeder genetic algorithm: I. continuous parameter optimization. Evol Comput 1:25–49

Muhlenbein H, Paas G (1996) From recombination of genes to the estimation of distributions I. Binary parameters. Parallel Problem Solving from Nature – PPSN IV, pp 178–187

Murthy CA, Chowdhury N (1996) In search of optimal clusters using genetic algorithms. Pattern Recognit Lett 17:825–832

Myers R, Montgomery D, Vining G, Borror C, Kowalski S (2004) Response surface methodology: a retrospective and literature survey. J Qual Technol 36(1):53–77

Ng R, Han J (1994) Efficient and effective clustering methods for spatial data mining. In: Proceedings of the 20th conference on VLDB, Santiago, Chile

Ong CS, Huang JJ, Tzeng GH (2005) Model identification of ARIMA family using genetic algorithms. Appl Math Comput 164:885–912

Ozaki T (1982) The statistical analysis of perturbed limit cycle processes using nonlinear time series models. J Time Ser Anal 3:29–41

Pasia JM, Hermosilla AY, Ombao H (2005) A useful tool for statistical estimation: genetic algorithms. J Statistical Comput Simul 75:237–251

Pelikan M (2005) Hierarchical Bayesian optimization algorithm. Springer, New York, NY

Peña D (1990) Influential observations in time series. J Bus Econ Stat 8:235–241

Peña D, Tiao GC (2003) The SAR procedure: a diagnostic analysis of heterogeneous data. Manuscript submitted for publication

Pepelyshev A, Poli I, VB M (2009) Uniform coverage designs for mixture experiments. J Stat Plan Inference 139:3442–3452

Piccolo D (1990) A distance measure for classifying ARIMA models. J Time Ser Anal 11:153–164

Pistone G, Riccomagno E, Wynn H (2000) Algebraic statistics: computational commutative algebra in statistics. Chapman & Hall/CRC, London

Pittman J, Murthy CA (2000) Fitting optimal piecewise linear functions using genetic algorithms. IEEE Trans Pattern Anal Mach Intell 22(7):701–718

Pizzi C, Parpinel F, Soligo M (2009) Spline regression for an evolutionary approach to experimental design. Working paper 25, European centre for living technology, Venice, 2nd Workshop of the ERCIM Working Group on Computing & Statistics, Cyprus

Poli I (2006) Evolutionary design of experiments. Working paper 18, European Centre for Living Technology, Venice, PACE Report

Poli I, Jones R (1994) A neural net model for prediction. J Am Stat Assoc 89(425):117–121

Poli I, Roverato A (1998) A genetic algorithm for graphical model selection. J Ital Stat Soc 2: 197–208

Price KV, Storn R, Lampinen J (2005) Differential evolution, a practical approach to global optimization. Springer, Berlin

Priestley MB (1988) Non-linear and non-stationary time series analysis. Academic Press, London

Rand WM (1971) Objective criteria for the evaluation of clustering methods. J Am Stat Assoc 66:846–850
Reeves CR, Rowe JE (2003) Genetic algorithms – principles and perspective: a guide to GA theory. Kluwer, London
Reinsel GC (1993) Elements of multivariate time series analysis. Springer, New York, NY
Riani M (2004) Extensions of the forward search to time series. Stud Nonlinear Dyn Econom 8(2), Article 2
Rissanen J (1987) Stochastic complexity. J R Stat Soc B 49:223–265
Rissanen J (2007) Information and complexity in statistical modelling. Springer, Berlin
Roberts GO, Gilks WR (1994) Convergence of adaptive direction sampling. J Multivar Anal 49:287–294
Robles V, Bielza C, Larrañaga P, González S, Ohno-Machado L (2008) Optimizing logistic regression coefficients for discrimination and calibration using estimation of distribution algorithms. TOP 16:345–366
Rosenblatt F (1958) The perceptron: a probabilistic model for information storage and organization in the brain. Psychol Rev 65:386–408
Roverato A, Poli I (1998) A genetic algorithm for graphical model selection. J Ital Stat Soc 7:197–208
Rudolph G (1997) Convergence properties of evolutionary algorithms. Verlag Dr. Kovač, Hamburg
Rumelhart DE, Hinton GE, Williams RJ (1986) Learning internal representations by error propagation. In: Rumelhart DE, McClelland JL (eds) Parallel distributed processing. MIT Press, Cambridge, MA, pp 318–362
Sabatier R, Reynés C (2008) Extensions of simple component analysis and simple linear discriminant analysis using genetic algorithms. Comput Stat Data Anal 52:4779–4789
Sahni S, Gonzalez T (1976) P-complete approximation problems. J Assoc Comput Mach 23:555–565
Sarle WS (1994) Neural networks and statistical models. In: Proceedings of the 19th annual SAS users group international conference. SAS Institute, Cary, NC, pp 1538–1550
Schmitt LM, Nehainv CL, Fujii RH (1998) Linear analysis of genetic algorithms. Theor comput sci 200:101–134
Schneider J, Kirkpatrick S (2006) Stochastic optimization. Springer, Berlin Heidelberg
Schwarz G (1978) Estimating the dimension of a model. Ann Stat 6:461–464
Sessions D, Stevans L (2006) Investigating omitted variable bias in regression parameter estimation: a genetic algorithm approach. Comput Stat Data Anal 50:2835–2854
Shapiro J (2001) Statistical mechanics theory of genetic algorithms. In: Kallel L, Naudts B, Rogers A (eds) Theoretical aspects of genetic algorithms. Springer, Berlin, pp 87–108
SI (2008) Statistical innovations, http://www.statisticalinnovations.com /products /DemoData /diabetes.dat
Slanzi D, De March D, Poli I (2009a) Evolutionary probabilistic graphical models in high dimensional data analysis. In: Mola F, Conversano C, Vinzi V, Fisher N (eds) European regional meeting of the international society for business and industrial statistics, Cagliari, Italy, TAPILA editore, pp 124–125
Slanzi D, De March D, Poli I (2009b) Probabilistic graphical models in high dimensional systems. In: Ermakov S, Melas V, Pepelyshev A (eds) Simulation. St. Petersburg VVM com., pp 557–561, Saint Petersburg, Russia
Slanzi D, Poli I (2009) Evolutionary bayesian networks for high-dimensional stochastic optimization. Working paper 26, European centre for living technology, Venice, 2nd Workshop of the ERCIM working group on computing & statistics, Cyprus
Slanzi D, Poli I, De March D, Forlin M (2008) Bayesian networks for high dimensional experiments. Working paper 20, European centre for living technology, Venice, workshop on Bayesian analysis of high dimensional data, 14–16 Apr 2008, Warwick, UK
Smith RE, Forrest S, Perelson AS (1993) Population diversity in an immune system model: implications for genetic search. In: Whitley DL (ed) Foundations of genetic algorithms 2. Morgan Kaufmann, San Mateo, CA, pp 153–165

Spears WM, De Jong KA (1991) An analysis of multi-point crossover. In: Rawlins GJE (ed) Foundations of genetic algorithms. Morgan Kaufmann, San Mateo, CA, pp 301–315
Statlib (2008) The data and story library (DASL). http://lib.stat.cmu.edu/DASL
Stock JH, Watson MW (2004) Combination forecasts of output growth in a seven-country data set. J Forecast 23:405–430
Storn R, Price K (March 1995) Differential evolution – a simple and efficient adaptive scheme for global optimization over continuous spaces. Technical Report TR-95-012, ICSI. ftp.icsi.berkeley.edu
Stützle T, Hoos HH (2000) Max–min ant systems. Future Gen Comput Syst 16(8):889–914
Subba Rao T (1981) On the theory of bilinear time series models. J R Stat Soc B 43:244–255
Sun ZL, Huang DS, Zheng CH, Shang L (2006) Optimal selection of time lags for TDSEP based on genetic algorithm. Neurocomputing 69:884–887
Symons MJ (1981) Clustering criteria and multivariate normal mixtures. Biometrics 37:35–43
Syswerda G (1989) Uniform crossover in genetic algorithms. In: Schaffer JD (ed) Proceedings of the 3rd international conference on genetic algorithms. Morgan Kaufmann, Los Altos, CA, pp 2–9
Tan Y, Wang J (2001) Nonlinear blind source separation using higher order statistics and a genetic algorithm. IEEE Trans Evol Comput 5:600–612
Teräsvirta T (1994) Specification, estimation and evaluation of smooth transition autoregressive models. J Am Stat Assoc 89:208–218
Theis M, Gazzola G, Forlin M, Poli I, Hanczyc M, Packard N, Bedau M (2008) Optimal formulation of complex chemical systems with a genetic algorithm. Working paper 19, European centre for living technology, Venice
Tolvi J (2004) Genetic algorithms for outlier detection and variable selection in linear regression models. Soft Comput 8:527–533
Tong H (1990) Non linear time series: a dynamical system approach. Oxford University Press, Oxford
Tsay RS (1986) Time series model specification in the presence of outliers. J Am Stat Assoc 81:132–141
Tsay RS (1988) Outliers, level shifts and variance changes in time series. J Forecast 7:1–20
Tsay RS, Peña D, Pankratz AE (2000) Outliers in multivariate time series. Biometrika 87:789–804
Tseng LY, Yang SB (2001) A genetic approach to the automatic clustering problem. Pattern Recognit 34:415–424
Turing AM (1950) Computing machinery and intelligence. Mind 59:433–460
Van Emden MH (1971) An analysis of complexity. Mathematical Centre Tracts, Amsterdam
Versace M, Bhatt R, Hinds O, Shiffer M (2004) Predicting the exchange traded fund DIA with a combination of genetic algorithms and neural networks. Expert Syst Appl 27:417–425
Vitrano S, Baragona R (2004) The genetic algorithm estimates for the parameters of order p normal distributions. In: Bock HH, Chiodi M, Mineo A (eds) Advances in multivariate data analysis. Springer, Berlin Heidelberg, pp 133–143
Vose MD (1999) The simple genetic algorithm: foundations and theory. The MIT Press, Cambridge, MA
Wang X, Smith KA, Hyndman RJ (2005) Characteristic-based clustering for time series data. Data Min Knowl Discov 13:335–364
Whitley D (1994) A genetic algorithm tutorial. Stat Comput 4:65–85
Winker P (2001) Optimization heuristics in econometrics: applications of threshold accepting. Wiley, Chichester
Winker P, Gilli M (2004) Applications of optimization heuristics to estimation and modelling problems. Computat Stat Data Anal 47:211–223
Wolpert DH, Macready WG (1997) No free lunch theorems for optimization. IEEE Trans Evol Comput 1:67–82
Wong CS, Li WK (1998) A note on the corrected akaike information criterion for threshold autoregressive models. J Time Ser Anal 19:113–124

Wu B, Chang CL (2002) Using genetic algorithms to parameters (d,r) estimation for threshold autoregressive models. Comput Stat Data Anal 38:315–330

Wu C, Hamad M (2000) Experiments. Wiley, New York, NY

Xie XS, Beni G (1991) A validity measure for fuzzy clustering. IEEE Trans Pattern Anal Mach Intell 13:841–847

Zani S (1983) Osservazioni sulle serie storiche multiple e l'analisi dei gruppi. In: Piccolo D (ed) Analisi moderna delle serie storiche. Franco Angeli, Milano, pp 263–274

Zemella G, De March D (2009) The optimisation of building envelopes with evolutionary procedure. Working paper 27, European Centre for Living Technology, Venice, 2nd workshop of the ERCIM working group on Computing & Statistics, Limassol, Cyprus

Zhou X, Wang J (2005) A genetic method of LAD estimation for models with censored data. Comput Stat Data Anal 48:451–466

Ziehe A, Müller KR (1998) Tdsep – and efficient algorithm for blind separation using time structure. In: Proceedings of the international conference on ICANN, perspectives in neural computing. Springer, Berlin, pp 675–680

Index